life's tough.

get over it & get on with it!

stop wasting time...you only have one life to live.

cynthia m. brenneke
www.ironworksfitness.org
cindy@ironworksfitness.org

211 north broadway, suite 980 • saint louis, mo • 63102
written by cynthia brenneke
exercises and stretches modeled by
cynthia brenneke, edward coleman, cheryl sept, brandon woods and nicholas viviano

First edition: December 2008
Second edition: October 2009
Third edition: October 2010

ISBN: 978-1-4507-3721-0

Visit our website: www.ironworksfitness.org

Printed in the United States of America

Dedication

This book is dedicated to my incredible family and friends.
I am truly lucky to have each
and every one of them in my life.

contact information

name

address

home phone

office phone

cell

fax

email

emerg. contact name/phone

emerg. contact name/phone

drivers license

blood type

allergies

passport #

accountant

bank

club

dentist

doctor

gyno

home insurance

auto insurance

health insurance

lawyer

mechanic

vet

We all have information we can't "live without."

This is the information you have stored in a computer or on your phone. You may think you are safe; however, I know through experience, the time will come when you drop your phone in the water or a thief will run away with your computer. And, though you may have backups, it may not be at your immediate disposal. So, for all of those really important numbers and such...write it down!!! Ten minutes may save you hours of frustration.

contents

meet the crew

edward coleman

cynthia brenneke

brandon woods

nicholas viviano

cheryl sept

Breakfast

Desserts

Soups

Protein Shakes

Appetizers/Snacks

Salads

My name is Dee Phillips. Until recently, I ate whatever I wanted, drank more than I should have, and played an online game for a minimum of 50 hours a week. I smoked a pack of cigarettes a day and happened to be more than 130 pounds overweight. Did I mention that I've been a Type 2 diabetic for the last 5 years? In other words, I had an extreme death wish, all at the age of 28. I got a wake-up call when I finally saw a doctor and was told my pancreas was failing, my kidneys were damaged, my A1C was 12.5 (that translates into an average blood glucose reading of about 400; it's supposed to be no more than 140 at the maximum), and my cholesterol was high. The short version of the diagnosis was that I was committing suicide.

I decided right there that I was not dying without a fight. I was furious that I'd eaten myself into the kind of medical problems people twice my age start to have. My resolve was born of pure fear. No 40th birthday bash, no watching my nephew graduate from college; I had apparently traded all that in for Doritos and every item on the menu at Hardee's (I'm not joking, I really have had every item on the menu, shakes included). I recalled briefly joining a gym years ago, run by Cindy. As it turned out, she was still around, so I joined and starting fighting for my life. I was not concerned with weight loss I just wanted better control of my diabetes. I had finally run out of excuses, it was literally "do or die" time.

Something amazing began happening within a month of doing cardio at lunch. My mood changed (I have a very short temper). My eating habits changed; I felt guilty if I had doughnuts for lunch like the old days (again, not joking, I should have bought stock in Krispy Kreme). Most surprising of all, I played fewer games on the computer and spent more time outside in the park. My blood glucose levels dropped. I've been going to Cindy's place for a few months now, and I never pass by without words of encouragement from her. I dare say her optimism is rubbing off on me.

And it all has been paying off. My A1C is 5.9, my cholesterol is well within normal (in fact, for the first time ever there is more HDL than LDL), and I've been taken off insulin. My pancreas is coming back from the brink. My clothes are starting to hang off me. I no longer threaten violence when I'm stressed. And I laugh myself silly at the stunned look on my doctor's face.

So use this journal, even if you don't have the health problems that I do. I'd much rather you make the decision to be healthy now than wait till you are knocking on death's door like I was. I have learned the hard way that making excuses for not doing what you are supposed to can get you killed. So make the effort to live. And bring a veggie plate to my 40th birthday party.

The economy is in shambles, morale is on the decline and one has to wonder what's going to happen to our country over the next few years. You may be one of the "lucky ones" who still has a career and your home, or you may be one of those not so lucky. Either way, this book is for you—for the next 365 days are going to be absolutely fantastic!

I say this as I sit at the small kitchen table in my quaint one room cabin, with the dogs and kittens playing at my feet. It's an absolutely gorgeous summer day. I have the door propped open so the summer breeze and song of the robins may enter freely. The peacocks put on a show for me, as they dance and display their beautiful tail feathers for the coy peahen. The sheep lay quietly under the giant oaks as their young run playfully through the forest maze. I find myself laughing out loud, as their antics are more entertaining than anything I've seen on TV for quite some time. I feel I am one of the luckiest people I know.

How I ended up in this situation is not important. For as with many Americans, I was simply touched, no hammered, by the fallen economy. When writing the 2010 edition of this journal I was perched on a leather couch with a movie playing on the big screen in the background. The four bedroom, three bath house that I had made my home was filled with more furniture and "things" than most large families would ever need.

When faced with the reality of having to downsize, I was horrified. I wondered, *"how could this happen to me, what did I do to deserve this?"* I cried, I screamed, and then I realized that it really wasn't so bad. After selling and giving away nearly everything I owned, I had an incredible feeling of liberation. The economy had forced me to do things I didn't realize I was capable of and gave me a new sense of pride. I had repeatedly told myself, as I reluctantly packed the boxes, *"everything happens for a reason"* and *"that which doesn't kill me, only makes me stronger"*. It's what I have preached for years and truly believed—and believe even more so now.

The falling of our economy has been a *reality check* for me and many others. The *things* we have will come and go—and their lack of importance is quickly revealed. Our body, our mind, our soul, our integrity—those are the things that we will have for the rest of our lives, and those are the things we should nurture and guard with all our might.

This journal is packed with the tools you need to take care of those things which are most important. Use it and not only will you be the healthiest person you can possibly be, but also the happiest and most optimistic. Make life the best it can be...your happiness and success depends on you!

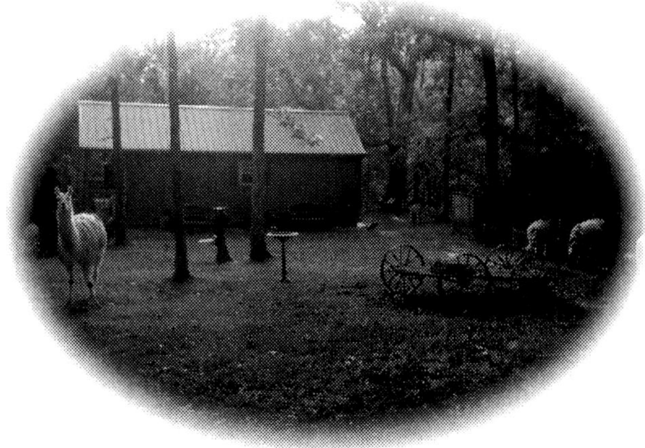

Many spend a lifetime looking for happiness and self-fullfillment—they struggle with everything from weight and health to their relationships with others. Looking for quick fixes and answers in all of the wrong places, they often give up and resign to a life of mediocrity.

What many don't realize is that the key to happiness lies within each of us. You've heard it before, but I will say it again, *"it's not what happens to you that matters, it's how you respond to that which happens."* It's up to you, and only you, to make your life the best it can possibly be— and with this journal in hand, you are well on your way!

With 365 pages for a one year journey, this journal will guide you to the success and happiness you have been seeking. You will learn not only how to feed your body, but also the importance of feeding your mind. Each page gives you a daily dose of positive thoughts to keep you going in the right direction. There are also exercises, health facts, websites, motivational quotations, thoughts and steps to help you grow and develop into the most remarkable person you will ever know.

To ensure success, use this journal to record your goals and your successes—BIG and small. Put your moods into writing and detail your day. The 10-20 minutes you use reading and writing in this journal on a daily basis are one of the best investments you can make in your future.

For those embarking upon a journey of weight loss this book is the perfect companion. Though many books and magazines romance you with stories of achieving the perfect buns, legs and abs, or promise diets that will help you lose 20-30 pounds, none of them will take you on a more successful journey than you are about to encounter with the aid of this journal. It has been designed to change your life physically, mentally and emotionally forever. It will motivate you to achieve goals you never thought possible and discover how great you truly are.

So, without hesitation, I encourage you to forego all procrastination and begin your new successful life today. Grab a pen and let the journey begin. Be sure to read the entire introduction to see how this journal is set up to work for you.

Every action you take affects your life.
Ask yourself each time you prepare to do something:
"Will this take me closer to my goal, or push me further away?"

Leading a successful life means living successfully at all levels: body, mind and soul. This journal has been set up to help you succeed at each of these levels. Begin your new journey by reading this entire introduction, and completing the *Desire Statement* on pages 6 and 7. It's also important to take your measurements, blood pressure, resting heart rate and stress heart rate. This information may be recorded on page 10.

For those using this journal to lose weight and create a health lifestyle you may want to make copies of pages 40 and 41. These charts can be used to chart your workouts and daily food and drink consumption. Of course this information may also be recorded directly in your journal pages.

Unlike most books this book should NEVER find its way to your bookshelf! Keep it at your side 24/7. Read the daily *quick reads* for motivation and reminders on how to lead a healthy lifestyle. Write in this book on a daily basis, record your goals, achievements and thoughts. And, of course, use it as a reference guide for eating, working out and staying motivated!

Each of the Journal's spreads contains *quick reads* —these are essential in keeping you motivated and on track for a healthy happy life!

Read it, live it, love the results.

These *read it, quick reads* give you the information you need to develop a positive attitude that will make you unstoppable in attaining that which you desire. You will also be given the *secrets* of staying young and healthy. Scientists once thought the secret to longevity was in our genes; however, new studies indicate that your age is greatly determined by your daily actions and attitudes.

Life's tough, get over it.

Bad things happen to everyone on a daily basis. It's not what happens to you that matters, but how you react to what happens. Keeping a positive attitude can dramatically change your life. I have learned that no matter what happens, if I think positive thoughts and focus on how the situation will help me grow, everything works out for the best. When you allow problems to affect you in a negative manner, you use these problems to become your excuse to procrastinate and fail at those things you desire. In these *life's tough, quick reads* you will soon realize everyone has problems—and many are much larger than the ones you face—yet each of these individuals have become very successful in achieving their desires.

Eating healthy tastes great!

More than ever, it seems that eating healthy has become a seemingly unattainable goal for many. With the multitudes of fad diets and quick weight loss solutions that have plagued the magazine and book racks over the years, many people are mystified as to what and how to eat. Review the facts and re-educate yourself on the value of healthy food, *(pages 19-31)* this will push you to make healthier choices in what you eat. In the *eating healthy, quick reads* you will find over 180 recipes that not only taste great, but are easy to prepare and healthy.

NOTE: The space for the recipes is restricted and the directions have been condensed, use common sense when preparing. Also, I seldom ever use salt in cooking, nor do I recommend it, so you will not see salt in the recipes, unless absolutely necessary. If you do use salt, you may want to use sea salt or a salt substitute as healthier alternatives. Also, when you use meats be sure to use lean cuts, and skinless.

Since you are in the process of reading and using this journal I would like to assume that "excuses" are not in your vocabulary. We all know it's wrong to assume; therefore, I will tell you up front "there is NO EXCUSE!" If you have an excuse for not being healthy and it's not listed this section, email me at: cindy@ironworksfitness.org. I assure you, I will rebuttal any excuse you feel is legitimate.

These are the Top 10 I have heard over the years;

10. I broke my toe. If you have a disabled body part, don't disable your entire body. Do the things you can, and you'll be back to 100% before you know it. A broken toe, or even a broken leg does not stop you from doing upper body exercises.

9. I can't eat healthy because I have kids and a husband. This makes NO sense at all! Your kids and husband should be eating healthy also! A healthy lifestyle protects everyone from disease. Most importantly, studies show that when children grow up eating healthy they eat healthier as adults and don't have the health issues that so many face.

8. I don't have the energy to workout. Well, duh! The more energy your body expends, the more it makes: meaning that people who workout have more energy than those who don't. When you sit around you have less energy than when you exercise. So, get up off the couch and MOVE!!

7. My knees hurt, I can't workout. The majority of people I have met with knee issues have them because of the extra weight they carry, which adds to the stress of their joints. Work out, eat healthy, get rid of the weight then the pain will usually vanish.

6. I want to enjoy life; I don't want to deprive myself of anything. As my father would say, *"people in hell want ice water."* When did we become so complacent that we decided it was okay to eat unhealthy foods despite the consequences? If gas tasted good, would you drink it? I would hope not. Though many don't hesitate to fill their bodies with foods that can cause nearly as much damage. When you eat healthy you are not depriving yourself—you are improving yourself!

5. I don't have time to workout. We all have time, it's a matter of prioritizing. When you watch TV in the evening, do the dumbbell exercises found in this book. If you take the kids to ball practice, walk around the park. See page 14 for many great ways to burn calories without *"working out."*

4. I'm too old so it doesn't matter. Nonsense! Studies show that people in their 80s and 90s are able to increase bone density and energy levels when they work out with weights. You're never too old!

3. I don't want to be sore. Sore is what you feel after a triple bypass or having a leg amputated due to diabetes. Get moving, get the weight off and your enthusiasm and well-being will far outweigh any muscles aches today and ward off the pain of illness and disease in later years.

2. It's in my genes, so it doesn't make a difference if I work out and eat healthy. Genetics and environment may increase the risk of personal weight gain; however, the choices you make about eating and physical activity contribute even moreso. If you were on a deserted island with only fruits and vegetables and had to rely upon walking for transportation, your genes couldn't possibly keep you overweight and unhealthy! Don't fool yourself, you are certainly not fooling me!

1. I just can't make myself do it. WHAT?!?? If your boss gave you a big project to work on, one in which your future relied upon, would you tell him *"I just can't do it"*. Of course not; you would give it your all. Your health and wellbeing is the biggest project you will ever face. If you fail, you will suffer a lifetime of consequences. Make changes now so you don't have regrets in the future. **YOU CAN DO IT!!!**

Throughout this journal you will find *quick reads* relating to the *success principles*, which Napolean Hill detailed in his book *Think and Grow Rich*–a book I highly reccommend.
These principles have not only influenced me, but are responsible for the success of millions of men and women throughout the world; you too can find your success in these principles.
Read through these carefully.

1. Desire This is the starting point for achieving your goals. You must have a strong desire to be healthy or you will not be able to achieve and maintain a healthy lifestyle.
Complete the Desire Statement on pages 6 and 7.

2. Faith In order to accomplish your goals, you must have faith in yourself. Throughout this journal we will explore ways to build your faith and self-confidence.

3. Auto-Suggestion By repeating your desire to be healthy, the subconscious mind will accept it as fact. You will be amazed at the control you have over your mind once you focus.

4. Specialized Knowledge In order to develop a plan of action for reaching your goals, you must have specialized knowledge. The pages of this journal are filled with everything you need to know about getting into the best shape possible and maintaining a healthy lifestyle. Read and remember.

5. Imagination It has been stated by many great philosophers that, *"whatever the mind can conceive and believe, it can achieve."* Limit your imagination and you limit your possibilities.

6. Organized Planning Just as you cannot build a house without a blueprint, you cannot lead a healthy life without a plan. Setting up long-term and short-term goals is all a part of the plan.

7. Decision When you make up your mind to begin a healthy lifestyle, stick with it. Many people fail because of the influence of others or procrastination. As *Nike* would say, *"Just do it!"*

8. Persistence This is a combination of willpower and desire that will give you the power to make it through the tough times. There will be times when you want to give up, when it all seems too difficult. That's when you reach deep inside, refuse failure and remain persistant.

9. The Power of the Mastermind When two great minds come together, solutions are found that may have never been discovered. Find a workout a buddy, someone with whom you can share ideas and discover great ways to lead a healthy life.

10. Enthusiasm To achieve a healthy lifestyle, you must have enthusiasm and determination.
I have never met an individual who has lost weight and kept it off if they did not have the enthusiasm to do it for themselves.

11. The Subconscious Mind Your subconscious mind is most influenced when envisioning a clear picture of having accomplished your goal. If you want to be slim and healthy, picture yourself slim and healthy, then live your life as if you were slim and healthy–do what slim and healthy people do.

12. The Power of the Brain Organized knowledge is power. Whether formally educated or self-educated, everything we achieve is a result of the knowledge we have and how we use it. When used to its fullest extent, your brain can bring to you all of that which you desire.

13. The Sixth Sense Master the above twelve principles and you will discover your sixth sense, a function of the subconscious mind. It's pulling into the parking space farthest from the building or reaching for a water instead of soda without thinking about it. You will be amazed at the healthy decisions which come naturally.

Get into The Arena

"It is not the critic that counts; not the man who points out how the strong man stumbles. Or where the doer of deeds could have done better. The credit belongs to the man who is actually in the arena, whose face is marred by dust and sweat and blood, who strives valiantly, who errs and comes short again and again, because there is no effort without error and shortcoming; who knows the great enthusiasms, the great devotions; who spends himself in a worthy cause; who at best knows in the end the triumph of high achievement. And at worst, if he fails, at least fails while daring greatly, so that his place shall never be with those cold and timid souls who know neither victory nor defeat."
– President Theodore Roosevelt, "The Man in the Arena" Paris, 1910

Make this your best year yet.

Make this your year to get into the arena, set goals and become healthier and happier than ever. Remember, your goals are the blueprint for your future.

Here, you will record your **desire statement**, indicating that which you desire most.
Then, throughout this journal, record the daily goals that will bring you closer to this desire.
When writing your desire statement and setting goals keep these things in mind:

1. Make sure the goal you are working towards is something you truly desire—it should not be a goal your family or friends set for you.

2. Don't reach for something that's not attainable. For example, try to lose thiry pounds in thirty days. Keep your goals within reason, you want to challenge yourself without making it impossible.

3. Your desire statement should be written with family, career, spirituality, physical health, social well-being and educational advancement all considered. Focusing on each of these six areas of life, will ensure the achievement of a goal that is truly worth reaching.

4. Write your desire statement in the positive, not the negative. Work towards that which you want, not away from what you don't want. Writing your desire statement and goals creates a set of instructions for your subconscious mind to carry out. As you will learn in reading this journal, the subconscious mind can't determine right from wrong, nor does it judge. It's only function is to carry out your instructions. Therefore, the more positive instructions you give, the more positive results you will receive.

Do not skip over these questions as they are essential to creating your healthy lifestyle.
It was Andrew Carnegie who developed these steps and Thomas Edison who placed his stamp of approval upon them as being the essential steps for the attainment of any definite goal.

1. What is it that you desire most? *Answer with detail.*

2. **List the steps necessary to achieve your desire.** *Keep in mind that you reap what you sow.*

3. **Date that you intend to possess that which you desire:** ____________

4. **Create a definite plan for carrying out your desire.** *Begin at once, don't procrastinate.*

5. **Write your *"Desire Statement."*** *This is a clear, concise statement of your responses to the preceding four steps. Example: I am healthier, happier and more energetic than ever weighing just 130 pounds and have having 22% body fat.*

6. **Read your "Desire Statement" out loud at least twice daily.**

Read this desire statement when you get up in the morning and again before you go to bed. As you read, you should see, feel and believe you already possess that which you desire. Keep the statement posted at your desk or as a screen saver on your computer. It's a simple, REQUIRED step, for BIG results.

Being healthy and fit is not about being sexy: it's about living a long, healthy life, enjoying retirement, being able to take vacations and playing with your grandchildren. I have heard it too many times... *"I don't need to lose weight; I just need to tone and tighten."* The numbers don't lie, when your BMI is over 30%, you need to do more than tone and tighten, you need to get rid of the FAT!
If you are carrying excess fat, you are slowly killing yourself. Start making lifestyle changes now that could save your life. Below is a checklist that will help you determine if you are at risk for obesity related illnesses. The way you live each day affects your health and your future, determine if you are at risk and make changes as necessary.

Place a check by each that applies to you.
Risk factors you can control

- ☐ **Obesity** • *Check your BMI as noted on page 10. A score of 30 or greater indicates you are obese.*
- ☐ **Physical Inactivity** • *Check if you don't exercise at least 20-30 minutes, 3 days every week.*
- ☐ **High Blood Pressure** • *Check if your blood pressure is higher then 135/85.*
- ☐ **Diabetes** • *Check if you've been told that you have diabetes.*
- ☐ **Blood Cholesterol Levels** • *Check if your HDL is less than 50 or your LDL is greater than 130.*
- ☐ **Smoking** • *Check if you smoke or you are exposed to second-hand smoke daily .*
- ☐ **Birth Control Pills** • *Check if you take birth control. (Combined with smoking, greatly increases your risk.)*
- ☐ **Excessive Alcohol Intake** • *Check if you consume more than one alcoholic beverage nightly.*
- ☐ **Stress** • *Check if you lead a high stress lifestyle.*
  Stress is a normal part of life, how you cope with stress can affect your heart. Using this journal, you will learn to cope with stress and not let it become detrimental to your health.
- ☐ **Family History** • *Check if your father or brother under age 55 or your mother or sister under age 65 has had a heart attack, stroke, angioplasty, cancer or bypass surgery.*
- ☐ **Older Age** • *Check if you are over 55 years old.*
- ☐ **Hormones & Menopause** • *Includes a complete or partial hysterectomy.*

If you have checked two or more of the risk factors listed above,
consult with your physician for a complete risk assessment.
You are at increased risk for many diseases and health conditions including:

- Hypertension (high blood pressure)
- Osteoarthritis
- Sleep apnea and respiratory problems
- Cancer (endometrial, breast, and colon)
- Dyslipidemia (high total cholesterol or high levels of triglycerides)
- Coronary heart disease
- Stroke
- Gallbladder disease
- Type 2 diabetes

If it's a healthy, happy life you want, one of the first things you need to do is record your *"starting point,"* this will allow you to monitor your improvements. Seeing these numbers improve over the months will keep you motivated.

Your weight and Body Mass Index (BMI).
Your weight should be checked once a week—on the same day and time each week.
To calculate your BMI, enter your numbers into this calculation;
(Weight in pounds) divided by [(height in inches) x (height in inches)] x 703
Example:
For an individual who is 5'5" (65") and weighs 155lbs, the formula would look like this:
155 divided by 4225 (which is 65x65), multipy by 703, this equals a BMI of 25.79.

Once you've determined your BMI, refer to this chart:
Below 18.5: Underweight • 18.5 - 24.9: Normal • 25 - 29.9: Overweight • 30 and above: Obese

Keep in mind that BMI is a poor indicator of body fat for athletes and those who have a muscular build. It may also underestimate body fat in older individuals and people who have lost muscle mass. Despite these drawbacks, the average person can check their BMI to get a rough idea of their health. The other option is to have your body composition done by a professional who can give you a more accurate assessment of your body fat.

If your BMI is higher than 25, you may be at risk for numerous health conditions including heart disease, type 2 diabetes, high blood pressure, high cholesterol, respiratory problems, joint injuries, osteoprosis and depression. Women who are underweight may experience an interruption of their menstrual cycle and bone loss.

Body measurements should also be taken, as they may be an indicator of risk for health related diseases. Measurements, which are taken on the right side of the body, should be checked once a month. With the help of a friend or family member, measure each of these body parts as indicated.
See image on page 13 for location of body part if you are unsure.
Chest: measure around the largest part of the chest.
Bicep: measure 4" up from the bend of the elbow.
Stomach: measure about 4" below your belly button, or where your stomach protrudes the most.
Waist: measure where you are the smallest. If you don't have a waist, measure at the navel line
Hips: measure at the widest area of the hips, stand with feet together.
Thigh: measure where they are the largest.
Calf: measure where they are the largest.

Waist-to-Hip Ratio
This is the proportion of fat stored on your body around your waist and hips.
Women should have a waist-to-hip ratio of 0.8 or less, men should be at 0.95 or less.
To determine your waist-hip ratio, divide your waist size by your hip size.
The higher the fat content in the abdomen, the higher your risk of heart disease.

In addition to recording your measurements you should also record your **resting heart rate** and **stress heart rate**. To measure your heart rate, locate the pulse on your wrist near the base of the thumb, then count the beats for one minute. It is best to check your *resting heart rate* first thing in the morning. To check *stress heart rate,* step up and down for one minute on a step approximately eight inches high (the height of an average step in your home), then take your heart rate. As your health improves these numbers will get lower.

Date						
Chest						
Biceps						
Forearm						
Waist						
Stomach						
Hips						
Thigh						
Calf						
Weight						
BMI						
Waist-Hip						
Clothing Size						
Resting HR						
Stress HR						

Date						
Chest						
Biceps						
Forearm						
Waist						
Stomach						
Hips						
Thigh						
Calf						
Weight						
BMI						
Waist-Hip						
Clothing Size						
Resting HR						
Stress HR						

The key to weight loss is quite simple, you must burn more calories than you consume.
I have repeatedly heard the excuse, *"I don't have time to workout"*. Yet, those same people have time for a cigarette break, a fifteen minute chat at the water cooler, and/or two to three hours watching TV. Stop making excuses and start following the *"rules"* below for a healthy, happy body. You'll be amazed at how much better you'll feel in just a week!

1. Keep A Training Journal. You may use this journal or make copies of pages 40 and 41 and put them in a binder. Use the exercise chart to record everything you do to burn calories. Use the food intake chart to track everything that goes into your mouth. Compare these two charts on a daily basis. Make sure the calories on your workout chart exceed those on the food intake chart. If you need to lose weight, it should be your goal to burn approximately 1000 more calories than you consume. You will have to burn a total of 3500 calories to drop one pound of body weight.

2. Set up a Detailed Exercise Plan. Plan your workouts for the week and stick with them. Write out specific strength and cardio workouts. Your cardio workouts may include cardio classes, walking, running, treadmill, bike, elliptical workouts or one of the activities listed on page 14. See page 12 for sample strength training workouts.

3. Maximize the Time You Have Available. Everyone has time to workout. If you don't have time for a "formal workout" try these tips; skip the elevator, climb the stairs. Don't email co-workers, deliver your message in person. Perform isometric exercises and stand at your desk when possible. In the evenings, play with your children and/or pets. If you *"must"* watch television, work out while watching—in this journal you will find several exercises which can be performed nearly anywhere—including your living room.

4. Workout with Resistance for Strength. For a lean healthy body, perform strength workouts at least three days a week, in addition to your cardio workouts. Many trendy workouts and equipment have come and gone, while dumbbell and band workouts remain the favorites as an easy, inexpensive way to get into great shape and strengthen muscles. Unlike machines, dumbbell exercises use the body's natural movement patterns and incorporate a greater range of motion. This also allows you to target specific areas of the body more effectively. Additionally, dumbbells and bands take up little space and cost far less then most other equipment. Forget the diamonds, it's dumbbells and bands that are a girl's best friend. On average you can burn 315-720 calories in an hour when weight training.

5. Don't Forget the Cardio. One of the most important things you can do for a healthy heart is regular cardio exercise—it's recommended that you do at least 30 minutes a day, five days a week. Here I have listed a few great cardio options with the number of calories you could burn in just one hour. Make sure you mix up your workouts to optimize results.
Biking 630-945 • Elliptical Trainer 648 • HealthRider 360 • Rowing 630-765
Ski machine 630 • Stair step machine 810 • Running 720-1350 • Walking 225-720

Play it safe.

Before starting your strength workout, read through the basic safety rules:

1. Start with 4-5 minutes of warm up and stretching. *Failing to do so can result in strains, tears or other injuries.*
2. Make sure you are performing the exercises properly— watch yourself in a mirror if possible. If you find that you cannot maintain proper form, try working out with lighter weights or no weight at all.
3. It is recommended that you have a workout partner with you at all times.
4. Check with your physician before beginning any workout routine.

Here you will find a few sample strength workouts.

The weights you choose and the number of repetitions and sets will depend upon your fitness level. If you're just getting started, I recommend doing one set of 10-12 repetitions with light weights (3-8lbs). These full-body workouts should be done three days a week, with one day between each workout. You will also want to vary the workouts. If you perform the same exercises for over a month your muscles will *"remember"* the workout and you will no longer get results. Also, make sure you go up in weights if you no longer feel the *"burn"* by the seventh or eighth repetition.

For more direction, check out our website, www.ironworksfitness.org, for the BLAST workout videos. These videos will take you through a full body workout with dumbbells or bands—it's just like being in class.

sample workout 1

legs/glutes

1. step ups *(page 103)*
2. lunge with knee lift *(page 144)*
3. step overs *(page 150)*
4. step with twist *(page 109)*

back

1. bent over dumbbell row *(page 170)*
2. straight arm pullovers *(page 155)*

chest

1. beginner push ups *(page 183)*
2. inside dumbbell press *(page 186)*

biceps

1. bicep curls *(page 214)*
2. hammer curls *(page 219)*

triceps

1. kickbacks *(page 237)*
2. overhead extensions *(page 231)*

shoulders

1. front raises *(page 251)*
2. lateral raises *(page 261)*

abdominals

1. regular crunches *(page 62)*
2. oblique twist *(page 74)*
3. reverse crunches *(page 63)*
4. pikes *(page 87)*

sample workout 2

legs/glutes

1. butt blaster *(page 122)*
2. butt blaster crossover *(page 123)*
3. butt blaster combo *(page 124)*
4. straight leg lifts *(page 126)*

back

1. lower back extension *(page 158)*
2. superwoman/man *(page 161)*
3. airplane *(page 156)*

chest

1. burpee *(page 188)*
2. butterfly chest presses *(page 193)*

biceps

1. cross body curls *(page 226)*
2. 21s *(page 227)*

triceps

1. tricep dips *(page 236)*
2. kickouts from chest *(page 240)*

shoulders

1. shoulder presses *(page 248)*
2. rear rotation *(page 271)*

abdominals

1. washing machine *(page 82)*
2. elbow to knee twisting *(page 67)*
3. elbow to knee *(page 68)*
4. t-stand *(page 90)*

sample workout 3

legs/glutes

1. dumbbell squat *(page 145)*
2. hack squat *(page 129)*
3. reverse lunge *(page 130)*
3. plié squat with flye *(page 141)*

back

1. one arm dumbbell rows *(page 171)*
2. upright row *(page 174)*

chest

1. suicide pushups *(page 195)*
2. straight arm flyes *(page 189)*

biceps

1. reverse curls *(page 222)*
2.concentration curls *(page 221)*

triceps

1. behind back press *(page 242)*
2. one arm side pushup *(page 243)*

shoulders

1. bent over lateral *(page 254)*
2. military press *(page 249)*

abdominals

1. planks *(page 85)*
2. plank with leg ext. *(page 86)*
3. kneeling elbow to knee *(page 83)*
4. toe reach *(page 81)*

Here you will find a list of the body parts referred to throughout this journal.

Biceps: The large muscles located to the front of the upper arms. This two 'headed' muscle flexes the forearm and draws it up.

Triceps: The smaller muscle located to the back of the upper arm. This three 'headed' muscle extends

Hips: The outward-projecting part of the pelvis, top of the femur and the overlying tissue. The triglycerides in our body tend to get stored as fat in this area.

Pectoral Muscle: The muscle underlying the breast area. Though it looks like two separate muscles, it's actually one continuous fan shaped muscle situated at the upper front of the chest wall.

Glutes: This area consists of three different muscles. The gluteus maximus, gluteus medius and gluteus minimus. The gluteus maximus is the largest gluteal muscle and the biggest muscle in the human body. This muscle forms the bulk of the buttocks. It acts to extend the upper leg, spread it, and turn it outward.

Abdominals: A group of six muscles in the front of the abdomen extending from the thorax to the pelvis. These muscles provide postural support—supporting the muscles of the spine while lifting and keeping abdominal organs, such as the intestines in place. They also assist in regular breathing movement.

Quadriceps: The large four 'headed' muscle of the thigh. This muscle extends down the femur, over the the kneecap and anchors into the top of the tibia, the large bone in the lower leg. The function of the quadriceps is to straighten the leg.

Hamstring: The hamstrings are prominent tendons located at the back of the knee. They are the sidewalls of the hollow behind the knee. Both hamstrings connect to muscles that flex the knee.The medial hamstring contributes to medial rotation of the leg at the flexed knee joint, whereas the lateral hamstring contributes to lateral rotation.

Calves: The fleshy hind part of the leg below the knee. The largest and most superficial muscle of the calf is the gastrocnemius muscle. The calf is responsible for the plantar flexion of the foot.

Back Muscles:

The back is made up of three major muscle groups. All of which are involved in nearly every activity you do, so it is important they're kept strong.

The **rhomboids**, posture muscles, are between the shoulder blades. These muscles aid in rotation, elevation and retraction of the shoulder blades.

The **latissimus dorsi**, also known as lats, are located on each side of the back. They work to extend, rotate and pull your arms toward your body.

The **erector spinae** is made up of three muscles that run the length of your back from your neck to your glutes. This muscle aids in flexion and extension of the upper body, as well as rotation.

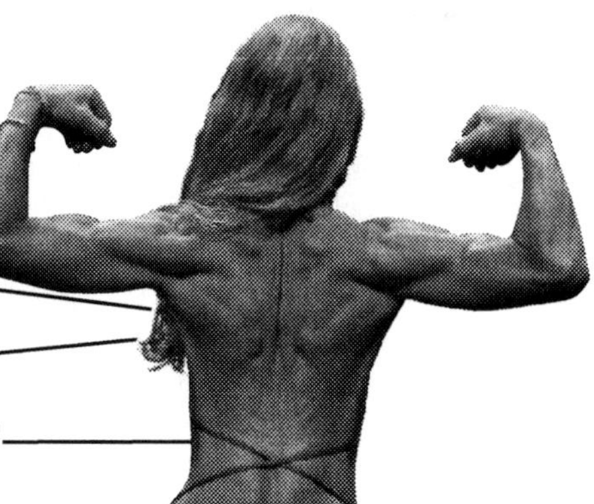

There are plenty of ways to burn calories without going to the gym—and they don't cost a dime. They simply require you getting off the couch and moving! Each activity listed below shows the calories the average 150 pound individual would burn in an hour for that activity.

Outdoor Activities

Digging	450
Gardening	360
Gardening and weeding	405
Mowing lawn with pushmower	540
Painting outside of home	450
Planting seedlings and shrubs	405
Raking lawn	387
Shoveling snow by hand	540
Sweeping outside	360

Indoor Activities

Crafts/standing, light effort	162
Paint, paper, remodel	405
Children's games, moderate	360
Children's games, vigorous	450
Cleaning house, general	270
Cooking/food preparation	180
Food shopping	207
Heavy cleaning	270
Reading: sitting	90
Standing in line	108
Vacuuming	315

Office Activities

Driving vehicle to work	180
Light office work sitting	135
Light office work standing	207
Riding in a bus to work	90
Typing	135

Sports

Basketball, playing a game	720
Basketball, shooting baskets	405
Billiards	225
Bicycling, mountain bike	765
Bicycling	720-1440
Bowling	270
Boxing, sparring	810
Boxing, punching bag	540
Dancing	270-432
Frisbee	270
Golf, carrying clubs	405
Golf, using cart	315
Golf, driving range	270
Golf, walking, pulling clubs	387
Gymnastics	360
Hacky sack	360
Handball	1080
Hiking cross-country	540
Hockey field & ice	720
Horseback riding	360
Ice skating	630
Jumping rope	900
Kayaking	450
Martial arts	900
Race walking	585
Racquetball	630
Rock climbing	990
Rollerblading	1125
Running, 5 mph/12 min/mile	720
Running, 10 mph/6 min/mile	1440
Running, cross-country	810
Running up stairs	1350
Scuba or skin diving	630
Skateboarding	450
Skiing cross-country	630-810
Skiing downhill	540-720
Sledding	630
Snorkeling	450
Soccer, competitive play	900
Softball or Baseball	450
Swimming	540-900
Table Tennis	360
Tai Chi	360
Tennis	450-720
Volleyball	270-720
Walk (5 mph/12 min/mi)	225-720
Water skiing	540
Water jogging	720

Walking is FREE and HEALTHY!!!

If there were a pill you could take in order to reap all of the benefits of walking you, like many others, would pay top dollar for the pill and make it one of the most popular prescriptions in the history of modern medicine! Unfortunately, the pill does not exist; however, your ability to walk does...and it's FREE without side effects. Start walking today and you will begin to see immediate results, as well as bestow upon yourself many long term benefits. When you improve your health you improve your life!

The benefits of walking include:

- Reducing your risk of many diseases, heart attacks and strokes
- Reducing your risk of hip fractures
- Reducing your risk of glaucoma
- Aids in managing your weight
- Burns fat and builds muscle
- Helps control your blood pressure
- Prevents depression, colon cancer, constipation, osteoporosis and impotence
- Lengthens lifespan
- Lowers stress levels
- Relieves arthritis and back pain
- Strengthens muscles, bones, and joints
- Reduces your risk of ever needing gallstone surgery
- Improves sleep
- Helps build great looking legs
- Elevates mood and sense of well-being

Count your Steps

To keep yourself motivated wear a pedometer on a daily basis, and record this information. You will find a spot on your daily journal entry pages.

Set a goal of steps each day.

The recommended number of steps taken daily is 6000 or more for health and 10,000 or more for weight loss. *Note that for optimal weight loss, an uninterrupted walk each day of 4000-6000 steps is recommended.*

Wear good shoes

Makes sure you wear good shoes when walking. Your feet are supporting the entire weight of your body. If you walk in flip flops, heals or worn sneakers you will soon be suffering in pain instead of rejoicing in health!

Walk tall for great results

Though most of us have been doing it for years, many still don't do it well. Follow these steps to get the most out of your walk.

- Walk with good posture. This will enable you to breathe easier and avoid back pain.
- Stand up straight, don't arch your back.
- Don't lean forward or lean back this puts strain on the back muscles.
- Keep your eyes forward, looking about 20 feet straight ahead.
- Keep your chin up and parallel to the ground.
- Relax your shoulders, letting them fall slightly back.
- Hold your stomach in, keeping the abdominal muscles tight.
- Rotate your hips forward slightly to keep your back from arching.

Consult your physician.

As with any physical activity, you should consult your physician before beginning a walking program.

This is particularly important if any of these apply to you:

- Sedentary for a year or more
- Heart trouble
- Sedentary and over age 65
- High blood pressure
- Pregnant
- Diabetes
- Chest pain
- Feel faint
- Suffer other medical conditions
- Suffer dizzy spells

This is the third year that I have published this journal and the third year I have managed to unintentially lose weight when doing reseach for the nutrition section.

I was thiry-two when I changed my lifesyle for the better. I was devastated over another failed relationship and a terrifying view of my backside in a dressing room mirror. I entered *"The Body for Life Challenge,"* a twelve-week body and life transformation program based upon eating healthy and working out. I celebrated happy hour one day a week instead of seven and began eating foods that nourished my body instead of tearing it down. It was the best thing I ever did for myself. In three months I changed my physique, health and attitude. Now, over ten years later I still work and eat healthy, generally keeping my weight at 133 and body fat at 13%. However, when spending hours researching the effects of food on the body, I subconsciencely eat even better and manage to drop a few pounds without even trying. I preach daily about the importance of eating healthy; however, reading what others have to say and studying the reseach seems to put my subconscious mind into overdrive. I actually shuddered one day last week when walked down the snack aisle. I had visions of *"free-radical"* bugs climbing on the packages...I practiacally ran back to the produce aisle. Hopefully, when you read through this next section you will have the same experience.

In my research, I am reminded that our bodies are like fine-tuned automobiles. We wouldn't dream of using an inferior fuel or skipping oil changes for a new Cadillac Escalade; however, we fuel our bodies with *inferior fuels* on a daily basis, and continuously neglect our internal maintenance. The sad part of this equation is that the automobile can be replaced, your body can't. You know how fat looks on your thighs, buns and belly, can you imagine how it looks wrapped around your organs and running through your bloodstream? Fat is not pretty—though it's unappealing appearance is of little consequence compared to the ghastly destruction it does to your internal organs.

The next several pages have been set aside to help you understand the importance of giving your body the fuel it needs to stay healthy. Too often we view eating healthy as a form of deprivation. However, once you familiarize yourself with the crucial health benefits of certain foods you will want to get as many of them into your diet as possible, leaving little room for *junk*.

The more you know about the foods you consume, the more likely you are to stay on track with your healthy eating plan. The information in these food charts is very limited. For more in-dept information you may check these websites: *The USDA Database* at *www.nal.usda.gov* and *The World's Healthiest Foods* at *www.whfoods.com.*

Note, the nutrition facts in this section are based upon a portion size of one cup unless otherwise noted. The information was taken from *The USDA Database* at *www.nal.usda.gov* and *The World's Healthiest Foods* at *www.whfoods.com.*

The key to eating healthy is to consume a diet composed of a variety of healthy foods; as there is no single type of food or single food group that can provide all of the vitamins and nutrients needed to keep your body in good health. Below are the *U.S. Food and Drug Administration's* recommended portions to maintain optimum health. *Note: caloric intake varies from person to person.*

Dairy
2 -3 cups

Products made with milk provide protein, vitamins and minerals, especially calcium. Choose non-fat milk and yogurt and cheeses made from skim milk. *See page 19.*

Equal to 1 cup serving
- 1 cup milk or yogurt
- $1\frac{1}{2}$ oz natural cheese
- 2 oz processed cheese

Health benefits of Dairy
- reduces the risk of developing osteoporosis
- may protect against metabolic syndrome
- can make your body stronger and treat illnesses
- may help prevent high blood pressure
- helps blood to clot
- keeps muscles and nerves working properly

Grains
6 servings

This includes whole grain breads, pastas, breakfast cereals, brown rice, wild rice, barley and popcorn. Make low-fat choices from foods in this group. *See page 21.*

Equal to 1 serving
- 1 slice bread
- 1 cup ready-to-eat cereal
- $\frac{1}{2}$ cup rice, pasta, or cooked cereal

Health benefits of Whole Grains
- reduces the risk of coronary heart disease
- increases energy
- may help with weight management
- eating grains fortified with folate before and during pregnancy helps prevent neural tube defects during fetal development

Protein
5.5 ounces

This category includes meat, poultry, fish, eggs, peanut butter, legumes, nuts, tofu and protein powders. *See pages 22 and 23.*

Equal to 1 oz serving
- 1 oz meat, poultry or fish
- 1 egg
- 1 tbs peanut butter
- $\frac{1}{4}$ cup cooked dry beans
- $\frac{1}{2}$ oz nuts or seeds

Health benefits of Proteins
- protects against bone loss in older people
- source of the cancer-protective B vitamin, niacin
- protects against Alzheimer's and cognitive decline
- increases energy and ability to produce muscle
- improves cardiovascular health
- source of selenium, important to overall health

Vegetables
2.5 cups or more

Vegetables are rich in nutrients and fiber, and low in fat and sodium. Many are excellent sources of vitamin A, vitamin C, folate or potassium. *See pages 24 and 25.*

Equal to 1 cup serving
- 1 cup vegetables
- 1 cup vegetable juice
- 2 cups leafy greens

Health benefits of Vegetables
- may reduce risk of stroke
- may reduce risk of cardiovascular diseases
- reduces risk for type 2 diabetes
- protects against certain cancers
- may reduce the risk of coronary heart disease
- may reduce the risk of developing kidney stones
- may help decrease bone loss

Fruits
2-3 cups

Fruits are also rich in nutrients and fiber, and low in fat and sodium, Though higher in carbs than vegetables, so limit the intake. *See pages 26 and 27.*

Equal to 1 cup serving
- 1 cup fruit
- 1 cup 100% fruit juice
- $\frac{1}{2}$ cup dried fruit

Health benefits of Fruits
- may reduce risk of stroke
- may reduce risk of cardiovascular diseases
- reduces risk for type 2 diabetes
- protects against certain cancers
- may reduce the risk of coronary heart disease
- may reduce the risk of developing kidney stones
- may help to decrease bone loss

Oils
up to 6 teaspoons

This group also includes, salad dressings, oils, cream, butter, margarine, sugars, soft drinks, candies and sweet desserts. These items should be eaten sparingly. *See pages 21 and 23.*

- 1 oz roasted nuts = 3tsp
- $\frac{1}{2}$ med. avocado = 3tsp
- 1 oz sunflower seeds = 3tsp
- 1 tbs mayonnaise=11/2tsp
- 2 tbs italian dressing=2tsp

Health benefits of Olive Oil
- reduces blood pressure
- inhibits the growth of some cancers
- benefits people at risk for or with diabetes
- lessens the severity of asthma and arthritis
- may help maintain a lower weight

One of the questions I am asked most often is, *"what do I eat?"*
In response, I have outlined a few different options for daily meals. Keep in mind that even when eating healthy foods, you must eat reasonable portion sizes. *A portion is about the size of your fist.* I seldom have time for preparing meals on a daily basis; therefore, when I do cook or bake I prepare extra large portions—and enjoy the luxury of leftovers. I also freeze portions for future use. When you make eating healthy easy, you are more likely to stick with a healthy lifestyle.

The FDA recommends the average daily caloric intake;
1,600 for most women and some older adults • 2,000 for average adult
2,200 for most men, active women, teenage girls and children • 2,800 for active men and teenage boys

	sample day 1	**sample day 2**	**sample day 3**
5:30am	green tea, coffee or water piece of fruit • 1 cup skim milk	green tea, coffee or water low carb yogurt	green tea, coffee or water protein bar
8:30am	green tea, coffee or water Strawberry Pineapple Protein Shake *(page 12)*	green tea, coffee or water two hard boiled eggs slice of whole wheat toast	green tea, coffee or water Mediterranean Veggie Scramble whole wheat toast *(page 32)*
11:30am	green tea, coffee or water Berry Chicken Salad *(page 286)* whole wheat crackers	green tea, coffee or water Thai Tuna Salad *(page 182)* whole wheat toast	green tea, coffee or water Black Bean Salad *(page 28)*
2:30pm	green tea or water 1/2 cup nuts and dried fruit	green tea or water Peach Jello Salad *(page 90)*	green tea or water low fat cheese stick and cup of carrots
5:30pm	green tea, water or skim milk Parmesan Chicken *(page 66)* sauteed veggies and 1/2 cup brown rice	green tea, water or skim milk Baked Salmon with Herbs & Red and Green Salad *(pages 200 and 68)*	green tea, water or skim milk Sloppy Joe—Turkey Style and Cucumber and Onion Salad *(pages 240 and 226)*
7:30pm	green tea or water low carb yogurt	green tea, coffee or water jello	green tea, coffee or water raw carrots and celery

For great tasting healthy meals, keep these ingredients in your cabinets and refriderator at all times.
Basil, bay leaves, black pepper, cayenne pepper, cinnamon. dill, ginger, oregano, parsley, paparika, rosemary, sage, thyme, honey, olive oil, tobasco sauce, minced garlic, onions, oatmeal, whole wheat pasta, brown rice, green tea bags, frozen bags of spinach, broccoli, peas and mixed vegetables, canned mushrooms, tomatoes, tomato paste, tuna, beans, chicken, skim milk, eggs, low fat cheeses and artificial sweenener.
Vary your fruits, vegetables and meats each week to make eating healthy exciting.

Foods you should SELDOM EVER add to your grocery list.
Bagels, beer/regular, bread/white, cakes, candy, sweetened cereals, chips, crackers
cookies, cold cuts, cream cheese, donuts, fried foods, granola, ice cream, mayonnaise, meats/fatty
muffins, pasta/white, pies, rice/white, full fat salad dressings, sherbet, soda, sour cream, and any item which contains TRANS Fats.

Do you read the Nutrition Facts labels? Do you know how many calories, carbs and fats are in the foods you are eating? When discussing *weight issues* with clients, I often hear *I only eat healthy stuff, I don't know why I can't lose weight.* Well, I do! More than likely you are eating WAY TOO MUCH! Even if a food is healthy you can't eat unlimited amounts of it...unless it's celery. A calorie is a calorie is a calorie. The reason you eat healthy foods is so you may get more nutritional bang out of your calories; therefore, having to consume fewer of them. This is key to losing weight and maintaining a healthy lifestyle.
This next section will cover reading labels and reviewing the nutritional values of the foods and drinks you should be consuming.

Nutrition Facts
Serving Size 1 cup (228g)
Servings Per Container 2

Amount Per Serving
Calories 250 Calories from Fat 110

	% Daily Value*
Total Fat 12g	18%
Saturated Fat 3g	15%
Trans Fat 3g	
Cholesterol 30mg	10%
Sodium 470mg	20%
Total Carbohydrate 31g	10%
Dietary Fiber 0g	0%
Sugars 5g	
Protein 5g	
Vitamin A	4%
Vitamin C	2%
Calcium	20%
Iron	4%

* Percent Daily Values are based on a 2,000 calorie diet. Your Daily Values may be higher or lower depending on your calorie needs.

	Calories:	2,000	2,500
Total Fat	Less than	65g	80g
Sat Fat	Less than	20g	25g
Cholesterol	Less than	300mg	300mg
Sodium	Less than	2,400mg	2,400mg
Total Carbohydrate		300g	375g
Dietary Fiber		25g	30g

Serving information.
This is very important because everything is based on one serving.

Nutrition information.
Remember this informaiton is based upon the serving listed. You will often find item servings in 2 or more. This makes the item look healthier at first glance. However if you plan to consume the entire product you must multiply these numbers by the serving total.
i.e. If you ate this entire product you would be consuming 500 calories! Try to choose products which are low in calories, fats and carbs, higher in dietery fiber and protein.

Dairy

Dairy foods are broadly defined as products derived from cow's milk, such as different types of milk, yogurts, and cheeses. These foods are great sources of protein, calcium, vitamin D and other essential nutrients. *The FDA recommends eating/drinking 2-3 cups daily.*

	Cal	Carb	Fat	Fbr	Prtn	In these Recipes	More information
low fat cheese	determined by brand selected					14, 54, 66, 176, 190, 306	
2% milk (8oz)	122	12.5	4.9	0	8.1	2, 24, 30, 32, 34, 64, 90, 100, 116, 118, 178, 202, 218	
1% milk	105	12.3	2.5	0	8.5	224, 242, 250, 262, 274, 284, 290, 322, 328, 336	
skim milk	91	12.3	.7	0	8.7		
goat's milk	168	11	10	0	9		
yogurt	determined by brand selected					22, 30,40, 46, 50, 64, 68, 76, 82, 96, 124, 134, 210, 212, 216, 250, 302	

low fat cheese: *protects against gout • boosts fat burning after a meal • strengthens teeth • helps prevent cancer specially good for bones of children, elderly people and pregnant and lactating women • reduces risk of osteoporosis*

2% milk, 1% milk, skim milk: *protects heart • increases energy • reduces migraines • promotes healthy thyroid • fights infections & arthritis promotes good bone and teeth health • improves skin • reduces risk of hypertension and some forms of cancer decreases risk of dehydration • reduces respiratory problems, obesity and osteoporosis*

goat's milk: *some people who can't tolerate cow's milk are able to drink goat's milk • contains anti-inflammatory compounds combats cancer • prevents bone loss • prevents arthritis • prevents migraines • reduces PMS symptoms*

yogurt: *provides '"good" bacteria in the digestive tract • prevents osteoporosis • reduce risk of high blood pressure guards against ulcers • strengthens bones • aids digestion • lowers cholesterol • supports immune system*

Drinks

Grabbing a juice is a great way to get a quick nutritional boost; however, make sure you read the nutritional label before making your purchase. Many juices are filled with sugars and additives that may cause more damage than good to your body. The nutritional values listed here are for one cup of non-sweetened juice; these may vary from one producer to another. *The FDA recommends eight glasses of fluids a day.*

	Cal	Carb	Fat	Fbr	Prtn	In these Recipes	More information
green tea	2	0	0	0	0		65
studies recommend drinking at least three cups a day • lower risk for a wide range of diseases, from simple bacterial or viral infections to chronic degenerative conditions, including cardiovascular disease, cancer, stroke, periodontal disease and osteoporosis. protects against death from all causes							
carrot juice	94.4	21.9	0.4	1.9	2.2		40, 242, 354
soothing influence on ulcers, colitis and other conditions involving stomach • alkalizer • antioxidant compounds help protect against cardiovascular disease and cancer • promote good vision, especially night vision							
cranberry juice	144.2	36.4	0.3	0.3	0		212
aids digestion • normalizes bowels • prevents bladder infections • reduces risk of urinary tract and kidney infections protects against viruses • combats herpes virus • acts as a natural probiotic • prevents the development of cavities prevents kidney stone formation • increases HDL (good) cholesterol • reduces LDL (bad) cholesterol							
grape juice	154.3	37.8	0.2	0.3	1.4		310, 324
stimulates bile secretion • helps burn fat • mild laxative • blood cleanser • reduces stress • reduces risk of cancers decreases risk of heart disease • reduces platelet clumping and blood clots • helps keep the heart muscle flexible may lower cholesterol • protective for persons with high blood pressure • may lower risk of Alzheimer's Disease protective against food-borne illness • reduces risk of all-causes of mortality							
grapefruit, pink	96.3	22.7	0.2	0.0	1.2		
protects heart • promotes weight loss • reduces strokes • combats prostate cancer • lowers cholesterol							
orange juice	109.6	25.0	0.7	0.5	2.0		
combats cancer • supports immune system • protects heart • straightens respiration • reduces stress							
pineapple juice	140	34.5	0.2	0.5	0.8		
strengthens bones • relieves colds • dissolves warts • prevents diarrhea • aids digestion							
prune juice	181.8	44.7	0.0	2.6	1.6		
high in antioxidants beneficial to tissues of the body • protects against cell damage • high-fiber based laxative							
tomato juice	41.3	10.3	0.1	1.0	1.8		
See tomatoes on page 25 for a full list of benefits.							
water	0	0	0	0	0	51146, 142, 219	51, 58, 146, 219, 203, 244
combats cancer • promotes weight loss • conquers kidney stones • smoothes skin transpsorts nutrients and oxygen into cells • moisturizes the air in lungs • helps with metabolism protects our vital organ • helps organs absorb nutrients • regulates body temperature • detoxifies protect and moisturizes joints • natural remedy for headaches • reducse the risk of cancer							
Harmful Effects and Symptoms of Dehydration (20% or more dehydrated there is a risk of death) tiredness • migraines • constipation • muscle cramps • irregular blood-pressure • kidney problems • dry skin							

Grains

Eating whole grains provides great health benefits. However, you must make sure that the product you are eating is truly whole grain. Foods labeled with the words *"multi-grain," "stone-ground," "100% wheat," "cracked wheat," "seven-grain,"* or *"bran"* are usually not whole-grain products. Color is also not an indication of a whole grain. Read the label and look for the words "Whole Grain". *The FDA recommends 6-11 ounces daily.*

	Cal	Carb	Fat	Fbr	Prtn	In these Recipes	More information
brown rice	216	44.7	1.75	3.5	0	104, 144, 282, 358	
combats cancer • protects heart • battles diabetes • reduces strokes • conquers kidney stones • prevents diarrhea beneficial for stomach and intestinal ulcers • great nutrient for the hair, teeth, nails, muscles and bones							
barley	149	32	1	1	4	166	166
promotes regularity • lowers cholesterol • protects against atherosclerosis • protects against heart disease decreases colon cancer • protects intestines • great cardiovascular benefits for postmenopausal women lowers risk of type 2 diabetes • protects against breast cancer • helps prevent gallstones • benefits arthritis sufferers helps repair of body tissue •							
oatmeal	129	22.4	2.13	3.7	5.43	100, 118, 252	
combats cancer • lowers cholesterol • prevents constipation • smoothes skin • battles diabetes • prevents heart disease good source of vitamin E, zinc, selenium, copper, iron, manganese, magnesium and protein							
wheat germ	determined by brand selected					212, 228, 360	
combats diseases including cancers • prevents constipation • lowers cholesterol • reduces strokes • improves digestion keeps reproductive organs working well in both males and females • reduces signs of aging • aids in weight loss reduces chances of birth defects • keeps hair strong and natural looking • fights against muscular dystrophy							
wheat bran	determined by brand selected						
combats colon cancer • prevents constipation • lowers cholesterol • reduces strokes • improves digestion							
whole wheat	determined by brand selected						
lowers type 2 diabetes risk • helps prevent gallstones • promotes gastrointestinal health • aids in weight loss reduces risk of cardiovascular disease • lessens chronic inflammation • prevents heart failure rich in fiber, vitamins, minerals, antioxidants, and healthy fats reduces risk of metabolic syndrome (a strong predictor of both type 2 diabetes and cardiovascular disease) combined with fish is highly protective against childhood asthma							

Other

	Cal	Carb	Fat	Fbr	Prtn	In these Recipes	More information
honey	64	17	0	0	0	30, 60, 70, 92, 134, 146, 198, 228, 232, 236, 238, 244, 250, 252, 294	*extra info on 100*
aids digestion • guards against ulcers • fights allergies • increases energy heals wounds • works as an anti-bacterial, anti-viral, anti-fungal substance • aids upper respiratory problems may promote better blood sugar control • improves athletic performance • a spoonful a day keeps free radicals at bay							
olive oil	119	0	14	0	0	Too many to list	181, 222
contains monounsaturated fat, a healthier type of fat that can lower your risk of heart disease by reducing the total and low-density lipoprotein, LDL cholesterol, levels in your blood reduces blood pressure • combats some cancers • reduces risk of diabetes • lessens asthma and arthritis symptoms							

Protein

Getting enough protein in your diet is essential for your overall good health. This category includes: meat, poultry, fish, eggs, peanut butter, legumes, nuts, tofu and protein powders.
Note, one egg, 1/2 cup beans or 1/3 cup nuts is equal to one ounce of protein. The FDA recommends 5.5 ounces of protein.

	Cal	Carb	Fat	Fbr	Prtn	In these Recipes	More information
lean beef *(4oz)*	193	0	11.64	0	20.43	222	

great cardiovascular benefits • fights certain cancers • improves immunity • reduces risk of osteoporosis
prevents damage to blood vessel walls which can contribute to atherosclerosis

	Cal	Carb	Fat	Fbr	Prtn	In these Recipes	More information
lean pork *(4oz)*	237	0	11.1	0	32.3		

may reduce heart disease and type two diabetes

	Cal	Carb	Fat	Fbr	Prtn	In these Recipes	More information
fish *(cod filet)*	84	0	1.22	0	16.91	86, 94, 132, 138, 140, 146, 210, 266, 350, 352	6, 86, 192, 308, 348 352, 354
salmon *(1/2 filet)*	362	0	21	0	39	102, 108, 120, 142, 200, 358	
tuna *(can light)*	265	0	2.6	0	80.36	76, 116, 160, 196, 190, 182, 302, 308	
shrimp *(4 lg)*	30	0	0	0	6	158, 186, 326, 340	6, 86, 192, 308, 326 348, 352, 354

high omega-3 essential fatty acids • combats cancer • improves blood flow • "brain food"
boosts memory • reduces inflammation • helps maintain immune and circulatory systems
help prevent erratic heart rhythms • reduces risk of arrhythmia • reduces heart attacks and strokes
prevents and controls high blood pressure • reduces strokes • protects those with diabetes • fends off dry eyes
protective against deep vein thrombosis, pulmonary embolism, blood clots • reduces risk of macular degeneration
protects skin against sunburn, and possibly, skin cancer • improves mood • reduces depression
protects against Alzheimer's and age-related cognitive decline • destroys Alzheimer's plaques
lowers risk of Leukemia, Multiple Myeloma, and Non-Hodgkins Lymphoma • protects against childhood asthma

	Cal	Carb	Fat	Fbr	Prtn	In these Recipes	More information
chicken *(breast)*	193	0	7.6	0	29.2		

combats cancer • protects heart • protects against bone loss • gives you energy • protects against alzheimer's
essential for thyroid hormone metabolism, antioxidant defense systems, and immune function • increases energy

	Cal	Carb	Fat	Fbr	Prtn	In these Recipes	More information
turkey *(breast)*	212	0	8.3	0	32.16	4	254
turkey *(lean,ground)*	193	0	11	0	22	(4oz burger) 240, 306, 338, 356	
turkey *(bacon/1oz)*	61	0	4	0	5	14, 184, 168, 180, 344, 340	

combats cancer • protects heart • optimizes insulin activity • induces DNA repair and synthesis in damaged cells
essential component of several major metabolic pathways, including thyroid hormone metabolism,
antioxidant defense systems, and immune function • converts proteins, fats, and carbohydrates into usable energy

	Cal	Carb	Fat	Fbr	Prtn	In these Recipes	More information
egg *(hard boiled)*	78	.56	5.3	0 6	.29	6, 10, 14, 18, 24, 32, 58, 120, 122, 138, 140, 152, 162 168, 178, 186, 196, 208, 228, 254, 256, 258, 260, 262 274, 280, 300, 320, 328, 334, 358, 364	

contains more essential vitamins and minerals per calorie than virtually any other food
improves brain function • prevents blood clots • protects against macular degeneration and cataracts
recent studies found no connection between egg consumption and heart disease or high cholesterol
Note: One egg equals one ounce of meat

	Cal	Carb	Fat	Fbr	Prtn	In these Recipes	More information
tofu *(1 slicefirm)*	52	2	2	0	6		

combats cancer • protects heart • lowers cholesterol • reduces arthritis symptoms • high in protein • builds muscle
reduces menopause symptoms • protects bones • rich in minerals for energy and antioxidant protection

Nuts

Nuts are one of the best plant sources of protein. They are also rich in fiber, phytonutrients and antioxidants such as Vitamin E and selenium. Unfortunately, they are also very high in calories and fat, so you will need to limit the amount you eat. *Note: 1/3 cup of nuts equals one ounce serving of protein.*

	Cal	Carb	Fat	Fbr	Prtn	In these Recipes	More information
almonds	824	27	73	4.2	30		
lowers cholesterol • reduces risk of heart disease • promotes optimal health • assists in weight loss							
cashews	784	44.8	63.48	4.8	20.96		
protects heart • high in antioxidants • increases energy • helps development of bones and blood vessels							
water chestnuts	120	30	0	4	2		
combats cancer • protects heart • promotes weight loss • lowers cholesterol • controls blood pressure							
peanuts	828	6	71	12.4	27		
protects against heart disease • promotes weight loss • combats prostate cancer • lowers cholesterol							
pecans	753	15.2	78.5	10.5	10		
protects against heart disease • promotes weight loss • combats prostate cancer • lowers cholesterol							
pistachio	699	33	56.6	12.7	26.3		
high in antioxidants • reduces risk of cancer and heart disease • high fiber food • reduces risk of macular degeneration							
walnuts	654	13.7	65.2	6.7	15.2		
combats cancer • protects heart • lifts mood • lowers cholesterol • boosts memory							

Legumes

Legumes (beans and lentils) are packed with nutrition, including protein, calcium, vitamins and minerals. Eat in place of refined carbohydrates, as they can prevent food cravings, prevent metabolic syndrome, prevent type 2 diabetes, protect against cancer, prevent obesity and protect against heart disease.
Note: 1/2 cup of beans equals a one ounce serving of meat.

	Cal	Carb	Fat	Fbr	Prtn	In these Recipes	More information
black beans	227	41	22	15	15.2		
combats cancer • protects heart • lowers cholesterol • increases energy level • stabilizes blood sugar • high in protein contains high level of antioxidants • improves flow of blood, oxygen and nutrients throughout body							
garbanzo beans	286	54.3	2.7	10.6	11.9		
(chickpeas) can lower cholesterol • improves blood sugar levels • great food for diabetics							
kidney beans	210	37.1	1.5	11	13.4		
combats cancer • protects heart • increases energy • stabilizes blood sugar • helps memory • lowers cholesterol							
lima beans	190	39.5	.5	11.6	11.9		
combats cancer • protects heart • lowers cholesterol • stabilizes blood sugar • increases energy							
navy beans	296	53.7	1	13.4	19.7		
combats cancer • protects heart • increases energy • stabilizes blood sugar • helps memory • lowers cholesterol							
soy beans *(Edamame)*	254	20	12	8	22		
great meat replacement • combats cancer • protects heart • lowers blood pressure lowers cholesterol • increases energy							

Vegetables

Vegetables provide essential nutrients for good health and the maintenance of your body. To maximize the availability of these nutrients, vegetables should be eaten raw or steamed lightly when possible. Vegetables are also generally low in carbs and calories. This enables you to eat larger quantities without risking additonal weight gain. *The FDA recommends 2½ or more cups daily.*

	Cal	Carb	Fat	Fbr	Prtn	In these Recipes	More information
asparagus	34	5.2	.16	2.8	2.95	194, 274	194, 274
detoxifying & diuretic effects • rids body of excess water • cleans out gastrointestinal tract							
broccoli	31	6	.34	2.4	2.57	52, 208, 284, 332	52, 284, 332, 360
combats cancer • strengthens bones • detoxifies body • prevents ulcers • saves eyesight may prevent some birth defects • wards off heart disease • reduces chance of stroke • combats anemia							
brussel sprouts	00	00	00	00	00		
combats cancer • excellent source of vitamin D and folic acid during pregnancy may prevent some birth defects • contains higher protein levels than most vegetables							
beets *(cooked)*	37	8	0	2	1	20	20
combats cancer • protects heart • pressure • strengthens bones • aids weight loss • controls blood							
cabbage	22	5.16	.09	2.2	1.14	154, 166	52, 260
contains anti-peptic ulcer factor • optimizes our cells' ability to disarm and clear free radicals and toxins lowers risk of cancer • lowers risk of lung cancer in smokers by 69% • protects heart • promotes weight loss helps hemorrhoids • prevents constipation							
carrots	35	8.25	.13	2.9	.64	154, 166, 242, 256	44, 175, 242, 354
combats cancer • saves eyesight • improves night vision • prevents constipation • promotes weight loss the richest vegetable source of the pro-vitamin A carotenes • protect against cardiovascular disease regulates blood sugar • may reduce chances of lung inflammation and emphysema							
cauliflower	25	5.3	.10	2.5	1.98	208, 260	52, 260
protects against prostate and breast cancers • banishes bruises • strengthens bones guards against heart disease and hypertension							
celery	16	3	.17	1.6	.70	6, 58, 68, 76, 112, 116, 148, 186, 204, 214, 262, 308, 330, 332	41, 204
may reduce blood pressure • combats obesity • may help reduce cold symptoms or severity of cold symptoms reduces severity of inflammatory conditions, such as asthma, osteoarthritis, and rheumatoid arthritis combats cancer • lowers cholesterol • reduces strokes							
collard greens	11	2.05	.15	1.3	.88		
a nutritional superstar • lessens many cancers, including breast and ovarian cancers							
cucumbers	68	3.78	.12	.6	.68	208, 260	52, 260
lowers blood pressure • smoothes skin • prevents water retention							
eggplant	20	4.67	.16	2.8	.83	18, 152, 256, 320	166
combats cancer • lowers cholesterol • protects brain and joints from free radical damage							

	Cal	Carb	Fat	Fbr	Prtn	In these Recipes	More information
green beans	34	7.83	.13	3.7	2.0	270, 326, 332	270, 360
maintains strong bones • reduces risk of blocked arteries, heart attack or stroke • controls blood pressure							
green peppers	30	6.91	.25	2.5	1.28	24, 148, 152, 158, 166, 168, 170, 174, 178, 204 206, 214, 222, 240, 254, 256, 262, 266, 288, 306 316, 326, 330, 332, 352, 362	284, 154
combats cancers • prevents constipation • lowers cholesterol • helps hemorrhoids • stabilizes blood sugar very powerful antioxidant • reduces risk of heart attack and stroke							
mushrooms	15	2	0	1	2	32, 38, 186, 206, 222, 234, 240, 270, 296, 300, 302, 342, 362	
combats cancer • controls blood pressure • lowers cholesterol • kills bacteria • strengthens bones							
onions	64	15	0	3	2	Too many to list	72
combats cancer • reduces risk of heart attack • kills bacteria • lowers cholesterol • fights fungus antibiotic and bactericidal effects • has soothing action on the respiratory system • diminishes risk of blood clots improves lung function, especially in asthmatics							
peas	117	21	1	7	8	14, 72, 248, 282, 344, 354	2
combats cancers • maintains strong bones • protects heart • increases energy							
potatoes	116	26	0	4	4	44, 48, 140, 202, 256, 272	40, 212, 284
combats cancer • controls blood pressure • protects heart • reduces stress • aids in building new cells							
romaine lettuce	8	2	0	1	1	20, 68, 356	154
protects heart • lowers cholesterol • reduces strokes • lowers blood pressure							
spinach	7	1.09	.12	.7	.86	6, 24, 38, 122, 180, 164, 234, ,258 280, 292 300, 302, 308, 312, 332	122, 154, 260, 274 332, 360
blood enricher • gland regulator • effective alkalizer and laxative • promotes gastrointestinal health protects against osteoporosis, heart disease and arthritis • functions as antioxidant and as anti-cancer agent contins anti-inflammatory nutrients • protects brain from oxidative stress • slows loss of mental function protective against eye diseases such as age-related macular degeneration and cataracts • increases energy							
sweet potato	114	27	0	4	4	16, 44	40, 44
combats cancer • lifts mood • strengthens bones and teeth • helps heart and kidney function improves vision, skin, nail, and hair health • helps fend off bacterial infections • regulates blood pressure keeps blood vessel walls and gums healthy							
summer squash	18	4	0	1	1		
reduces risk of heart attack and stroke • reduces blood pressure • lowers cholesterol							
tomatoes *this is actually a fruit, though often thought of as a vegetable.*	25	5.02	.30	1.4	1.83	6, 14, 18, 28, 32, 50, 52, 102, 128, 144, 148 152, 168, 174 184, 240, 288, 300, 308, 316, 320 330, 342, 356	40, 58, 154, 188, 284 320, 354
neutralizes free radicals and cuts the risk of cancers • lowers cholesterol • natural antiseptic • prevents diarrhea reduces risk of heart attack • keeps bones strong • helps prevent hemorrhages • can dissolve gallstones improves texture of skin and adds glow • has blood purifying properties • protects liver from cirrhosis reduces risk of macular degenerative disease • soothes eye irritation • prevents night blindness when applied topically, tomato pulp can help heal sunburn, wounds and sores • reduces urinary tract infections							

Fruits

Fruits provide the nutrients essential for good health and the maintenance of your body. Eating fruits provides incredible health benefits: however, they are generally higher in carbs and calories. So, even though healthy, you must limit your portions. *The FDA recommends 2-3 cups daily.*

	Cal	Carb	Fat	Fbr	Prtn	In these Recipes	More information
apples (med)	72	19.6	.23	3.3	.36	34, 54, 68, 88, 118, 112, 118, 156, 230, 298, 252, 328, 338	212, 230, 252, 360
protects heart • prevents constipation • prevents diarrhea • improves lung capacity • cushions joints • reduces strokes protect post-menopausal women from osteoporosis and may increase bone density • strengthens bones reduces the risk of asthma in children when mother eats apples • may protect from Alzheimer's disease lowers LDL ("bad") cholesterol • reduces risk of some cancers • aids in management of diabetes • promotes weight loss							
apricots (med)	74	17.4	.6	3.1	2.2		
protects heart • reduces risk of cataracts and macular degeneration • helps lower cholesterol							
avocados *(med)*	227	11.75	20.96	9.2	2.67	10, 50, 158, 168, 288	10, 288
battles diabetes • lowers cholesterol • reduces strokes • smoothes skin • lowers incidence of heart disease inhibits growth of prostate cancer • protects against macular degeneration and cataracts • controls blood pressure							
banana *(med)*	105	27	.39	3.1	1.29	2, 40, 70, 134, 136, 212, 232, 250, 268, 276, 324	2, 40
protects heart • quiets a cough • controls blood pressure • prevents diarrhea • strengthens bones keeps nervous system in good shape • minimizes risk of kidney stones • minimizes loss of calcium reduces risk of osteoporosis • acts as mood enhancers or mild sedatives • maintains healthy immune response							
blackberries	62	13.84	.71	7.6	2	192	212, 360
combats cancer • protects heart • boosts memory • prevents constipation • stabilizes blood sugar							
blueberries	84	21.45	.49	3.6	1.10	192, 212, 238, 276, 286	238, 212, 318
combats cancer • protects heart • boosts memory • prevents constipation • stabilizes blood sugar • lowers cholesterol effective immune builder and anti-bacterial • neutralizes free radicals • reduces signs of aging • reduces belly fat promotes urinary tract health • preserves vision • lowers risk of age-related macular degeneration prevents and heals neurotic disorders • heals damaged brain cells • restores health of central nervous system improves learning capacity and motor skills • strengthens cardiac muscles • improves digestion • acts as anti-depressant							
cantaloupe	54	13	.30	1.4	1.34	30	284
combats cancer • saves eyesight • lowers cholesterol • supports immune system • controls blood pressure reduces fever • fights obesity • reduces risk of rheumatism and arthritis • prevents skin diseases and constipation reduces abdominal and stomach gas • prevents blood deficiencies • minimizes disorders of the kidneys and bladder							
cherries	74	18.7	.23	2.5	1.24	192	360
combats cancer • protects heart • ends insomnia • slows aging • shields against alzheimer's							
cranberries	51	13	0	5	0	84, 236, 246, 312	212
aids digestion • normalizes bowels • prevents bladder infections • reduces risk of urinary tract and kidney infections protects against viruses • combats herpes virus • acts as a natural probiotic • prevents the development of cavities prevents kidney stone formation • increases HDL (good) cholesterol • reduces LDL (bad) cholesterol							
grapefruit *(lg)*	104	26	0	4	2		2, 95, 320
protects heart • promotes weight loss • reduces strokes • combats prostate cancer • lowers cholesterol							

	Cal	Carb	Fat	Fbr	Prtn	In these Recipes	More information
grapes *(purple)*	104	27.3	.24	1.4	1.09	4, 112, 134, 216, 204, 324	310, 324
stimulates bile secretion • helps burn fat • mild laxative • blood cleanser • reduces stress • reduces risk of cancers decreases risk of heart disease • reduces platelet clumping and blood clots • helps keep the heart muscle flexible may lower cholesterol • protective for persons with high blood pressure • may lower risk of Alzheimer's Disease protective against food-borne illness • reduces risk of all-causes of mortality							
honeydew	61	15.45	.24	1.4	.92	30	2
combats cancer • supports immune system • protects heart • enhances blood flow							
kiwi *(lg)*	56	13.34	.47	2.7	1.04	164, 236	
combats cancer • strengthens immune system • fights depression • stabilizes blood sugar • reduces impotence benefits respiratory tract • reduces syptoms of colds • protects from age-related macular degeneration lowers cholesterol • prevents asthma • prevents wheezing and coughing • protects dna from mutations							
mango *(med)*	135	35.19	.56	3.7	1.06	82, 134, 148, 158, 294	44
combats cancer • supports immune system • protects heart • enhances blood flow • prevents constipation							
orange *(med)*	69	17.56	.21	3.1	1.27	36, 70, 62, 134, 148, 236, 228, 232, 276, 244, 302, 324, 310	2, 58
combats cancer • supports immune system • protects heart • strengthens respiration • reduces stress							
peaches	60	14.69	.39	2.3	1.40	192, 212, 250	2
combats cancer • prevents constipation • reduces strokes • helps hemorrhoids • aids digestion reduces risk of macular degeneration							
pears *(med)*	103	27.52	.21	5.5	.68	324	
combats cancer • prevents constipation • kills bacteria and viruses • protects colon • aids with gout							
pineapple	109	28	0	2	1	12, 36, 74, 76, 90, 104, 134, 192, 216, 204, 218, 324, 340	216
strengthens bones • relieves colds and coughs • dissolves warts • prevents diarrhea • aids digestion effects growth of bones in young people • strengthens bones in older people							
pomegranates *(4" round)*	234	52.7	3.4	11.3	4.7		
helps stop blood clots • can increases blood flow from the heart • slows growth of tumors reduces risk of breast cancer							
plums	76	18.8	.46	2.3	1.15		212
assists with absorption of iron • helps eyesight • boosts memory • lowers cholesterol							
prunes/dried	418	111.15	.66	12.4	3.79		2
slows aging • prevents constipation • lowers cholesterol • protects against heart disease • boosts memory							
strawberries	46	11	.43	2.9	.96	2, 12, 26, 36, 40, 70, 192, 212, 238, 232, 286	212, 284, 360
combats cancer • protects heart • reduces blood pressure • reduces risk of rheumatism, gout, and cataracts nourishes brain cells increasing brain health and function • prevents constipation • removes tartar from teeth							
watermelon	46	11.48	.23	.6	.93		2, 58, 320
protects prostate • promotes weight loss • lowers cholesterol • reduces strokes • controls blood pressure great source of antioxidant, lycopene • reduces risk of rheumatoid arthritis • increases energy removes ammonia from body • reduces severity of asthma • reduces risk of colon cancer • protects heart							

Herbs & spices

Herbs and spices have more disease-fighting antioxidants than most fruits and vegetables–
be sure to add them to your foods for extra health benefits and great taste!

	In these Recipes	More information
basil	6, 14, 46, 86, 102, 200, 296, 308, 316, 332, 354	
protects heart • fights bacteria • anti-inflammatory • aids with rheumatoid arthritis and inflammatory bowels offers the same anti-inflammatory effects as medical marijuana without the mental and neurological side effects		
bay leaves	246	
apply to rheumatic joints to relieve pain • add to bath for body aches • promotes digestion • normalizes blood sugar antifungal and antibacterial properties when applied to skin • bay leaf tea can relieve colds and headaches		
black pepper	28, 32, 44, 68, 102, 128, 188, 226, 248, 296	
has antioxidant and antibacterial properties • improves digestion • prevents intestinal gas		
cayenne pepper	172, 242	
fights cancer • helps inflammatory pain • clears congestion • boosts immunity • protects heart • promotes weight loss		
chili pepper	24, 130, 160, 188, 240, 266, 288, 330, 352	
combats cancer • aids digestion • clears sinuses • boosts immune system • soothes a sore throat		
cinnamon	76, 84, 100, 114, 118, 188, 228, 230, 236, 244, 246, 250, 328	100
prevents blood clots • boosts brain • protects heart• stabilizes blood sugar levels • stops bacteria and fungus growth		
dill	6, 20, 48, 50, 138, 308	
protects against free radicals and carcinogens (smoke) • prevents bone loss • prevents bacteria growth • aids in digestion		
garlic	Too many to list.	72, 202
combats cancer • lowers cholesterol • controls blood pressure • kills bacteria • fights fungus		
ginger	18, 74, 182, 278, 252, 352	129
decreases motion sickness and nausea • may relieve pain and swelling associated with arthritis		
oregano	6, 14, 44, 52, 88, 94, 102, 196, 248, 274, 308, 320	
combats cancer • protects heart • potent anti-oxidant • lowers cholesterol • stops bacteria growth		
parsley	48, 66, 72, 94, 102, 140, 160, 184, 200, 220, 242, 262, 272, 284, 332, 344, 354	
vitamin rich herb (A, B and C) • decreases stomach gas • combats rheumatic pain		
paprika	220	
contains capsaicin, whose anti-inflammatory and antioxidant effects may lower the risk of cancer		
rosemary	62, 74, 310, 338	
aids in digestion • improves blood circulation when applied externally		
sage	338	
a life giving tea and general health tonic		
thyme	62, 132, 200, 184, 266, 296, 316, 320	
natural medicine for respiratory problems • used as a gargle and disinfectant • preserves foods • kills bacteria in foods		

Minerals

The foods we eat contain a host of vitamins, minerals and other nutrients that keep our bodies strong and healthy. The next few pages will be dedicated to explaining the importance of each—when you know why you eat healthy foods you will be more inclined to do so.

	Benefits	Food Sources
calcium	*strong bones and teeth • blood clotting muscle and nerve function*	*green leafy vegetables • sardines with bones • tofu*
chloride	*aids digestion*	*foods with salt*
chromium	*carbohydrate metabolism*	*vegetables • whole grains • brewer's yeast*
copper	*blood cell and connective tissue formation*	*grains • legumes • shellfish*
flouride	*strengthens tooth enamel*	*flouridated water • fish • tea*
iodine	*maintains proper function of thyroid*	*milk • grain • iodized salt*
iron	*carries oxygen in blood • energy metabolism*	*red meat • fish • poultry • whole grains • legumes dark green leafy vegetables*
magnesium	*aids nerve and muscle function • strong bones*	*legumes • nuts • grains • green vegetables*
manganese	*bone and connective tissue formation fat and carbohydrate metabolism*	*spinach • nuts • pumpkin • tea • legumes*
potassium	*controls acid balance in the body works with sodium to maintian fluid balance*	*vegetables • fruits • meats • milk*
selenium	*helps vitamin e protect cells and body tissue protect cells from free-radical damage enables thyroid to produce thyroid hormone lowers risk of joint inflammation*	*button mushrooms • shiitake mushrooms • cod shrimp • snapper • tuna • halibut • calf's liver salmon • brazil nuts*
signs you are low selenium	weakness or pain in the muscles • fingernails whitening discoloration of the hair or skin	
sodium	*fluid balance • nervous system function*	*salt • foods which contain salt*
zinc	*heals wounds • promotes growth • increases appetite*	*seafood • meats • nuts • legumes*

Vitamins

	Benefits	Food Sources
vitamin d	*calcium absorption • bone and tooth growth*	*sunlight • fortified milk • eggs • fish*
vitamin e	*protects cells from damage • antioxidant*	*vegetable oils • green leafy vegetables wheat germ • whole grain products*
vitamin k	*reduces clotting of blood protects bones from fractures prevents postmenopausal bone loss prevenst calcification of your arteries*	*spinach • brussels sprouts • swiss chard • green beans asparagus • broccoli • kale • mustard greens green peas • carrots*
signs you are low vitamin k	excessive bleeding—heavy menstruals, bleeding gums, nose bleeds easy bruising • bone fractures or bones weakening	

Vitamins

	Benefits	Food Sources
vitamin a	*heals woulds • promotes growth • increases appetite*	*seafood • meats • nuts • legumes*
b vitamins		
biotin	*fat, protein and carbohydrate metabolism*	*whole and enriched grains • vegetables • meats*
folate	*red blood cell development • tissue growth & repair*	*green leafy vegetables • oranges • beans*
flavonoids	*protects blood vessels from rupture or leakage* *prevents excessive inflammation in body* *nervous system function • enhances power of vitamin c* *protect cells from oxygen damage*	*apples • apricots • blueberries • pears • raspberries* *strawberries • black beans • cabbage • onions • parsley* *pinto beans • tomatoes*
signs you are low flavonoids	red or sore tongue • tingling or numbness in feet easy bruising • excessive swelling after injury frequent colds or infections • frequent nose bleeds • nervousness	
pantothenic	*fat, protein and carbohydrate metabolism*	*wholes and enriched grains • meats • vegetables*
riboflavin	*fat, protein and carb metabolism • healthy skin*	*dairy products • wholes and enriched grains*
thiamin b1	*carb metabolism • maintains healthy nervous system* *maintains energy supplies • supports heart function*	*asparagus • romaine lettuce • mushrooms • spinach* *sunflower seeds • tuna • green peas • tomatoes* *brussels sprouts • eggplant*
signs you are low thiamin	loss of appetite • "pins and needles" sensations feeling of numbness, especially in the legs muscle tenderness, particularly in the calf muscles	
niacin b3	*stabilizes blood sugar • helps body process fats* *supports genetic processes in cells*	*salmon • chicken breast • asparagus • halibut • venison* *crimini mushrooms • tuna*
signs you are low niacin	generalized weakness or muscular weakness lack of appetite • skin infections • digestive problems	
vitamin b6	*protein metabolism needed for normal growth*	*meats • poultry • fish • beans • grains* *dark green leafy vegetables*
vitamin b12	*supports red blood cell growth • improves skin* *helps metabolize protein, carbohydrate and fats* *allows nervous system to develop properly • prevents anemia*	*best source: calf's liver • snapper* *other: meats • poultry • fish • dairy products*
signs you are low b12	red or sore tongue • tingling or numbness in feet • nervousness heart palpitations • depression • memory problems	
vitamin c	*maintains healthy gums, teeth and blood vessels* *builds collagen • reduces risk of cancer* *helps protect cells from free radical damage* *regenerate vitamin e • improve iron absorption*	*parsley • broccoli • bell pepper • strawberries* *lemon juice • papaya • cauliflower • kale • oranges* *mustard greens • brussels sprouts*
signs you are low vitamin c	slow healing wounds • frequent colds or infections lung-related problems	

Other nutrients

	Benefits	Food Sources
carotenoids	*protects cells from damaging effects of free radicals* *enhances functioning of immune system* *helps reproductive system function properly*	*carrots, sweet potatoes, spinach, kale, collard greens* *tomatoes*
choline	*keeps cell membranes functioning properly* *allows nerves to communicate with muscles* *prevents build-up of homocysteine* *reduces cardiovascular disease and osteoporosis* *reduces chronic inflammation*	*soybeans, egg yolk, butter, peanuts, potatoes* *cauliflower, lentils, oats, sesame seeds and flax seeds*
signs you are low choline	fatigue • insomnia • nerve-muscle problems poor ability of the kidneys to concentrate urine accumulation of fats in the blood	
coenzyme q	*helps prevent cardiovascular disease* *stabilizes blood sugar* *helps reproductive system function properly*	*fish, organ meats (liver, heart, or kidney)* *germ portion of whole grains*
dietary fiber	*regulates bowles • normalizes blood sugar levels* *helps maintain normal cholesterol levels* *helps maintain healthy weight*	*turnip greens • mustard greens • cauliflower* *collard greens • broccoli • swiss chard • raspberries* *whole grains*
signs you are low fiber	constipation • high blood sugar levels high cholesterol levels	
glutamine	*maintains health of intestinal tract* *helps produce glutathione, a key antioxidant nutrient* *ensures proper acid-base balance in body* *helps maintain muscle mass*	*cabbage, beets, beef, chicken, fish, beans* *dairy products*
signs you are low glutamine	frequent colds and flus • low muscle mass intestinal dysbiosis, e.g., irritable bowel syndrome	
lycopene	*protects cells from damaging effects of free radicals* *slows the development of atherosclerosis*	*watermelon, tomatoes, pink grapefruit, guava*
omega-3 fatty acids	*lowers amount of lipids in bloodstream* *reduces inflammation throughout body* *reduces blood clots • maintains fluidity of cell membranes* *inhibits thickening of the arteries • helps prevent cancers* *improves body's ability to respond to insulin*	*salmon • cod • tuna • fish oil capsuls* *cod liver oil (3 tsp per day)*
signs you are low omega-3s	suffering from cardiovascular disease or type 2 diabetes fatigue • dry, itchy skin • brittle hair and nails joint pain • inability to concentrate • depression	
tryptophan	*helps regulate appetite • improves sleep* *elevates mood*	*red meat • dairy products • nuts • seeds • bananas* *soybeans and soy products • tuna • shellfish • turkey*
signs you are low tryptophan	depression • anxiety • irritability • impatience impulsiveness • inability to concentrate • insomnia slow growth in children • unexplained weight changes overeating and/or carbohydrate cravings • poor dream recall	

Here I have put together a list of some of the *"better choices"* from fast food restaurants.
Note, simply because something is on this list does not mean it has my endorsement as something you *should eat*. It's simply the healthiest of the options which are available.

Some basic rules to follow when eating out:

- Request dressings and sauces to be served on the side
- Choose broth based soups over cream based
- Choose lean cuts of meat, avoid processed meats
- Skip mayonnaise, order with mustard instead
- Avoid super-sized specials, unless you plan to share
- Avoid fried foods
- Order low fat dressing for your salad
- Order sandwiches on whole grain bread
- Don't order with extra cheese
- Skip dessert.

McDonalds

	Cal	Carb	Fat	Fbr	Prtn
breakfast					
egg mcmuffin	300	30	12	2	18
scrambled eggs	170	1	11	0	15
desserts					
apple dippers	100	23	.5	0	0
yogurt parfait (with granola)	160	31	2	0	4
yogurt parfait (no granola)	130	25	2	0	4
kiddie cone	45	8	1	0	1
salads *no dressing // see dressing info below*					
southwest (no chicken)	140	20	4.5	6	6
southwest (grilled chix)	320	30	9	6	30
caesar salad (no chicken)	90	9	4	3	7
caesar salad (grilled chix)	220	12	6	3	30
fruit & walnut	210	31	8	2	4
side salad	20	4	0	1	1
dressing					
low fat balsamic dressing	40	4	3	0	0
sandwiches					
cheeseburger	300	33	12	2	15
hamburger	250	33	9	1	12
mcchicken	360	40	16	2	14
filet-o-fish	380	38	18	2	15

Taco Bell

	Cal	Carb	Fat	Fbr	Prtn
side dishes					
pinto's & cheese	170	19	6	9	10
pinto's fresco style	130	20	2.5	9	7
burritos					
chili cheese	370	40	16	4	16
grilled chicken	430	46	18	3	8
bean	370	55	10	11	14
gordita bajas					
beef	350	30	18	4	13
chicken	320	29	15	3	16
steak	310	28	15	3	14
tacos					
grilled chx soft	270	21	14	2	14
grilled steak soft	250	20	14	2	11
soft beef taco	210	21	9	3	10
taco	170	12	10	3	9
fresco style tacos					
crunchy taco	150	13	7	3	7
soft taco with beef	180	22	7	3	8
ranchero chix soft	160	21	4.5	2	9
grilled steak soft	160	21	4.5	2	9

Panera Bread

	Cal	Carb	Fat	Fbr	Prtn
breakfast					
egg and cheese grilled	380	43	14	na	18
desserts					
apple	80	21	0	na	0
salads • *use low fat dressings*					
classic cafe salad	170	18	11	na	2
soups • *low fat versions*					
chicken noodle	110	10	4	na	8
chicken tortilla	190	24	6	na	10
black bean	170	29	4	na	10
garden vegetable	160	28	3.5	na	5
sandwich • *smoked turkey breast 1/2 size*					
on sourdough	225	35	1.5	na	17

Subway

	Cal	Carb	Fat	Fbr	Prtn
breads *choose one of the 6 inch subs*					
honey oat bread	260	49	3	5	9
wheat bread	210	42	2	4	8

condiments
choose the honey mustard, yellow mustard, brown mustard or sweet onion sauce
load with lettuce, tomatoes, onions, green peppers, pickles and olives

main topping
choose the ham, roast beef, turkey or veggie

	Cal	Carb	Fat	Fbr	Prtn
mini subs					
ham	180	31	2.5	3	10
roast beef	200	30	3.0	4	15
turkey	190	31	2.5	3	12
veggie	150	30	1.5	3	6

Chick-fil-A

	Cal	Carb	Fat	Fbr	Prtn
wraps					
chargrilled chix	410	50	12	9	33
chicken caesar	460	47	15	8	39
spicy chicken	410	48	12	8	35
salads/sides					
chargrilled and fruit salad	230	23	6	4	22
chargrilled chx	180	11	6	4	22
southwest	240	18	9	5	22
fruit cup	100	27	0	3	1
hearty chx soup	220	30	6	3	12
sandwiches					
chargrilled chix	300	38	3.5	3	23

Dairy Queen

	Cal	Carb	Fat	Fbr	Prtn
sandwiches					
hamburger	350	33	14	1	17
grilled chix	330	48	11	1	24
grilled chix wrap	200	9	13	1	12
shredded chix	290	30	7	1	30
salads/sides					
side salad	50	11	0	3	2

Burger King

	Cal	Carb	Fat	Fbr	Prtn
breakfast					
breakfast muffin	400	24	9	na	17
sandwiches *order with NO mayo*					
cheeseburger	310	28	15	na	16
hamburger	260	27	11	na	14
whopper jr.	260	28	11	na	14
bk veggie burger	340	46	8	na	23
tendergrill chix	360	40	5	na	55
salads *with fat free ranch dressing*					
side salad	190	31	6	na	6
tendergrill grdn	350	33	3.5	na	36

KFC

	Cal	Carb	Fat	Fbr	Prtn
wraps/sandwiches *no sauces on sandwiches*					
kfc snacker	210	3	32	2	13
tndr rst fillet wp	240	8	23	1	20
tndr grill fillet wp	240	8	23	1	19
grill fillet sand	200	4.5	32	2	32
chicken					
grill chix wing	80	5	1	0	9
grill chix breast	210	8	0	0	34
grill chix thigh	160	11	0	0	16
grill chix drum	80	4	0	0	11
salads *no dressing or croutons // dressing info below*					
grill chix caesar	210	7	5	2	33
grill chix blt	230	8	7	3	34
house side	15	0	2	1	1
dressings					
light italian	10	.5	2	0	1
fat free ranch	35	0	8	0	1
sides					
green beans	20	0	3	1	1
mshed pot/no gravy	90	3	15	1	2
3" corn on cob	70	.5	16	2	2
three bean salad	70	0	14	3	3

Arbys

	Cal	Carb	Fat	Fbr	Prtn
salads					
farmhouse chix	260	10	14	3	24
side salad	70	4	5	1	4
soups					
chix noodle	80	11	2	1	6
vegetable soup	90	10	4	1	2
potato soup	170	23	7	2	6
sandwiches					
grilled rst chx	406	40	16	3	24
arby's melt	320	38	11	2	18
arby's q	370	51	10	3	19
ham & swiss	300	37	8	2	18
roast beef	350	37	13	2	13

Wendy's

	Cal	Carb	Fat	Fbr	Prtn
salads					
garden side	25	5	0	2	1
caesar side	60	5	0	2	4
apple pecan salad	350	29	12	5	37
-light ranch dressing	100	4	9	0	2
-fat free french	80	19	0	1	0
sandwiches					
grilled chicken	370	42	7	2	34
jr. cheeseburger	270	27	11	1	15
jr. hamburger	230	26	8	1	12
grilled chix wrap	260	25	10	1	20
homestyle chix wrp	320	29	16	1	15
spicy chix wrp	310	30	15	2	15
sides					
large chili	340	32	10	8	28
small chili	220	22	3	6	18
mandarin oranges	90	21	0	1	1
plain baked potato	270	61	0	7	7

Hardees

	Cal	Carb	Fat	Fbr	Prtn
breakfast					
country ham biscuit	440	36	26	0	14
sides					
side salad	191	7	7	2	7
sandwiches					
cheeseburger	350	32	19	1	16
hamburger	310	32	15	1	14

Starbucks

	Cal	Carb	Fat	Fbr	Prtn
choose nonfat *"tall" (12 fl oz) options*					
caffè latte	100	0	15	0	10
cappuccino	60	0	9	0	6
iced caffè latte	70	0	10	0	6
iced skinny latte	60	0	9	0	6
skny cin dolce latte	90	0	14	0	9
skinny flavored latte	90	0	14	0	9

On page 4 I didn't list the excuse I hear most—or disagree with most.
"It's too expensive to eat healthy."

Funny thing, when I'm on a tight budget I lose weight! So, I know for a fact this excuse is completely invalid. To prove my point I will use two full pages (36-37) to validate this answer.
If you read through and disagree I urge you to email me with your reason: cindy@ironworksfitness.org

Tips to eating healthy without spending a fortune.
1. Prepare your meals at home. And when you do, prepare large meals so that you can have leftovers throughout the week. Or freeze them for future use.
2. Shop the local Farmer's Markets. You can often get produce much cheaper here than you will at the grocery stores.
3. Buy discounted fruits and vegetables. I have often purchased ripe or slightly overripe fruit and vegetables for half of what I would normally pay. Then I take my find home, clean it and freeze it. Frozen fruit is excellent for smoothies and the frozen veggies work great in soups and egg scrambles.
4. Buy frozen fruits and vegetables on sale. Watch your sale papers, you can often purchase frozen fruits and vegetables for half of what fresh costs—and they still have great nutritional value.
5. Eat oatmeal for breakfast. Compared to other cereals it cost pennies a bowl.
6. Keep hard boiled eggs in the refridgerator. At $2/dozen this healthy treat costs less than 20¢!
7. Enjoy jello. You can even freeze it if you want! Another great food that costs less than 20¢ a serving.

Grocery shop intelligently, this is key to maintaining a health lifestyle.
- Go to the store with a list organized according to the categories: produce, meats, dairy, grains, drinks, etc.
- Don't go down the aisles containing cookies, chips or other unhealthy items, skip the tempation.
- Don't shop on an empty stomach, doing so will increase your chances of impulse buying.
- Try new healthy foods and recipes, you may find a new food you absolutely love!

Tips for cooking at home
- Prepare the recipes in this journal. (See pages 38 and 39 for complete list)
  Make it your goal to try each and every one—you might find something new you love!
- Prepare large portions and take leftovers to the office for lunch.
- Use herbs, spices and lemon juice instead of salt.
- Use non-stick cooking sprays and olive oil instead of vegetable oils.
- Never fry foods. Instead, broil, roast, bake, grill, stew or poach.
- Use lean cuts of meat. Always remove skin from chicken and turkey, cut off any fat.
- Use low-fat dairy items and light mayonnaise.
- Use frozen foods, as opposed to canned, when you can't use fresh.
- ALWAYS read labels.

The pricing and nutritional information on the next two pages was gathered from Dierberg's in Saint Louis, MO on September 3, 2010. The product and portion sizes are the same for compared products, unless otherwise noted.

Instead of this,	Sz	Cal	Fat	Prtn	Cost	**eat this!**	Sz	Cal	Fat	Prtn	Cost
From the deli:											
italian tortilla pasta salad	lb	-	-	-	5.99	4 bean salad	lb	-	-	-	3.99
chicken alfredo	lb	-	-	-	5.49	chicken parm	lb	-	-	-	4.99
corned beef	lb	-	-	-	9.49	turkey breast	lb	-	-	-	7.99
ham	lb	-	-	-	7.99	chicken breast	lb	-	-	-	7.49
cheddar cheese	lb	-	-	-	6.99	mozzerella cheese	lb	-	-	-	6.99
angel hair pasta	lb	-	-	-	3.99	spinach linguini	lb	-	-	-	3.99
dressings/toppings											
marzetti balsamic reg.	2tbs	90	8	0	1.49	marzetti balsamic light	2tbs	30	3	0	1.49
italian regular	2tbs	90	8	0	1.49	fat free italian	2tbs	15	0	0	1.49
hidden valley ranch	2tbs	140	14	1	3.18	ranch fat free	2tbs	30	0	0	3.28
kraft sand. shop mayo	2tbs	40	3.5	0	2.99	french's spicy mustard	2tbs	20	0	0	1.50
real bacon bits/1	1tbs	25	1.5	3	5.78	dry rstd sunflower seeds	1tbs	45	4	2	1.55
concord grape jelly	1tbs	50	0	0	2.79/18oz	low sugar version	1tbs	25	0	0	2.09/15.5oz
pasta/rice dishes											
newman's alfredo sauce	1/4 c	90	8	1	2.77	tomato & basil	1/4 c	45	2.25	1	2.77
ragu classic alfredo	1/4 c	110	10	1	1.99/16oz	tomato, garlic & onion	1/4 c	40	1.25	1	1.99/26oz
rice-a-roni chicken	1 c	230	1	7	1.18	whole grain version	1 c	190	1.5	6	1.18
riceland white rice	1/4 c	160	0	3	1.29	whole grain version	1/4 c	150	1	3	1.29
chichi's tortillas	1 trt.	160	3.5	4	2.19/8ct	whole wheat version	1 trt.	170	4	5	2.19/8ct
refried beans traditional	1/2 c	90	0	5	1.27	spicy fat free version	1/2 c	90	0	5	1.27
soups											
creamy chix mushroom	-	100	6	2	1.47	healthy request chix noodle	-	60	2	3	1.47
cream of mushroom	-	70	2.5	2	1.53	beefy mushroom	-	50	2	3	1.49
wheat thins original	-	140	5	1	2.00	reduced fat	-	130	3.5	2	2.00
bread											
plain bagels	1	260	2	9	2.49/6ct	english muffins	1	100	5	5	1.99/8ct
drinks											
coke	1	140	0	0	3.49/12ct	diet coke	1	0	0	0	3.49/12ct
pepsi	1	150	0	0	3.49/12ct	diet pepsi	1	0	0	0	3.49/12ct
						water	1	0	0	0	4.99/24ct
						green tea bags	1	0	0	0	3.99/40 bags
						folgers coffee	1	0	0	0	8.99/2lbs

Cut expenses & calories!

Instead of this, eat this!

	Sz	Cal	Fat	Prtn	Cost		Sz	Cal	Fat	Prtn	Cost
meats											
chix of the sea tuna/oil	¼c	100	6	10	.99	in water	¼c	50	5	11	.99
hamburger patties	1	330	29	17	4.19/6	chicken breasts	1	193	7.6	29	4.99/6
bacon	2 slices	80	7	4	4.19/1lb	turkey bacon	2 slices				
pork kielbasa	2oz	180	15	6	3.99	turkey kielbasa	2oz	80	6	9	1.99
beef brats	1	220	19	10	2.99	turkey brats	1	110	6	10	2.99
dairy											
land o lakes butter	-	90	10	0	2.18	light version	-	50	5	0	1.83
cottage cheese	½c	110	5	14	1.99	low fat version	½c	90	2.5	14	1.99
sour cream	2 tbs	60	5	1	2.00	low fat version	2 tbs	40	2.5	2	2.00
milk vitamin D	1c	150	8	8	3.35/gal	skim milk	1c	90	0	8	3.35
cheddar cheese	¼c	110	9	7	2.90	mozzarella cheese	¼c	80	6	8	2.90
vanilla ice cream	½c	160	9	2	3.99/1.75qt	vanilla yogurt	½c	120	2	3	2.29/qt
snacks											
chocolate chip cookie	1	80	4	1	3.19/13oz	reduced fat oreos	1	50	1.25	0	3.19//18oz
vanilla wafers	-	140	1.5	1	2.99	reduced fat wafers	-	120	2	1	2.99
reeses candy bar	1	210	13	5	.89	apple	1	72	.23	.36	.40
hershey's candy bar	1	210	13	3	.89	banana	1	105	.39	1.29	.30
kitkat candy bar	1	210	11	3	.89	peach	1	60	.39	1.40	.50
brown cow ice cream bars	1	120	7	2	2.49/12ct	northstar cherry pops	1	60	0	0	.99/6ct

Instead of this,	**eat this!**
bacon	*ham*
bagel	*english muffin*
baked potato	*baked sweet potato*
bran muffin	*bran flakes*
bread	*low carb tortilla shell*
cake	*fat free jello*
chai tea latte	*green tea*
cheese dip	*salsa*
cheddar cheese	*light mozzarella*
cole slaw	*lettuce salad*
cookies	*blueberries*
cream based soups	*broth based soups*
doritos	*peanuts*
donuts	*orange*
eggs and cheese	*scrambled egg whites*
french fries	*fruit and yogurt parfait*
fried foods	*baked foods*

Instead of this,	**eat this!**
hamburger	*bocca burger*
ice cream	*light yogurt*
margarita	*gin and diet tonic*
mayonaise	*mustard*
M&Ms	*strawberries*
mocha	*coffee with cream*
potato chips	*raw vegetables*
reg. salad dressing	*low-fat vinaigrette*
soda	*green tea*
steak	*cod fillet*
sweetened cereals	*oatmeal*
sub sandwich	*protein shake*
sugar	*honey*
snack mix	*popcorn*
potato salad	*three-bean salad*
white pasta	*wheat pasta*
white rice	*brown rice*

It's important to keep track of your workouts and calories burned.
Make copies of this page and put them in a binder or folder. You may even want to pre-date the charts, so you are not tempted to skip days. Each is set up for two days of activities.

Cardio Workout

DATE								
EXERCISE	Time	Mileage	Calories	Notes	Time	Mileage	Calories	Notes
Regular Bike								
Recumbent Bike								
Elliptical								
TreadMill								
Walking Outside								
Stairs								

Strength Workout *(you can burn 315-720 calories in an hour)*

DATE												
EXERCISE	REPS	WEIGHT	REPS	WEIGHT	REPS	WEIGHT	REPS	WEIGHT	REPS	WEIGHT	REPS	WEIGHT

One of the essential steps to leading a healthy lifestyle is to record what you eat and drink on a daily basis. I can't stress it enough: *if it goes in your mouth, you must write it down.* I often hear the excuse: *"I don't have time to write it down,"* my response is: *"It takes more time to eat something than it does to write it down–so, if you have time to eat it, you DO have time to write it down!"*

Date:	Water For The Day (X out for each 8ozs)	1	2	3	4	5	6	7	8
	FDA Recommendations (X out for each one met)	Dairy	Grains	Protein	Vegetables			Fruits	Oils

Time:		Calories
Time:		
Time:		
Time:		
Time:		
Time:		

Date:	Water For The Day (X out for each 8ozs)	1	2	3	4	5	6	7	8
	FDA Recommendations (X out for each one met)	Dairy	Grains	Protein	Vegetables			Fruits	Oils

Time:		Calories
Time:		
Time:		
Time:		
Time:		
Time:		

- Make sure you start each day with breakfast, then eat six SMALL meals every 2½ to 3½ hours
- STOP eating at least three hours before going to bed
- Try not to eat carbs later in the day, eat them early
- Use meal replacement bars/shakes–be sure to read labels, all are not created equal
- Keep track of calories consumed and calories burned

Books

The last time I actually "read" a book was over twenty years ago, *(gasp!)* Taking the time to sit and read is nearly impossible. However, I do keep up with reading by "listening to books." This I can do nearly anywhere and anytime. Whether I'm driving, working out or simply doing work around the house, there's always time to listen. Audio books may be purchased at most book stores, online and downloaded directly to your computer or picked up from the library. There's so much you can learn from reading and listening, it's a free education you can't afford to pass up. Picking just a few to share was very difficult, I do hope you enjoy them as much as I did.

Some of my favorite books:

Think & Grow Rich // *Napolean Hill* // My all time favorite book, a must read for everyone.
Create Your Greatest Life // *Les Brown* // How to create the life you always wanted.
Excuses Begone! // *Wayne Dyer* // How to change lifelong, self-defeating thinking habits.
Success Mastery Academy // *Brian Tracy* // Incredible motivational audio book.
Who Moved My Cheese? // Spencer Johnson //An amazing way to deal with change in your work and in your life.
Awaken the Giant Within // Anthony Robbins // A great motivational book.
How to Stay Motivated: The Goals Program // Zig Ziglar // Learn to set and achieve goals.
Healing Children Naturally // *Michael Savage*// A must have for all parents.
Spark // *John J Ratey* and Eric Hagerman// The revolutionary new science of exercise and the brain.
Body For Life // *Bill Phillips* // A 12-week challenge that changed my life over ten years ago.
Stop The Insanity // *Susan Powter* // Change the way you look and feel forever.
Make The Connection // Bob Greene and Oprah Winfrey // Ten steps to a better body and a better life.

Smart phone apps

Technology is a wonderful thing...even more impressive when you can use it to improve your life! Here you will find some great smart phone apps that put essential information at your fingertips!

Diet and Nutrition

Restaurant Nutrition Provides nutritional information for thousands of restaurants.
Food Network Nighttime Access great healthy recipes and instructional videos through the *Food Network.*
Shopping List Free Portable shopping list tool.
Nutrisystem Enjoy the ease and convenience of Nutrisystem from your iPhone.
LoseIt A great way to budget your calorie consumption with calories burned.
SparkPeople Complete health and fitness tracking for the iPhone.
MyNetDiary A diet and exercise program for the iPhone. Record calories consumed and burned.
Limeade Gives a health assessment and helps develop personalized fitness goals.
FitSync Access training programs, log your workouts and compare your progress to others. *$4.99*
SpeedoMeter A calculation tool that measure how fast you run or walk.
RunKeeper A tool that tracks your mileage using GPS.
iTreadmill Helps you keep track of how many steps you've taken, how far you've walked, your average speed and the amount of calories you've burned. *99¢*
iFitness Take exercises with you on the go as if you have your own personal trainer. *$1.99*
BMI calculator Gives information on your Body Mass Index.

Websites

Here, you will find a list of my favorite websites.
Each contains great information that will help you lead a healthy, happy life!

www.ironworksfitness.org //My personal website.
www.bodybuilder.com // Information, motivation and supplementation.
www.webmd.com // Better information for better health.
www.thedailyplate.com // An easy way to track what you are eating each day.
www.livestrong.com // Dare to change your life. A great health, fitness and lifestyle website.
www.fitnessmagazine.com // The website of Fitness magazine.
www.prevention.com // The website of Prevention magazine.
www.yogajournal.com // A great source for Yoga moves.
www.nutritiondata.self.com // An health and fitness information packed site from SELF.

Notes

Keep track of you own favorites here...

Now that you know what to do...
master your body and mind
on a daily basis — You are going to love the results!

Studies show that when you start your day with stretching you will be more energized and ready to tackle that which comes your way. Stretching also:
1) Increases range of motion, essential for daily activities.
2) Improves circulation and energy levels by increasing blood flow to your muscles.
3) Improves your posture and minimizes aches and pains.
4) Reduces stress, by relaxing tense muscles which often go hand-in-hand with stress.
In this section you will find several stretches which may be performed anywhere at any time.

A year from now you will wish you had started today.
–Karen Lamb

DATE

Steps Walked:
Cardio Workout:
Strength Training:
Calories Consumed:
Calories Burned:
Difference:
Weight / Body fat:

Write it down & get it done.

1
2
3
4
5
6
7
8
9
10

Read it, live it, love the results.

Read/use this book daily!
This journal has been written to help you stay on track with a healthy lifestyle. If you place it on your bookshelf, you will not reap its benefits–similar to a treadmill which is used to hang clothes. You are responsible for your future, everything you do today will take you closer to your goals or further from them. Which direction do you want to go? The choice is up to you.

Life's tough, get over it, he did!

Fitness, exercise and nutritional expert **Jack LaLanne** was addicted to sugar and junk foods when he was a child. He was very troubled and prone to rages, even attempted to burn down his family's home. At age fifteen, he heard a talk on health and nutrition and decided this is where he would place his focus. LaLanne became a successful bodybuilder, in addition to winning numerous awards, including a star on the Hollywood Walk of Fame and Hall of Fame.

All you need is the plan, the road map, and the courage to press on to your destination.
— Earl Nightengale

neck rotation

Standing or sitting tall, go through each of the stretches, holding each for 10 to 30 counts. Turn your head to the right, stretching your chin toward your shoulder. Bring your head back to center and touch your chin to your chest. Turn your head to the left, stretching your chin toward your shoulder. Look up at the ceiling, pushing your chin towards the ceiling, Repeat as necessary.

DATE

Steps Walked:
Cardio Workout:
Strength Training:
Calories Consumed:
Calories Burned:
Difference:
Weight / Body fat:

Eating healthy tastes great!

Strawberry Banana Shake
½ box sugar free strawberry gelatin
OR 1 cup strawberries
1 banana
16 oz cup of ice
½ cup skim milk
2 scoops vanilla protein

Place all ingredients in blender and blend until smooth.
I recommend that women use soy protein and men use whey protein.

Read it, live it, love the results.

Eat bananas, peaches and apricots to keep your blood pressure down.
Research indicates potassium is the mineral which helps control blood pressure. Bananas are often considered the perfect source of potassium, however, apricots, peaches, cantaloupe, grapefruit juice, honeydew melon, pears, watermelon, nectarines, orange juice, pomegranate, prunes, and raisins are also excellent sources.

Write it down & get it done.

1
2
3
4
5
6
7
8
9
10

torso stretch
Stand with feet together, raise hands overhead and stretch as far as you can without bending your torso. Hold for 10-30 counts. To stretch the obliques, reach hands to right, then to the left. Make sure your feet remain planted on the floor.

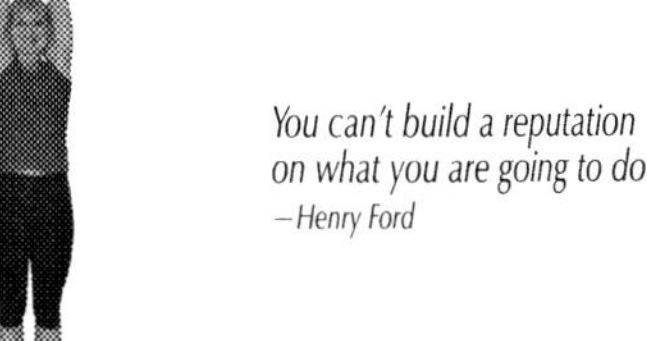

You can't build a reputation on what you are going to do.
– Henry Ford

DATE

Steps Walked:
Cardio Workout:
Strength Training:
Calories Consumed:
Calories Burned:
Difference:
Weight / Body fat:

Write it down & get it done.

1
2
3
4
5
6
7
8
9
10

Read it, live it, love the results.

Prioritize your tasks.
List each of your responsibilities in this book on a daily basis, then sort them, listing the top priority as "1" and so on down the list. Complete the most important tasks first. When you have a list to follow you will get more done throughout the day.

Life's tough, get over it, he did!

Conservative radio host, political commentator and author of twenty-five books including; *"Healing Children Naturally"*, **Dr. Michael Savage**, is the only member of the U.S. media ever blacklisted and banned from a Western nation. This ban has made him the *"poster child"* for free speech – not only for Americans, but for people around the globe. The ban of course has not stopped Dr. Savage from using his right to free speach – instead, it fueled his fire.

Nature arms each person with some faculty which enables them to do easily some feat impossible to any other.
– Ralph Waldo Emerson

basic stretch

Lie face up on the floor with legs extended straight out and toes pointing down. Extend your arms straight up, interlocking your fingers, with your palms pointing toward the ceiling. Keeping your arms straight, slowly lower your hands until they rest on the floor behind your head. Hold for 10-30 counts.

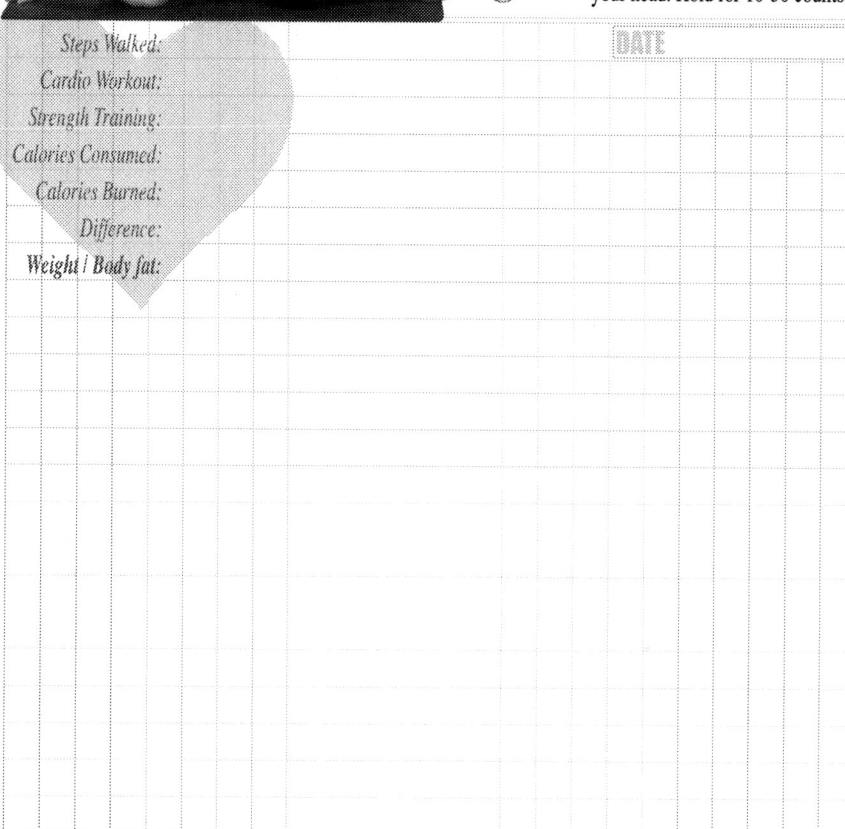

Eating healthy tastes great!

Fruit and Cheese Salad

$^{3}/_{4}$ cup concord seedless grapes
3 fresh apricots, cut into eighths
3 dried figs, sliced medium thick
$^{1}/_{2}$ pound mixed salad greens
2 tbs fresh lemon juice
salt, cracked black pepper and extra virgin olive oil to taste
3 oz goat or gorgonzola cheese
$^{1}/_{4}$ pound sliced turkey breast, cut into bite-size pieces
Toss all ingredients, except cheese. Top with cheese, serve chilled.

Read it, live it, love the results.

Fruits and vegetables are key to maintaining your health.

When you eat from a rainbow of colorful fruits and vegetables you enable your body to fight against the free radicals which threaten your health. In general the darker the green or the more vibrant the color the richer their antioxidant content. Some incredible sources of antioxidants are: broccoli, spinach, red bell peppers, cranberry juice and sweet potatoes.

Write it down & get it done.

1
2
3
4
5
6
7
8
9
10

forearm stretch
Kneel on the floor with your palms flat on the floor, fingers pointing away from your body. Keeping your back straight, bend forward and slowly turn your hands so your fingers are pointing towards you, then lower your buns to your heels, feeling the stretch in your forearms. Hold here for 10-15 counts.

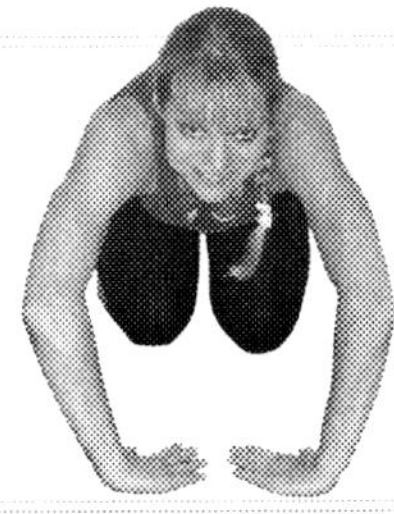

Opportunity is missed by most people because it is dressed in overalls and looks like work.
– Thomas Edison

DATE

Steps Walked:
Cardio Workout:
Strength Training:
Calories Consumed:
Calories Burned:
Difference:
Weight / Body fat:

Write it down & get it done.

1
2
3
4
5
6
7
8
9
10

Read it, live it, love the results.

Use this daily journal to record more than just your food intake and daily activites. Record your thoughts and emotions. Each day there are millions of thoughts that rush your mind, some quite remarkable. However, if you do nothing to record these thoughts and ideas, they may escape you forever. Take the time to write down those things which are noteworthy, in the future you will be glad you did.

Doors open, when you work hard.

Olympian swimmer **Michael Phelps** was diagnosed with Attention-Deficit Hyperactivity Disorder (ADHD) as a child. Influenced by his sisters and as an outlet for his energy, he began swimming at age seven. He excelled as a swimmer, and by the age of ten held a national record for his age group. Today he is the winner of fourteen career Olympic Gold medals—the most by any Olympian.

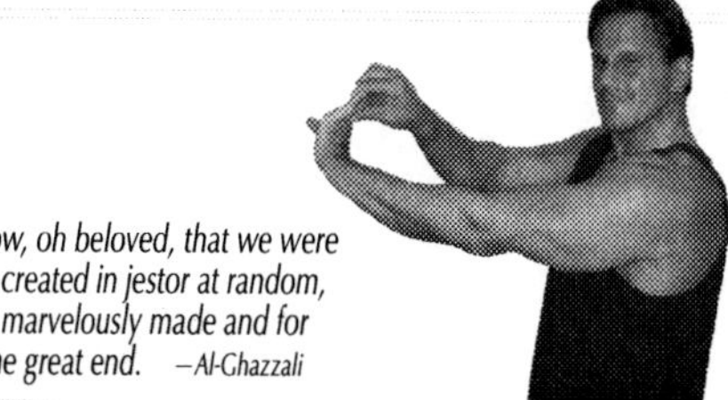

Know, oh beloved, that we were not created in jestor at random, but marvelously made and for some great end. —*Al-Ghazzali*

forearm stretch II

Extend your right arm straight out front with palm down. With the left hand, grasp the fingers of the right hand and pull back gently, stretching the wrist and forearm. Hold for 10-30 counts, relax, then repeat this stretch on the left side.

	DATE
Steps Walked:	
Cardio Workout:	
Strength Training:	
Calories Consumed:	
Calories Burned:	
Difference:	
Weight / Body fat:	

Eating healthy tastes great!

Low Fat Chicken Salad

4 cooked chicken breasts, chopped
2 hard-boiled eggs, chopped
2 cups spinach, chopped
2 tbs onion, finely chopped
$^{1}/_{2}$ cup each diced: tomatoes, dill pickles, celery and cucumber
1 cup fat-free mayonnaise
1 tbs dijon mustard and minced garlic
1 tsp oregano and basil
Combine all ingredients, mix well and serve over a bed of spinach or lettuce.

Read it, live it, love the results.

Vitamin B12 can give you energy when you need it most.

Vitamin B12 has many benefits, including its ability to speed up metabolic activities and increasing your energy level. Perhaps, even more importantly, it regulates DNA production and red blood cells formation. Those who suffer from anemia, may do so as a result of a B12 deficiency.
B12 is commonly found in meats, fish, milk, eggs, and cereals.

Write it down & get it done.

1
2
3
4
5
6
7
8
9
10

tricep stretch

Raise right arm straight up, so your upper arm is near your ear. Bending your elbow, let your hand fall to the back of your neck. With the other arm, reach behind your head and place your hand on top of the bent elbow. Gently pull down and back, holding for 10-30 counts. Repeat this stretch on the left arm.

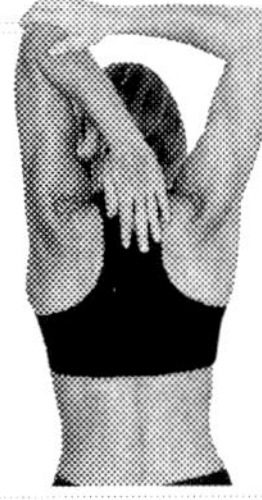

When your values are clear, your decision-making is easy.
– Walt Disney

DATE

Steps Walked:
Cardio Workout:
Strength Training:
Calories Consumed:
Calories Burned:
Difference:
Weight / Body fat:

Write it down & get it done.

1
2
3
4
5
6
7
8
9
10

Read it, live it, love the results.

Move, to reduce your risk of diabetes.

A recent study revealed that individuals who exercised more than four times per week have half the risk of developing diabetes, than those who don't exercise at least four times a week. Diabetes, as with many diseases, is "self-inflicted" when you choose to do nothing to lead a healthy lifestyle.

Life's tough, get over it, he did!

The founder of Hallmark Cards, **Joyce C. Hall**, actually began working at the age of eight to help support his family. Hall's father would say; *"The Lord will provide."* Hall felt, *"It's a good idea to give the Lord a little help."* In 1913, Hall and his brothers operated a store selling postcards and greeting cards. The store burned in 1915 and a year later Hall bought an engraving business and began printing his own cards. The business grew from there.

If you live your life today, just like yesterday, your tomorrow will be the same as today. Make that change today so tomorrow your life will be what it ought to be.
– unknown

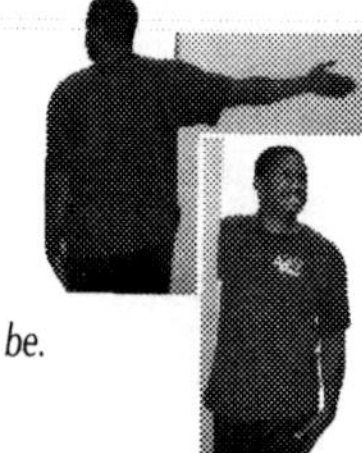

bicep & chest stretch

Place the right palm, inner elbow and shoulder against a wall. Holding your arm in this position, slowly turn your body to the left, feeling the stretch in your biceps and chest muscles. Hold here for 10-15 counts, then repeat with the other arm. When you raise your arm on the wall and repeat the stretch, you will then stretch your chest.

	DATE
Steps Walked:	
Cardio Workout:	
Strength Training:	
Calories Consumed:	
Calories Burned:	
Difference:	
Weight / Body fat:	

Eating healthy tastes great!

Spanish Chicken Breasts
4 chicken breasts
1 onion, sliced
6 oz can tomato paste
1/2 cup sweet pickle juice
pepper to taste
Preheat oven to 350ºF.
Place breasts in baking pan. Sprinkle with pepper. Place onion on breasts, Spread paste on top then pour pickle juice around the breasts. Bake 55-60 minutes, until chicken is done.

Read it, live it, love the results.

Don't view eating healthy as punishment.
Eating healthy makes you feel fantastic! Not only does eating healthy help you lose weight and decrease your risk of disease, it also increases your energy level and improves your self-esteem. Overall, eating healthy makes you feel great. When you change the way you think about food, you will change the way you eat!

Write it down & get it done.

1
2
3
4
5
6
7
8
9
10

stretch

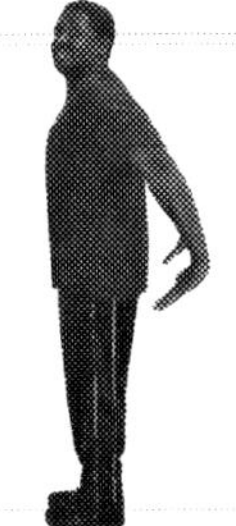

shoulder stretch
Standing tall with feet together, push your arms straight back with palms facing down. Hold here for 5-10 counts focusing on the shoulder and tricep muscles. Repeat 5-10 times.

I long to accomplish a great and noble task, but it is my chief duty to accomplish small tasks as if they were great and noble.
—Helen Keller

DATE

Steps Walked:
Cardio Workout:
Strength Training:
Calories Consumed:
Calories Burned:
Difference:
Weight / Body fat:

Write it down & get it done.

1
2
3
4
5
6
7
8
9
10

Read it, live it, love the results.

Look great without the help of a doctor and plastic surgery.
Skip the plastic surgery and engage in regular exercise, it's the key to slowing the aging process. Hundreds of studies show that exercise increases stamina, muscle strength, balance and bone density— all which normally deplete with age. Exercise, and your body will age slower. There's no need for plastic surgery when you look great naturally.

Doors open, when you work hard.

Author of the *Harry Potter* series, **J.K. Rowling,** first thought of Harry in 1990, while riding a train. *"Harry just strolled into my head fully formed."* In the years ahead she wrote in the quiet moments while her daughter napped. Ironically, she had a very hard time finding a publisher; however, she never gave up. Eventually, the publisher *Scholastic* took interest and her book became a huge success.

My parents always told me that people will never know how long it takes you to do something. They will only know how well it is done. –Nancy Hanks

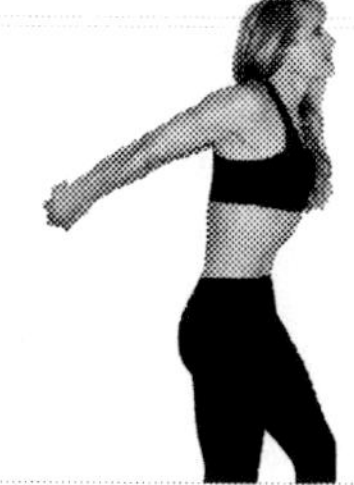

chest stretch
Stand tall with your feet shoulder-width apart. Clasp your hands behind your back and gently press them upward, keeping your arms straight. Look up towards the ceiling as you hold this stretch for 10-30 counts.

	DATE
Steps Walked:	
Cardio Workout:	
Strength Training:	
Calories Consumed:	
Calories Burned:	
Difference:	
Weight / Body fat:	

Eating healthy tastes great!

Guacamole Egg Scramble
2 eggs • 1 tablespoon water
Seasoned salt and pepper to taste
½ avocado • ½ tsp lemon juice
4 drops hot pepper sauce
1 tomato, diced

Mix eggs and water, cook until nearly done. Peel and mash avocado until chunky, add remaining ingredients and mix well. Add mixture to eggs and finish cooking.

Read it, live it, love the results.

Enjoy an avocado at least once a week for great health benefits.
Research shows that when a woman eats one avocado a week, it balances hormones, sheds unwanted birth weight, and prevents cervical cancers.
There are over 14,000 photolytic chemical constituents of nutrition in each avocado. Modern science has only studied and named about 141 of them.

Write it down & get it done.

1
2
3
4
5
6
7
8
9
10

stretch

behind head chest stretch

Stand tall with feet shoulder-width apart, shoulders back, chest out and abs in. Place hands behind your head, interlocking your fingers. Gently pull your elbows back as far as possible. Hold for 10-30 counts, relax, then repeat 2-5 times.

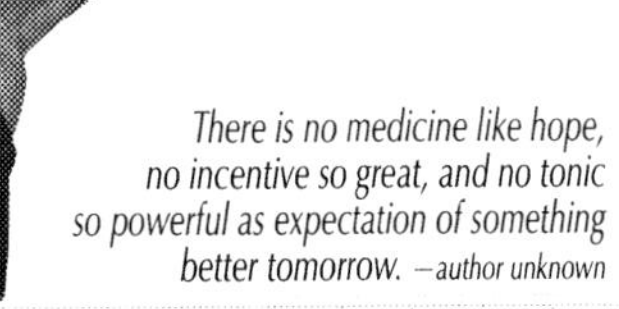

There is no medicine like hope, no incentive so great, and no tonic so powerful as expectation of something better tomorrow. –author unknown

DATE

Steps Walked:

Cardio Workout:

Strength Training:

Calories Consumed:

Calories Burned:

Difference:

Weight / Body fat:

Write it down & get it done.

1
2
3
4
5
6
7
8
9
10

Read it, live it, love the results.

Get rid of the sugar and you'll get rid of the weight.

One of the best things you can do to drop excess body fat is to decrease your intake of sugar. Start gradually by decreasing high sugar foods like donuts, candy bars, cakes, pies, hard candy, fudge, soft drinks and processed fruit juices.

Hard work equals great success.

The founder of Kentucky Fried Chicken **Colonel Sanders** was convinced his chicken was the best. Determined to make it a commercial success he traveled by car, city to city, frying chicken for restaurants, earning just 5¢ for each piece. His strong desire, devotion and hard work eventually led to the opening of Kentucky Fried Chicken in 1952– at the age of 62. He soon became one of the most recognizable people in the world.

I shall live badly
if I do not write,
and I shall write badly
if I do not live. – Francoise Sagan

wall chest stretch

Stand perpendicular to a wall with feet shoulder-width apart. With elbow bent at 90-degrees, place the inside of your bent arm on the wall with the elbow at shoulder height. Pressing firmly, turn your body away from positioned arm. Hold stretch for 10-30 counts, relax, then repeat with the other arm. Note: When you place the elbow lower you will stretch the upper chest more. Place the elbow higher and you will feel the stretch in your lower chest area.

	DATE
Steps Walked:	
Cardio Workout:	
Strength Training:	
Calories Consumed:	
Calories Burned:	
Difference:	
Weight / Body fat:	

Eating healthy tastes great!

Strawberry Pineapple Protein Shake

½ box sugar free strawberry gelatin
OR 1 cup strawberries
½ cup pineapple (no syrup)
16 oz cup of ice • ½ cup water
2 scoops vanilla protein powder

Place all ingredients in blender and blend until smooth.
I recommend that women use soy protein and men use whey protein.

Read it, live it, love the results.

Don't blame your genes.
Your genes don't fully determine your health and wellness—it's you who determines your health.
If you find yourself blaming your weight on your genes, you need to change your thoughts. You are in control. By eating healthy and working out, you will become healthier and happier. Don't fool yourself—you can change how you look and feel simply by making healthy choices.

Write it down & get it done.

1
2
3
4
5
6
7
8
9
10

lying back stretch

Lie face up on the floor, bringing both knees into your chest. Hold the knees closely by wrapping your hands around your legs just below the knees. Curling your hips slightly off the floor, hold for 10-30 counts, release, then repeat the stretch 2-5 times.

The great question is not whether you have failed, but whether you are content with failure.
–William Shakespeare

DATE

Steps Walked:
Cardio Workout:
Strength Training:
Calories Consumed:
Calories Burned:
Difference:
Weight / Body fat:

Write it down & get it done.

1
2
3
4
5
6
7
8
9
10

Read it, live it, love the results.

Never give up on that which you desire most!
The *"Desire Statement"* you recorded on page nine of this journal will come true for you, as long as you never give up! There will be days when you fail; however, everyone fails, it's the successful who get back up and continue in their journey.
Only those who don't get back up become failures.

Be the change you want to see.

Regarded as the greatest writer in the English language, poet and playwright **William Shakespeare** didn't actually publish any of his plays. It wasn't until 1623, seven years after Shakespeare's death, that John Heminges and Henry Condell, Shakespeare's friends and members of his theater company posthumously published thirty-six of his plays.

Accept what comes to you totally and completely so that you can appreciate it, learn from it, and then let it go.
—author unknown

lying back stretch
Lie on the floor, face up with legs extended straight out. Bring the right knee to your chest holding it as close as possible using both hands. Hold for 10-30 counts, relax, then perform the stretch bringing the other knee to your chest.

	DATE
Steps Walked:	
Cardio Workout:	
Strength Training:	
Calories Consumed:	
Calories Burned:	
Difference:	
Weight / Body fat:	

Eating healthy tastes great!

Seven-Layer Salad
10 cups mixed greens
1/2 cup low fat mayonnaise
1/2 cup fat free sour cream
oregano, basil & garlic to taste
6 strips turkey bacon, chopped
1/2 cup of each; chopped onion, diced tomatoes, frozen sweet peas, and light mozzarella cheese
3 hard-boiled eggs, chopped
Thoroughly mix mayonnaise, sour cream & spices, then combine with remaining ingredients.

Read it, live it, love the results.

Good health is not a matter of luck.
You may think healthy, fit people in their seventies and older are lucky to have their health. What you don't see is the walking, biking, workouts and healthy eating habits they developed through the years. In their desire to remain healthy, they have succeeded by making health a priority in their lives. As a result they can truly enjoy life as long as they live.

Write it down & get it done.

1
2
3
4
5
6
7
8
9
10

spinal twists

Sit on the floor with your legs extended straight out. Bring your right knee up crossing the right foot over the left knee. Reach your right hand through your right leg and place your left hand on the floor behind you as you twist to the left as far as possible. Hold for 10-30 counts then repeat the stretch on the other side.

Life is only traveled once, today's moment becomes tomorrow's memory. Enjoy every moment, good or bad, because the gift of life is life itself...
– author unknown

DATE

Steps Walked:
Cardio Workout:
Strength Training:
Calories Consumed:
Calories Burned:
Difference:
Weight / Body fat:

Write it down & get it done.

1
2
3
4
5
6
7
8
9
10

Read it, live it, love the results.

Don't smoke or overexpose your skin to the sun.
Studies show the two worst environmental factors which contribute to the early signs of aging are smoking and ultraviolet (UV) radiation from the sun. Overexposure to sunlight causes wrinkles, freckles, liver spots and dry, rough dull skin. Smoking ages the skin by constricting tiny blood vessels and reducing blood flow, causing wrinkles and aged skin.

Life's tough, get over it, he did!

One of the greatest geniuses in art history **Pablo Picasso** was dyslexic. He had a love for art at a very early age, however, the difficulty he faced reading the orientation of letters made school nearly impossible and would trouble him for most of his life. At age 16, his father sent him to Madrid's Royal Academy, the foremost art school. Yet his difficulties accepting formal instruction led him to stop attending class soon after enrollment. Despite this he never gave up on his art.

Your mind is a tool you can choose to use in any way you wish.
– author unknown

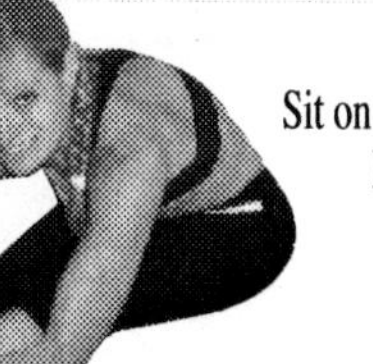

lower back reach

Sit on the floor with your legs straight out in front of you. Reach for your feet keeping your chin up and lower back slightly arched. Try not to round the back or tuck your chin—this decreases the effectiveness of the stretch. Hold for 10-30 counts.

	DATE
Steps Walked:	
Cardio Workout:	
Strength Training:	
Calories Consumed:	
Calories Burned:	
Difference:	
Weight / Body fat:	

Eating healthy tastes great!

Sweet Potato Fries

Avoid fried foods and try this healthier french fry instead, it's quick and simple.

Peel and cut sweet potatoes into french fry shapes. Place on a cookie sheet with a small amount of extra virgin olive oil. Sprinkle with seasoning salt.
Bake at 425°F for 20-30 minutes.

Read it, live it, love the results.

Develop a burning desire.

The morning after the Great Chicago Fire merchants met to discuss rebuilding or departing. All left Chicago, except one. He pointed to the remains of his store and said, *"Gentlemen, on that very spot I will build the world's greatest store, no matter how many times it may burn down."* The store he built still stands today as a towering monument to the power of Marshal Field's burning desire.

Write it down & get it done.

1
2
3
4
5
6
7
8
9
10

stretch

basic lower back stretch
On the floor, support yourself on your hands and knees with your hands directly under your shoulders. While keeping your hands in place, sit back onto your heels feeling the stretch along your back. Hold for 10-30 counts.

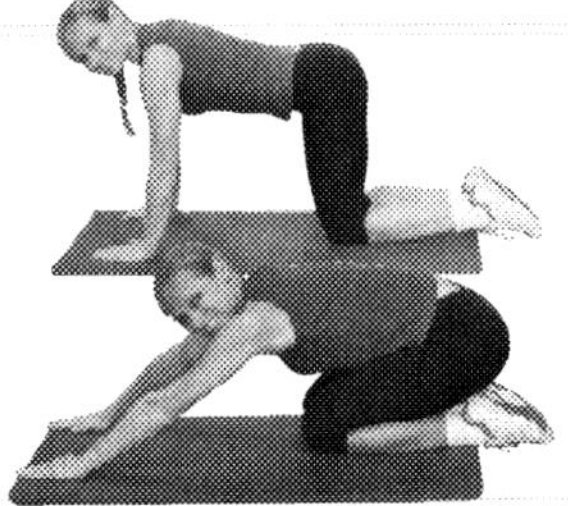

I never could have done what I have done without the habits of punctuality, order, and diligence, without the determination to concentrate myself on one subject at a time.
– Charles Dickens

DATE

Steps Walked:
Cardio Workout:
Strength Training:
Calories Consumed:
Calories Burned:
Difference:
Weight / Body fat:

Write it down & get it done.

1
2
3
4
5
6
7
8
9
10

Read it, live it, love the results.

A few simple rules of life.

- Don't compare your life to others.
- Don't overdo it.
- Don't take yourseld too seriously
- Dream more while you are awake.
- Forget issues of the past and don't remind others.
- No one is in charge of your happiness except you.

Life's tough, get over it, he did!

One of the most popular English novelists of the Victorian era **Charles Dickens** was born into a moderately well off family. However, this changed when his father was imprisoned for debt he aquired to retain his social position. At the age of twelve, Charles began working ten hours a day in Warren's boot-blacking factory, earning just six shillings a week. With this money he paid for his lodging and helped support his family who were incarcerated in the debtors' prison.

Find something in life that you love doing. If you make a lot of money, that's a bonus, and if you don't, you still won't hate going to work.
—Jeff Foxworthy

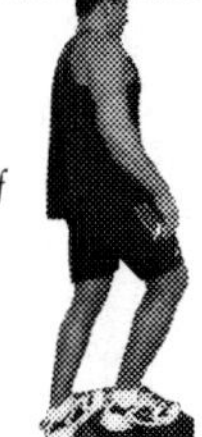

basic calf stretch

Stand on a step with the heel of your right foot hanging off the edge of the step. If necessary, hold a chair or the wall to balance. Drop the right heel below the level of the step until you feel the calf stretching. Hold for 10-30 counts, then repeat with your left.

Steps Walked:

Cardio Workout:

Strength Training:

Calories Consumed:

Calories Burned:

Difference:

Weight / Body fat:

DATE

Eating healthy tastes great!

Curried Eggplant Bisque

1 onion • 2 tsp grated fresh ginger
4 tsp curry powder
2 tomatoes, chopped
1 eggplant, peeled and diced
2 cups chicken bouillon
1/4 cup chutney • Chives

In large saucepan sauté onion, then add remaining ingredients, except chives. Cook for 20 minutes. Purée in blender. Serve either hot or cold.
Sprinkle with chives.

Read it, live it, love the results.

Act upon your dreams.

Though you may dream of a healthy lifestyle, dreaming alone will not bring it to you. You must act upon the dream, develop a desire that becomes an obsession and do all you can to make it come true. Using this journal, plan step by step how to acquire your dream. Then, back those plans with persistence which sees no failure. With this persistence, you will achieve all of your dreams.

Write it down & get it done.

1
2
3
4
5
6
7
8
9
10

leaning calf stretch

Depending upon your height, stand 2-4 feet from a wall. Lean in placing your hands on the wall shoulder-width apart. Gently push your hips forward while keeping your legs straight and heels flat on the floor.
Hold for 10-30 counts.

Leading a successful life means living successfully at all possible levels—body, mind and soul.
—Earl Nightengale

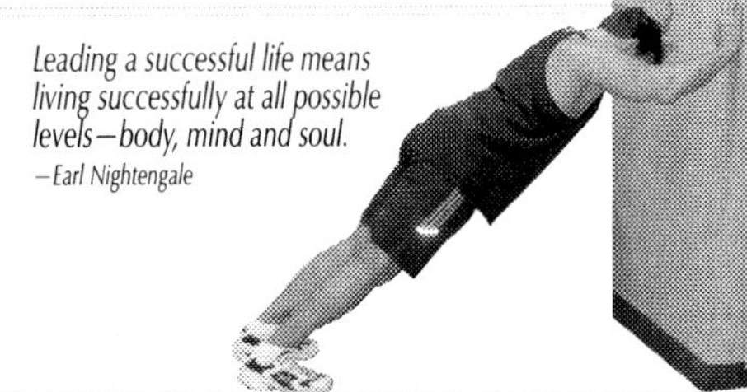

DATE

Steps Walked:
Cardio Workout:
Strength Training:
Calories Consumed:
Calories Burned:
Difference:
Weight / Body fat:

Write it down & get it done.

1
2
3
4
5
6
7
8
9
10

Read it, live it, love the results.

Stay active and in touch with family and friends.
One of the most comprehensive Alzheimer's studies being performed in Sweden follows everyone over the age of seventy-five living on one of the islands of greater Stockholm. This study indicates that those who are aging well have various things in common, one being, they tend to have high quality social support from family and friends.

Doors open when least expected.

Actor and film producer **Tom Cruise** grew up poor, moving city to city as his father looked for work. He never spent much time at any one school and due to dyslexia was often put into the remedial classes. As a result of academic problems, he focused on athletics and competed in many sports. However, a knee injury derailed his hopes of a promising athletic career.
Had this not happened he may have never pursued a career in acting.

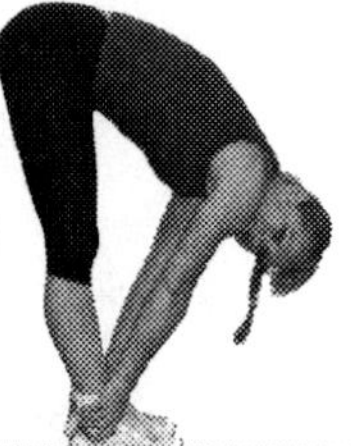

If we keep doing what we're doing, we're going to keep getting what we're getting.
–Stephen Covey

forward bends

Stand tall with your feet together. Bend down holding your legs as far down as possible. Pulling down bring your head as close as possible to your legs. Hold for 10-30 counts, stretching the hamstrings and back.

	DATE
Steps Walked:	
Cardio Workout:	
Strength Training:	
Calories Consumed:	
Calories Burned:	
Difference:	
Weight / Body fat:	

Eating healthy tastes great!

Dawn's Bayonne Beet Salad
4 beets, quartered
(you may also use canned beets)
1/2 cup light crumbled feta cheese
1 tsp fresh dill
4 tbsp balsamic, olive oil dressing
4 cups romaine lettuce

Roast fresh beets in foil, just as you would a baked potato. Once roasted and cooled, combine beets with feta, dill and balsamic olive oil dressing. Serve over romaine lettuce.

Read it, live it, love the results.

Eat beets to beat that rundown feeling.
Studies show that eating beets, which are a very condensed nutition food, can help strengthen fragile capillaries and, thus, restore weak heart valves and normalize varicose veins. They are also recommended to maintain a healthy liver, build blood and as a general "get-up" for a rundown body. *Diabetics should consult their physician before eating.*

Write it down & get it done.

1
2
3
4
5
6
7
8
9
10

lunge stretch

Stand with feet shoulder-width apart, arms resting at sides with palms facing in. Keeping your shoulders back, chest out and abs in, step forward 2-3 feet with your right foot. As you plant your right foot bend the right knee to about 90-degrees, coming down so that the left knee touches the floor. Place your hands on the floor near your right foot, then lean forward to get the maximum possible stretch in the thighs. Hold for 10-30 counts, straighten your right leg, locking your knee as you stretch the hamstrings of the left leg, then hold for another 10-30 counts. Return to starting position, then stretch on the other leg.

DATE

*If we did all the things we were capable of doing,
We would literally astound ourselves.* – Thomas Edison

Steps Walked:
Cardio Workout:
Strength Training:
Calories Consumed:
Calories Burned:
Difference:
Weight / Body fat:

Write it down & get it done.

1
2
3
4
5
6
7
8
9
10

Read it, live it, love the results.

Don't rely on quick fixes.
Studies show that medications taken regularly may rob calcium from bones, causing osteoporosis. This is particularly true of steroids, medications for thyroid problems, some drugs for rheumatoid arthritis, heart and gastrointestinal diseases and antiseizure medications. You should always know the long term effects of drugs—you are responsible for your health.

Life's tough, get over it, he did!

One of the most prolific inventors ever **Thomas Edison** was thrown out of school when he was twelve because he was thought to be dumb. He was noted to be terrible at mathematics, unable to focus, and had difficulty with words and speech. Despite his poor performance in school he never gave up on himself. Edison became one of the most brilliant scientists and inventors ever.

The truth that makes men free is for the most part the truth which men prefer not to hear.
– Herbert Sebastian Agar

lateral hip stretch
Sit on the floor with your legs straight out in front of you. Bending your left knee place the left foot over the right knee. With your left hand on the outside of the left knee, gently pull the knee toward your left shoulder, twisting your body to the right until you feel the stretch in your right hip. Hold for 10-30 counts then repeat on the opposite side.

	DATE						
Steps Walked:							
Cardio Workout:							
Strength Training:							
Calories Consumed:							
Calories Burned:							
Difference:							
Weight / Body fat:							

Eating healthy tastes great!

Chocolate Mocha Protein Shake
½ cup cold coffee • 16 oz cup ice
½ cup low fat vanilla yogurt
2 scoops chocolate protein

Place all ingredients in blender and blend until smooth.
I recommend that women use soy protein and men use whey protein.

Read it, live it, love the results.

Caffeine does have benefits.
Though the effects are often short term, studies show that caffeine can energize and help you focus and concentrate. Most people resort to a cup of coffee for their *caffeine fix,* however, it can also be found in chocolate, energy drinks and some medications. Keep in mind that more is often less: overdo it on caffeine and you may find yourself jittery and uncomfortable.

Write it down & get it done.

1
2
3
4
5
6
7
8
9
10

basic hips stretch

Lie on the floor face up with your legs straight out. Interlacing your fingers behind your right upper thigh pull your right knee toward your chest and hold. Hold for 10-30 counts then repeat the stretch pulling the left knee into your chest.

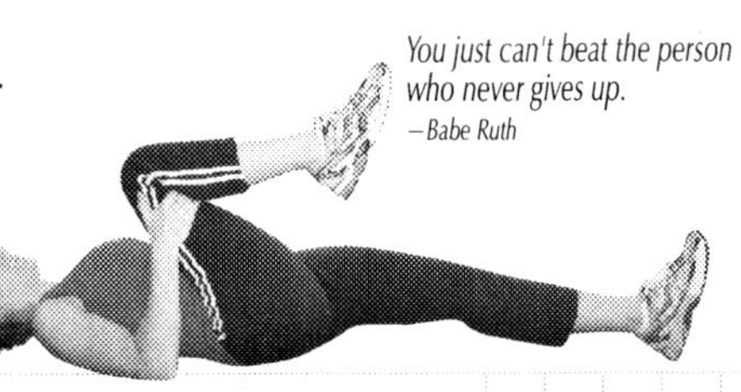

You just can't beat the person who never gives up.
—Babe Ruth

DATE

Steps Walked:
Cardio Workout:
Strength Training:
Calories Consumed:
Calories Burned:
Difference:
Weight / Body fat:

Write it down & get it done.

1
2
3
4
5
6
7
8
9
10

Read it, live it, love the results.

Eat a calcium rich diet for healthy bones.

Studies show that calcium is a very important part of your diet in building healthy bones. Some experts feel that women should take a calcium supplement of 1,200 to 1,500 mg a day. Men should get no more than 1,000 to 1,200 mg a day from all sources. Without healthy bones, you may spend later years in pain or perhaps immobilized with bone degenerative diseases.

Doors open when least expected.

Baseball's superstar **Babe Ruth** had a rough childhood. His parents worked long hours leaving Babe to care for himself, often running wild in the streets and causing problems. When Babe was seven, his father took him to St. Mary's Industrial School for Boys, a reformatory and orphanage. Here he signed over custody. During his twelve years there Babe seldom saw his parents, though he did learn to play baseball.

You cannot dream yourself into a character: you must hammer and forge yourself into one.
—Henry D. Thoreau

hip roll

Lie on the floor face up with knees bent and feet flat on the floor. Press your knees down to the right as far as possible and hold for 10-30 counts. Repeat this stretch on the left side holding for the same count.

	DATE
Steps Walked:	
Cardio Workout:	
Strength Training	
Calories Consumed:	
Calories Burned:	
Difference:	
Weight / Body fat:	

Eating healthy tastes great!

Spinach and Green Chile Eggs
4 egg whites
½ cup skim milk
4 oz can diced green chilies
1 cup red bell pepper, diced
1 cup shredded spinach leaves
2 tbs fat free sour cream
pepper to taste

Mix all ingredients, except eggs and milk, sauté 5-6 minutes. Add egg and milk mix, finish cooking.

Read it, live it, love the results.

Set your goals and don't stray from them.
If you want to achieve a healthy lifestyle set goals to take you in this direction. Break your larger goals into smaller goals with realistic deadlines and write them down. Strive for a healthy lifestyle and don't ever give up. No one can stop you from reaching your goals except for you. The key is to never give up. Remember, winners never quit and quitters never win.

Write it down & get it done.

1
2
3
4
5
6
7
8
9
10

hamstring stretch using a step
Standing 2-3 feet from a step, place your right foot on the step. Keeping your left leg straight, bend forward along the right leg and take hold of it as far down as possible. Pull gently to get the maximum stretch in your hamstrings. Hold for 10-30 counts, relax, then repeat the stretch on the left.

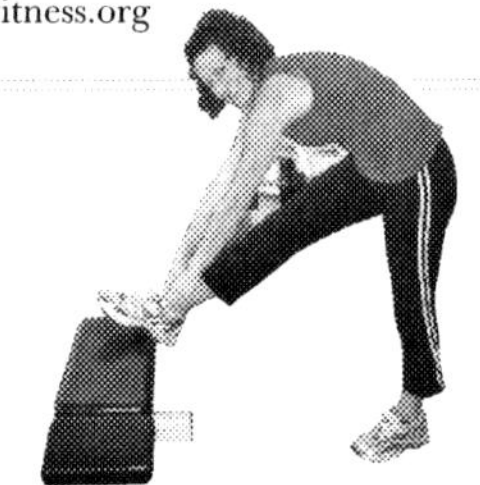

We design our lives through the power of choices.
– Richard Bach

DATE

Steps Walked:
Cardio Workout:
Strength Training:
Calories Consumed:
Calories Burned:
Difference:
Weight / Body fat:

Write it down & get it done.

1
2
3
4
5
6
7
8
9
10

Read it, live it, love the results.

Anything worth having takes hard work and time to achieve. There are no *"get rich quick"* schemes or *"easy way outs."* If your goal is to lose twenty pounds and create a healthy lifestyle, face the reality that it may take three to six months to make this happen. The key is to never give up, the results will come if you give it time.

Life's tough, get over it, he did!

One of Hollywood's top comedian actors **Jim Carrey** didn't always have it so easy. When he was a teen, his family fell on hard times and was forced to live in a tent or their Volkswagen van, and at times Carrey worked eight hours a day after school to help pay the bills. He had once written a check for twenty million, hoping to eventually cash it—today he *can* cash that check.

Be faithful to that which exists nowhere but in yourself.
–Andre Gide

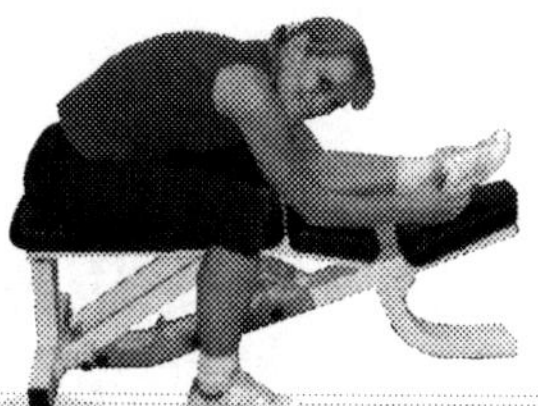

basic hamstrings stretch

Sit on a bench with your right leg extended out flat and your left foot flat on the floor. Rest your hands on your right knee, then slowly slide your fingers toward your toes reaching as far as possible and holding for 10-30 counts. Repeat the stretch on the left leg.

DATE

Steps Walked:
Cardio Workout:
Strength Training
Calories Consumed:
Calories Burned:
Difference:
Weight / Body fat:

Eating healthy tastes great!

Cabbage Tomato Skillet
5 cups cabbage, shredded
2 cups tomatoes, diced
1 cup onion, diced
1/4 cup light butter

Melt butter in large skillet. Stir in rest of ingredients. Cover, bring to a boil and cook 5 minutes, stirring often if necessary. Uncover and simmer a few minutes to reduce liquid, then serve.

Read it, live it, love the results.

Strawberries are a powerhouse of health, enjoy some today!
Strawberries are an excellent source of vitamins C, B5, B6 and K. They also contain manganese, folic acid, potassium, riboflavin, copper, magnesium and omega-3 fatty acids, in addition to significant levels of phytonutrients and antioxidants, which fight free radicals. These antioxidant properties are believed to be linked to what makes the strawberry bright red.

Write it down & get it done.

1
2
3
4
5
6
7
8
9
10

seated hamstring & lower back stretch

Sit on the floor with legs spread open to form a "*V*" with heels on the floor and toes pointed upwards. Place your hands on the floor and reach forward as far as possible. Hold here for 10 counts, then *walk* your hands over to the right leg, and reach down as far as possible. Hold for another 10 counts. Then *walk* your hands over to left leg and hold for another 10 counts.

I really believe in the philosophy that you create your own universe. I'm just trying to create a good one for myself.
–Jim Carrey

DATE

Steps Walked:
Cardio Workout:
Strength Training:
Calories Consumed:
Calories Burned:
Difference:
Weight / Body fat:

Write it down & get it done.

1
2
3
4
5
6
7
8
9
10

Read it, live it, love the results.

Have your bone density tested. Men should have a bone density test performed when they turn sixty-five or sooner if there is a family history of osteoporosis. Women should be checked at the onset of menopause or when stopping hormone therapy. Know your body so that you can take better care of it. Early detection may help you avoid osteoporosis and bone breaks in later years.

Be the change you want to see.

We all make mistakes we must live with. One of baseball's greats former New York Yankee **Mickey Mantle** spoke very highly of his father. He once stated; *"No boy ever loved his father more."* Sadly, he never shared this with his father, who died of cancer at the age of thirty-nine, just as young Mickey was starting his career. Mantle said one of the great heartaches of his life was that he never told his father he loved him.

If we don't care of our health today,
we will have to take of a disease tomorrow.
Let your food be your medicine,
let your medicine be your food.
– Hippocrates

seated forward hamstring stretch

Sit on the floor with your legs straight out front. Keeping your legs together, bend forward at your waist and reach down as far as possible. Hold for 10-30 counts.

	DATE
Steps Walked:	
Cardio Workout:	
Strength Training:	
Calories Consumed:	
Calories Burned:	
Difference:	
Weight / Body fat:	

Eating healthy tastes great!

Black Bean Salad

$^1/_2$ cup chopped onion
3 tbs minced garlic
15 oz can black beans, drain and rinse
1 cup frozen corn, thawed
8 cherry tomatoes, quartered
$^1/_2$ cup diced red bell pepper
2 tbs pumpkin seeds, chopped
$^1/_4$ cup cilantro, chopped
2 tbs olive oil
3 tbs fresh lemon juice

Mix all ingredients and refridgerate.

Read it, live it, love the results.

Have faith that you can accomplish that which you seek. Remember, you would never have had the desire to do something unless it was meant for you to accomplish. It will be difficult at times to have faith in yourself; however, when you maintain faith in yourself and the 13 principles discussed at the beginning of this journal, success will be inevitable. It's up to you.

Write it down & get it done.

1
2
3
4
5
6
7
8
9
10

extension stretch

Sit on the floor with legs spread open to form a "*V*", heels on the floor with toes pointing upwards. Lean forward reaching down on the legs as far as possible. Drop your chest towards the floor and hold for 10-30 counts, stretching the hamstrings and back.

A pessimist is one who makes difficulties of his opportunities and an optimist is one who makes opportunities of his difficulties.
– Harry S. Truman

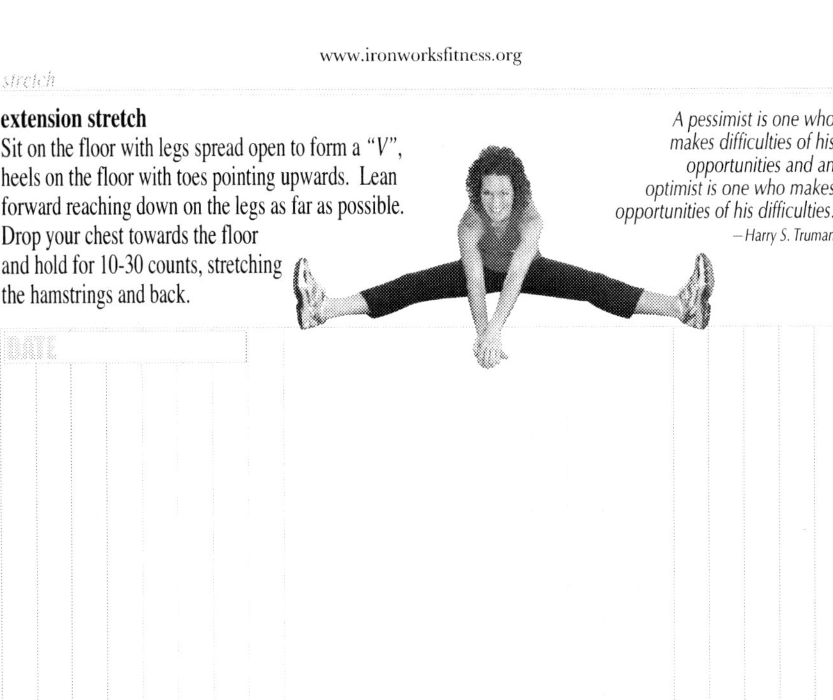

DATE

Steps Walked:
Cardio Workout:
Strength Training
Calories Consumed:
Calories Burned:
Difference:
Weight / Body fat:

Write it down & get it done.

1
2
3
4
5
6
7
8
9
10

Read it, live it, love the results.

Focus on eating healthy foods. What you eat matters more than you can imagine. Filling up on empty calories, such as candies, chips and fried foods, taxes your body's systems and zaps your energy reserves. Whereas, when you eat whole grains, lean proteins, fresh fruits and vegetables, you will energize your body and improve your overall health.

Life's tough, get over it, he did!

Our thirty-third President **Harry S. Truman** was prevented from entering college due to financial difficulties. Instead, he held a number of jobs, then returned to work on the family farm in 1902. He worked here until he entered military service in 1917. The war transformed Truman, bringing out his leadership qualities. His war record and rank of Colonel made possible his political career.

Many of life's failures are people who did not realize how close they were to success when they gave up.
—author unknown

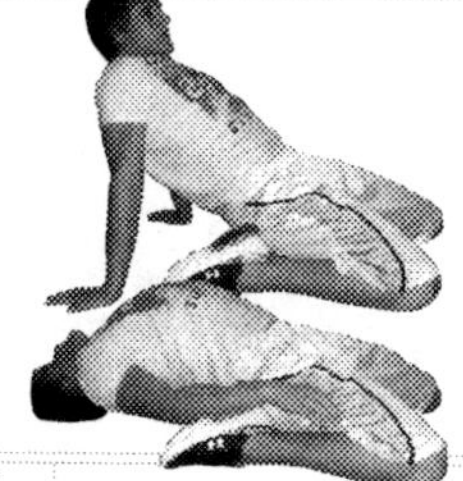

seated quad stretch
Kneel on floor with your feet separated far enough apart so that you can sit between them. Put your hands on the floor behind you and lean back as far as possible, feeling the stretch in the quadriceps. Hold this stretch for 10-30 counts.

	DATE
Steps Walked:	
Cardio Workout:	
Strength Training:	
Calories Consumed:	
Calories Burned:	
Difference:	
Weight / Body fat:	

Eating healthy tastes great!

Melon-Raspberry Shake
1 cup cubed cantaloupe or honeydew melon
1 cup raspberries, fresh or frozen
6 oz fat free strawberry yogurt
2 tbs skim milk • 1 tbs Splenda®
2 scoops vanilla protein

Place all ingredients in blender and blend until smooth.
I recommend that women use soy protein and men use whey protein.

Read it, live it, love the results.

Be self-confident.
Many people fail due to their lack of self-confidence. To build self-confidence you must tell yourself you have the ability to achieve whatever it is you desire. Tell yourself, "I am persistent," and promise yourself that you will stop at nothing. Focus on these dominating thoughts for at least thirty-minutes a day and they will eventually become a reality.
Keep all thoughts positive.

Write it down & get it done.

1
2
3
4
5
6
7
8
9
10

basic quad stretch
Stand tall, holding a chair or wall for support. Bending your right knee, grab your right foot with your right hand and pull the foot so that your heel presses against your buttocks. Hold for 10-30 counts, relax, then repeat the stretch on the left leg.

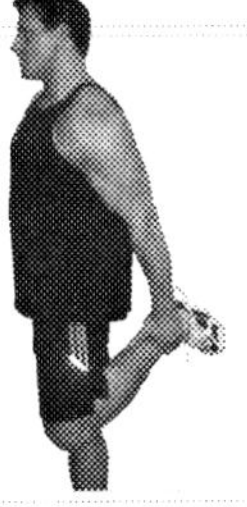

The gratification comes in the doing, not in the results.
—James Dean

DATE

Steps Walked:
Cardio Workout:
Strength Training
Calories Consumed:
Calories Burned:
Difference:
Weight / Body fat:

Write it down & get it done.

1
2
3
4
5
6
7
8
9
10

Read it, live it, love the results.

Know what your moods trigger. If frustration sends you to the cookie jar, create a list of alternative things to do and refer to this list when you get frustrated. It's never too late to change your bad habits...an old dog CAN learn new tricks!

Doors open, when you work hard.

Two-time Oscar-nominated actor **James Dean** didn't start out a great actor. In 1950, then a budding new actor, he had landed a role in the UCLA theater production of Macbeth. Reports stated that he, *"played the world's worst Malcolm."* Despite this, James Dean had a vision for himself and he never gave up on his dream to become an actor. Today he is known as one of the *"Legendary Greats."*

All that mankind needs for good health and healing is provided by God in nature. The challenge to science is to find it.
– Paracelsus, the father of Pharmacology

yoga

Since Yoga affects every part of the physical being, including the glands, organs, muscles, nervous system and skeletal system, the reasons for practicing it are many. Listed here are just a few good reasons for practicing: improved balance and flexibility, increased strength, improved muscle tone and reduced back pain.

	DATE
Steps Walked:	
Cardio Workout:	
Strength Training:	
Calories Consumed:	
Calories Burned:	
Difference:	
Weight / Body fat:	

Eating healthy tastes great!

Mediterranean Veggie Scramble
4 egg whites with 1/4 cup skim milk
1/4 cup mushrooms, diced
1/4 cup onion, diced
1/4 cup yellow pepper, diced
1/4 cup zucchini
1/4 cup cherry tomatoes
5 black olives, diced
2 tbs light Feta cheese

Mix all ingredients, except eggs and milk, sauté 5-6 minutes. Add egg and milk mix, finish cooking.

Read it, live it, love the results.

Practice yoga to ease back pain. The University of Washington perfomed a study on 101 people with lower-back pain. These individuals either practiced yoga or simply stretched once a week for three months. It was discovered practicing Yoga is twice as effective as stretching for back pain relief. So, if you have back pain, join a class or purchase a Yoga DVD, you might be amazed with the results.

Write it down & get it done.

1
2
3
4
5
6
7
8
9
10

corpse pose

Lie face up on the floor with legs open and rotated out with your arms laying palms up, slightly separated from your body. Rotate your spine by turning your head from side to side, centering it. Hold this position as you stretch outward through your entire body. Holding the pose for several minutes, breathe deeply and slowly from your abdomen as you still your mind and concentrate on the breaths and your body. Upon completion of this pose, bend your knees, then using your legs push yourself onto one side and push yourself into a sitting position.

DATE

I feel very adventurous. There are so many doors to be opened, and I'm not afraid to look behind them.
– Elizabeth Taylor

Steps Walked:
Cardio Workout:
Strength Training
Calories Consumed:
Calories Burned:
Difference:
Weight / Body fat:

Write it down & get it done.

1
2
3
4
5
6
7
8
9
10

Read it, live it, love the results.

Focus on setting, rearranging, evaluating and strengthening the purpose of your goals.
If you know where you want to be in life, you must set goals to get there. There are two ways to face the future: one is with apprehension, the other anticipation.
It's unfortunate that most people face the future with apprehension. When you set goals and have plans you can look forward to the future with anticipation.

Life's tough, get over it, she did!

Two-time Academy Award-winning actress **Liz Taylor** known for her acting skills and beauty, had a career that started off horribly. At the age of ten she received a small part in a movie which didn't go well and her contract was dropped. It was a devistating start; however, she never gave up. Next, she landed a part in the first Lassie movie, the critics took notice and, the rest is history.

It is during our darkest moments that we must focus to see the light.
– Taylor Benson

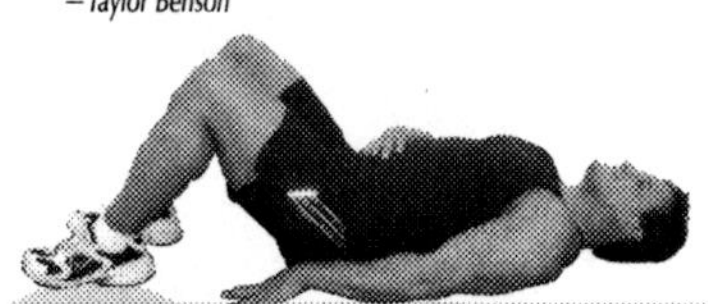

supine breathing

Lie on the floor, face up with knees bent and feet flat on the floor. Place your right hand on the floor palm down at your side with your left hand on your lower belly. Inhale, expanding through the ribcage and exhale pressing the bellybutton towards the spine. Relax the muscles in your shoulders and face as you continue to inhale and exhale for 5-7 breaths.

DATE

Steps Walked:

Cardio Workout:

Strength Training:

Calories Consumed:

Calories Burned:

Difference:

Weight / Body fat:

Eating healthy tastes great!

Grape Nuts Breakfast Bars

3 cups Grape Nuts cereal
1 cup 2% milk
1 cup applesauce unsweetened
1 cup raisins or craisins
2 tsp vanilla extract

Preheat oven to 350ºF.
Mix all ingredients, then pour in nonstick 9-in square baking dish.
Bake for 35 minutes, or until firm.
Cool and cut into 12 squares.

Read it, live it, love the results.

Eating raisins can help postmenopausal women maintain healthy bones.

Boron, a mineral that is critical to our health, is of special interest to women. Studies have shown that boron provides protection against osteoporosis and reproduces many of the positive effects of estrogen therapy in postmenopausal women. Raisins are among the top 50 contributors to total dietary boron in the U.S. diet.

Write it down & get it done.

1
2
3
4
5
6
7
8
9
10

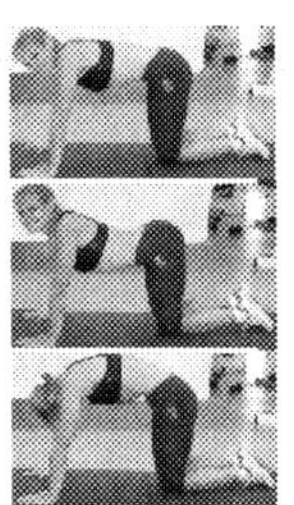

cat stretch

On the floor, support yourself on hands and knees—with knees under hips and hands under shoulders. With palms flat and fingers spread, contract your abs as you bring your head, neck and back in alignment. Inhale and look up as you press the sitting bone toward the ceiling and draw shoulders back and down away from your ears. Hold here 2-3 counts, then exhale and push chin to chest as you pull your belly towards your spine rounding your back. Hold here 2-3 counts then inhale and repeat 5-8 times.

DATE

Opportunities multiply as they are seized; they die when neglected. Life is a long line of opportunities. –John wicker

Steps Walked:

Cardio Workout:

Strength Training

Calories Consumed:

Calories Burned:

Difference:

Weight / Body fat:

Write it down & get it done.

1
2
3
4
5
6
7
8
9
10

Read it, live it, love the results.

Participate in Yoga.
A German study of twenty-four women showed that Yoga can reduce stress by nearly a third, which, as a result, helps smooth away wrinkles.
In an Indian study of 104 people, oxidative stress levels dropped by nine percent after just ten days of yoga. Reducing oxidative stress helps rejuvenate your skin's glow and keep you looking younger than ever.

Be the change you want to see.

One of the greatest orators in American history **Martin Luther King Jr.,** is best known for the 1963 *March on Washington* where he delivered his *"I Have a Dream"* speech. He had a vision of a color blind society and worked to end racial segregation and racial discrimination through civil disobedience and other non-violent means. In 1964, he became the youngest person to receive the *Nobel Peace Prize* for his work.

It's like most anything. If you want to be a loser, there's always a way to dwell on the negative. If you want to win, there's always a way to think positively. –Tony La Russa

thread the needle

From the *cat stretch*, sit back on your heels then reach forward as far as possible and touch your forehead on the floor. Hold this position, then inhale as you reach through the right arm and chest with your left hand—palm up. Exhale and rotate the upper back to extend the left arm even further out. Hold here for 3-5 breaths then repeat on the other side.

	DATE
Steps Walked:	
Cardio Workout:	
Strength Training:	
Calories Consumed:	
Calories Burned:	
Difference:	
Weight / Body fat:	

Eating healthy tastes great!

Fruity Blast Protein Shake

1/2 box sugar free strawberry gelatin *or 1 cup strawberries*
1/2 cup pineapple *(no syrup)*
1 small orange, no seeds
16 oz cup of ice • 1/2 cup water
2 scoops vanilla protein

Place all ingredients in blender and blend until smooth.
I recommend that women use soy protein and men use whey protein.

Read it, live it, love the results.

Know your desire.

The desire you place in your subconcious mind will eventually seek to become a reality through some practical means. If it is your desire to become healthier, you will find your body rejecting foods with no nutritional value and craving those high in nutrients, such as fruits and vegetables. When you change the way you think, you will change the way you eat.

Write it down & get it done.

1
2
3
4
5
6
7
8
9
10

full body plank
Lie on the floor face down with elbows resting on the floor next to your chest. Push your body into a pushup position on hands and toes. Keeping your body in a straight line from head to toe, contract your abs, holding this position for 4-8 breaths.

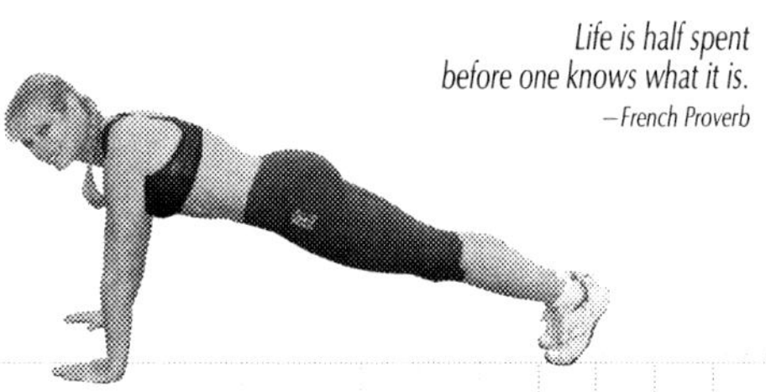

Life is half spent before one knows what it is.
—French Proverb

DATE

Steps Walked:
Cardio Workout:
Resistance Workout:
Calories Consumed:
Calories Burned:
Difference:
Weight / Body fat:

Write it down & get it done.

1
2
3
4
5
6
7
8
9
10

Read it, live it, love the results.

Moisturize your skin daily.
With cleansing, your skin is often stripped of protective oils, leaving it dry, dull and wrinkled. To maintain a great complexion, apply moisturizer daily—particularly after showering or washing your face. Despite the hype, there's no need to spend a fortune—some skin care professionals even recommend white petroleum jelly or hair conditioner.

Your level of success is up to you.

Baltimore Oriole's **Calvin Edwin "Cal" Ripken Jr.,** earned the nickname *Iron Man* for doggedly remaining in the lineup despite numerous minor injuries and for his reliability to *show up* to work every day. He is perhaps best known for breaking New York Yankees first baseman Lou Gehrig's record for consecutive games played, a record many deemed unbreakable. He's also a 19-time All-Star and member of the 3000 hit club.

The truly successful person inspires others to do more than they have thought possible for themselves. – Denis Waitley

side plank

From the plank position twist your body to the right supporting yourself with your right hand as you extend the left straight up in the air. Your left foot should rest on the right. Making sure you keep your body in line, look up at your hand. Hold this pose for 3-5 breaths then repeat on the other side.

	DATE
Steps Walked:	
Cardio Workout:	
Strength Training:	
Calories Consumed:	
Calories Burned:	
Difference:	
Weight / Body fat:	

Eating healthy tastes great!

Spinach Dip with Mushrooms

10 oz package frozen spinach thawed, chopped and squeezed dry
$1^1/_2$ cups fat free sour cream
1 cup fat free mayonnaise
1 cup mushrooms, diced
3 green onions, diced

Combine all ingredients, mix well, cover and refrigerate. Serve chilled with a variety of raw vegetables.

Read it, live it, love the results.

Build your desire upon truth and justice.

Eliminate hatred, envy, jealousy, selfishness and cynicism from your life. No matter how strong your desire is to achieve something, never hurt another in order to reach your goals. Reaching a goal by hurting another will only hurt you in the long run.

Write it down & get it done.

1
2
3
4
5
6
7
8
9
10

bow pose

Lie on the floor face down with arms at sides and palms facing up. Bend your knees bringing your heels as close as possible to your buttocks. Reach back and grab each of your ankles letting your weight rest on your stomach, not the pelvis. Continue breathing regularly as you raise your knees further gently pulling the ankles closer to your buttocks. Hold here for 10-15 counts.

The fruits of life fall into the hands of those who climb the tree and pick them.
—Earl Tupper

DATE

Steps Walked:
Cardio Workout:
Resistance Workout:
Calories Consumed:
Calories Burned:
Difference:
Weight / Body fat:

Write it down & get it done.

1
2
3
4
5
6
7
8
9
10

Read it, live it, love the results.

Lose weight and increase flexibility when you practice yoga. The University of Washington conducted a 10-year study of 15,500 men and women over the age of 45. Study participants who regularly practiced yoga lost up to five pounds and those who didn't gained up to thirteen and one-half pounds. Practicing yoga also increases your flexibility and the lubrication of your joints, ligaments and tendons.

Doors open, when you work hard.

The inventor of Tupperware, **Earl Tupper** started out with a landscaping and nursery business. Unfortunately, the *Great Depression* forced his business into bankruptcy. He then got a job with DuPont Chemical Company, molding plastics. Eventually, he left this company and founded the Tupperware Plastics Company. Within 3 years he had 9,000 people selling tupperware at home parties.

The road less traveled is the one most feared, but is the one the successful choose to take.
—Latossha Joseph

cobra lift

Lie on the floor face down with elbows bent and palms down near chest. Supporting your upper body with your elbows, keep your head straight and elbows tucked into your sides with your toes, hip bones, and ribs on the floor. Contract your back muscles and slowly curl your chest off the floor holding for two counts at the top peak. Then, slowly lowering to floor, repeat using a full range of motion without moving anything but your torso and arms. Perform 10-15 reps.

	DATE
Steps Walked:	
Cardio Workout:	
Strength Training:	
Calories Consumed:	
Calories Burned:	
Difference:	
Weight / Body fat:	

Eating healthy tastes great!

Strawberry Banana Nut Parfait
$1\frac{1}{2}$ cups fat free strawberry yogurt
2 cups Banana Nut Cheerios® cereal
1 banana, sliced
1 cup strawberries, sliced
2 tbs toasted coconut

In four tall glasses alternate layers of yogurt, cereal, banana and strawberries. Top each serving with coconut. Serve immediately.

Read it, live it, love the results.

To maintain a healthy blood pressure eat a diet rich in potassium.
Studies show that diets rich in potassium may help to maintain a healthy blood pressure.
Fruits and vegetables high in potassium include: bananas, sweet potatoes, tomato paste, tomato puree, beet greens, white potatoes, white beans, lima beans, cooked greens, carrot juice and prune juice.

Write it down & get it done.

1
2
3
4
5
6
7
8
9
10

wheel pose

Lie on the floor, face up with arms at sides, palms down, knees bent with feet flat on the floor. Reach back placing your hands on the floor beside your head with fingertips near shoulders. Slowly lift your hips until thighs are parallel with the floor and the crown of your head is resting on the floor.
Hold this position 2-3 counts then, keeping your knees together, press up until your body is fully extended. Keeping the angle of your wrists and hands at 90-degrees, stretch the legs without tightening the buttocks while keeping the shoulders relaxed.

DATE

The second mile, the one for which you're not paid, generally yields more returns in the long run than the first mile. –Napoleon Hill

Steps Walked:
Cardio Workout:
Strength Training:
Calories Consumed:
Calories Burned:
Difference:
Weight / Body fat:

Write it down & get it done.

1
2
3
4
5
6
7
8
9
10

Read it, live it, love the results.

Know that you can!
You should expect only the best from yourself—if you don't, no one else will. Set your standards high and don't let yourself down. Living your dream life should be your ultimate goal. Put everything you have into achieving this goal and you won't be disappointed. There will be times when things don't turn out as desired or anticipated; however, this doesn't make you a failure, you must never give up.

Success is the reward of hard work.

Chemist **Robert Chesebrough** was nearly broke when he discovered oil well workers applying a gooey waste product to wounds. In 1870, after experimenting and refining the material, he marketed Vaseline. He drove a horse and buggy around giving jars to anyone who promised to apply it to cuts and burns. Soon, he employed twelve salesmen to help sell the product and later founded the company that would became *Chesebrough-Ponds*.

There are two things to aim at in life; first to get what you want, and after that to enjoy it. Only the wisest of mankind has achieved the second.
—Logan Pearsall Smith

locust pose
Lie on floor face down, arms next to your body with palms facing up. Gently lift your head, upper body, arms and then legs. Keeping your arms parallel to the floor rest your abs and lower ribs on the floor. Hold here for 30 to 60 counts.

	DATE
Steps Walked:	
Cardio Workout:	
Strength Training:	
Calories Consumed:	
Calories Burned:	
Difference:	
Weight / Body fat:	

Eating healthy tastes great!

Easy Mexican Dip
1 can black beans, drained
1 can of white corn, drained
1 can of Rotel® Tomatoes
2 avocados, peeled and diced

Drain and mix each of the ingredients. Enjoy with Baked Tostado Scoops®.

Read it, live it, love the results.

Enjoy the morning sun.
Studies show that sunlight offers natural vitamins that are also needed for the development of the skin—especially for the regeneration of new skin cells. So, if it's younger skin you are seeking, spend more time under the morning sun and nourish your body.

Write it down & get it done.

1
2
3
4
5
6
7
8
9
10

cresent pose

Kneel with lower legs and toes on floor, back straight, shoulders back, chest out and abs in. With the left foot remaining stationary, step forward with the right until your thigh is parallel to the floor. You may increase the stretching of your leg muscles in the front part of your left hip by bending your front leg more and more. With thumbs hooked together, raise arms upwards, pulling the thumbs apart as you straighten the left leg, lifting your body from the floor, distributing the weight equally between the legs. If possible look upwards at fingertips.

DATE

Dream lofty dreams, and as you dream, so you shall become. Your vision is the promise of what you shall someday be; your ideal is the prophecy of what you shall at last unveil. –James Allen

Steps Walked:

Cardio Workout:

Strength Training:

Calories Consumed:

Calories Burned:

Difference:

Weight / Body fat:

Write it down & get it done.

1
2
3
4
5
6
7
8
9
10

Read it, live it, love the results.

Eat a ton of fruits and vegetables. Despite the billions of dollars that have been spent on the 'war on cancer', modern cancer treatment still revolves around the extremely unpleasant, 'slash-and-burn' treatments of chemotherapy and radiotherapy. *Prevention is better than a cure.*

When you eat healthy you may avoid a future that could prove gloomy and painful.

Be the change you want to see.

Senior citizen and competitive runner **Winnie Hopfe** decided to kick it into high gear for her retirement. Winnie does not feel that she is *"old"* and certainly does not look or act old. Instead of sitting in a rocker, Winnie stays active. She runs in seven or eight competitive events each year, often leaving women half her age in the dust. She has also taken up kayaking and spent a weekend water-tubing in the Adirondacks.

Have the courage to say no. Have the courage to face the truth. Do the right thing because it is right. These are the magic keys to living your life with integrity. –W. Clement Stone

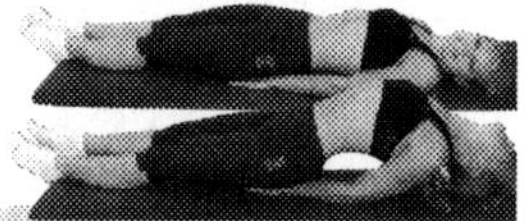

fish pose

Lie on floor face up with legs extended out straight and palms face down under your thighs. Pressing through your elbows, inhale and arch your back as you drop your head back until the top is on the floor. Keep your weight resting on your elbows with your legs and lower torso relaxed. Hold here for 30-60 counts, then gently lift your head and place flat on the mat.

DATE

Steps Walked:

Cardio Workout:

Strength Training:

Calories Consumed:

Calories Burned:

Difference:

Weight / Body fat:

Eating healthy tastes great!

Baked Sweet Potatoes

3 large sweet potatoes, *peeled and cut into medium pieces*
oregano and black pepper to taste
olive oil
Preheat oven to 350ºF.
Coat sweet potatoes with olive oil and sprinkle with spices. Place potates in baking dish coated with olive oil. Bake for 60 minutes or until soft.

Read it, live it, love the results.

Fight cancer with sweet potatoes, corn, carrots, pumpkin, mango and melon.

These yellow/orange foods contain beta-carotene, lycopene, and luteina, all varieties of carotenoids. Carotenoids are the pigments that give fruits and vegetables color. Most importantly, they act as antioxidants with strong cancer-fighting properties. Add them to your diet and you'll build a cancer-fighting army within your body.

Write it down & get it done.

1
2
3
4
5
6
7
8
9
10

mountain pose Is one of the most important poses in yoga, it's the start and finish point of all standing poses. The mind is quiet, the body strong and still, like a mountain. Stand with your feet hip width apart, toes spread and pointing straight ahead. Distribute your weight evenly through your feet from the toes to the heels. Without locking the knees, contract the front thigh muscles and lift the kneecaps. Contract the hamstrings forcing hip and buttocks to level the pelvis. Hips should be directly over your knees and knees directly over ankles. Slowly inhale extending your spine, lifting the ribcage, opening the chest and dropping the shoulders down. Extend your neck keeping your jaw and eyes soft and shoulder blades pressed into the back to support your ribcage. Breathe slowly and softly.

DATE

I hated every minute of the training, but I said; Don't quit, suffer now and live the rest of your life as a champion.
–Muhammad Ali

Steps Walked:
Cardio Workout:
Strength Training:
Calories Consumed:
Calories Burned:
Difference:
Weight / Body fat:

Write it down & get it done.

1
2
3
4
5
6
7
8
9
10

Read it, live it, love the results.

Plan ahead when eating out. When eating out it's often difficult to stay on track. In order to avoid binging, choose your meal ahead of time. Most restaurants have their menus available online many with calorie content. Check them out and make a responsible decision before you go. When at the restaurant you may get caught up in the great smells and the sight of others' entrees... don't tempt yourself.

Life's tough, get over it, he did.

Martial artist, action star and television and film actor **Chuck Norris** describes his childhood as downbeat . He was non-athletic, shy, and scholastically mediocre. While other kids taunted him about his mixed ethnicity, he could only daydream about beating them up. Ironically, he is now known for his action roles, tough image and roundhouse kick.

The happiest person is the person who thinks the most interesting thoughts.
—Timothy Dwight

wind relieving pose

Lie on the floor face up with arms at sides, palms down and legs flat on the floor. Raise your left knee, wrapping your hands around the knee and gently pulling it into your chest. Holding your knee in place, raise your head, touching your forhead to the knee. Breathe deeply for 15-30 counts, release and repeat with the right leg.

	DATE
Steps Walked:	
Cardio Workout:	
Strength Training:	
Calories Consumed:	
Calories Burned:	
Difference:	
Weight / Body fat:	

Eating healthy tastes great!

Turkey and Tomato Panini
3 tbs low fat mayonnaise
2 tbs nonfat plain yogurt
2 tbs Parmesan cheese
2 tbs chopped fresh basil
1 tsp lemon juice
8 slices whole wheat bread
8 oz thinly sliced turkey
8 tomato slices
Mix the first five ingredients, spread evenly on 4 slices of bread, top with turkey, tomato and other slice of bread. Grill on both sides.

Read it, live it, love the results.

Eating turkey may reduce your chances of getting cancer.
The skinless white meat of turkey is not only low fat and an excellent source of protein, but it also contains excellent anti-cancer properties. Scientific studies have suggested that the selenium in turkey, which is an essential component required for thyroid hormone metabolism, antioxidant defense systems, and immune function, can also bring down cancer incidence.

Write it down & get it done.

1
2
3
4
5
6
7
8
9
10

warrior pose II

Stand in the Mountain Pose, then move your left foot to the left until your feet are three to four feet apart. Raise your arms parallel to the floor, then turn your head to the left. Turn the left foot 90-degrees to the left and the right foot about 45-degrees to the left, then rotate your torso to the left. Bending the left knee, lower your body until the left thigh is parallel to the floor and the knee is directly above the foot. Hold here for 30-60 counts.

A man's health can be judged by which he takes two at a time—pills or stairs.
—Joan Welsh

DATE

Steps Walked:
Cardio Workout:
Strength Training:
Calories Consumed:
Calories Burned:
Difference:
Weight / Body fat:

Write it down & get it done.

1
2
3
4
5
6
7
8
9
10

Read it, live it, love the results.

When you go out to eat, ask for a "doggie bag" with your meal. Much like the waistlines of many, restaurant portions are getting bigger and bigger. A great way to cut calories is to ask for the *doggie bag* when your meal arrives. Immediately, put half of your meal in the container and eat only that which remains on your plate. Your waistline will thank you!

Doors open, when you work hard.

Billionaire **Oprah Winfrey** was born to a poor teenaged single mother. Winfrey was raped at the age of nine and fourteen. As a result, she gave birth to a son who died in infancy. While in high school she landed a job in radio, then, at nineteen, co-anchored the local evening news. After turning around the failing *AM Chicago* show, Oprah's career took off. She launched her production company and became internationally syndicated.

warrior pose III

Stand in the Mountain Pose, then with palms facing each other, raise arms straight overhead. Keeping your arms locked in this position, move your left foot backward as you lean forward keep your back straight until your left foot, back, and arms form a diagonal line. Lift your left leg as you straighten your right leg and keep your arms parallel to the floor. Your raised leg, upper body and arms should all be parallel to the floor. Holding this position, stretch your arms and legs giving length to the spine as you breathe through your belly.

Although the world is full of suffering, it is full also of the overcoming of it.
—Helen Keller

	DATE
Steps Walked:	
Cardio Workout:	
Strength Training:	
Calories Consumed:	
Calories Burned:	
Difference:	
Weight / Body fat:	

Eating healthy tastes great!

Herbed Roasted Potatoes
2 pounds russet potatoes, *peeled and cut into 3/4 -inch chunks*
1 tbs olive oil
2 tbs chopped fresh parsley & dill
freshly ground pepper to taste

Preheat oven to 450ºF. Place potatoes in a large roasting pan with oil, salt and pepper. Bake 30 to 35 minutes on upper rack, turning 2-3 times. Toss with herbs.

Read it, live it, love the results.

Think positive.
Nothing good can come out of a subconscious mind that is filled with negative thoughts. Focus on filling your mind with positive thoughts. Take the time to read or listen to motivational books, interact with upbeat people and listen to positive music.
Do all you can to fill your mind with positives, it will make a significant difference in your attitude *and* your future.

Write it down & get it done.

1
2
3
4
5
6
7
8
9
10

chair pose

Stand in the Mountain Pose, then with palms facing raise arms straight overhead. Keeping your arms locked in this position, exhale and bend your knees as you bend your upper body forward at about 45-degrees. Let the weight of your upper body rest on your pelvis as you relax the calf muscles. The weight of your body should be directed into the ground.

Lack of activity destroys the good condition of every human being, while movement and methodical physical exercise save it and preserve it.
–Plato

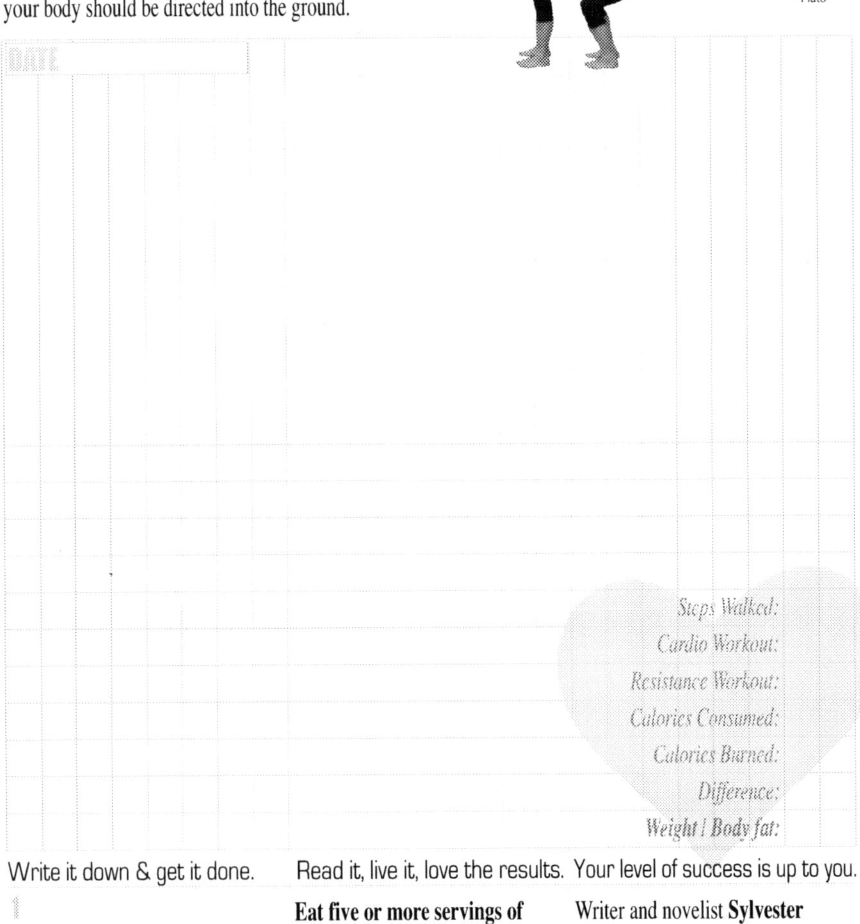

Write it down & get it done.

1
2
3
4
5
6
7
8
9
10

Read it, live it, love the results.

Eat five or more servings of fruits and vegetables daily.
If you make just one change in your diet for a longer, healthier life, this is the change you need to make. A small percentage of Americans eat the recommended five daily servings—yet diets rich in fruits and vegetables have consistently been found to help protect against heart disease, cancer, stroke, diabetes, cataracts and macular degeneration.

Your level of success is up to you.

Writer and novelist **Sylvester Stein** took up running at the age of 51. People doubted him, saying he started too late. That was 33 years ago and now at 84 he has became a British and European champion sprinter, the *World Champion Veteran* runner for the 200m and the winner of two gold medals. Proof that it's never too late to get started. Stein's most recent book, *"Who Killed Mr Drum?"*, was published in 2000.

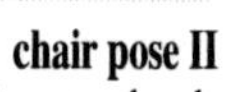

chair pose II

Stand in the Mountain Pose, then with palms facing, bring your hands together in front of your chest in prayer position. Bending at the waist, bring your upper body down parallel to the floor. Then lengthen the back by stretching out your neck. Look straight downwards at a spot on the floor as you breathe through your belly towards the chest bone, where you have your hands placed. Hold posture for 10-15 counts.

Passivity is the culprit.
Think of yourself as the victim,
you become the victim.
—from Law & Order

DATE

Steps Walked:
Cardio Workout:
Strength Training:
Calories Consumed:
Calories Burned:
Difference:
Weight / Body fat:

Eating healthy tastes great!

Chopped Chicken Salad
1 tbs of each:
reduced-fat sour cream, plain lowfat yogurt, lemon juice, chopped fresh dill and Dijon mustard
1/2 cup of each:
diced bell peppers, halved cherry tomatoes and cucumber slices
1/8 ripe avocado
4 cooked chicken breasts, diced
Combine all ingredients and refrigerate. Serve with pita bread or over lettuce/spinach.

Read it, live it, love the results.

Change your thoughts and you will change your life.
"If you think you are beaten, you are. If you think you dare not, you don't. If you want to win, but think you can't, it's almost certain that you won't. If you think you'll lose, you will. Success begins with a fellow's will—It's all in the state of mind."
–Napolean Hill

Write it down & get it done.

1
2
3
4
5
6
7
8
9
10

standing forward bend
Stand in the Mountain Pose, then bend your knees and drop down to a squatting position. Keeping your back straight, bend forward so your belly touches your thighs. Keeping your weight on the front part of your heels, relax your groins and slowly stretch your chest to your knees without losing the support of your lower back. Touch the ground or grab your ankles as you stretch downward and straighten your knees. Hold for 30-60 counts.

There's something really great and romantic about being poor and sleeping on couches.
– Ben Affleck

DATE

Steps Walked:
Cardio Workout:
Strength Training:
Calories Consumed:
Calories Burned:
Difference:
Weight / Body fat:

Write it down & get it done.
1
2
3
4
5
6
7
8
9
10

Read it, live it, love the results.

Don't make excuses, remember, "If it is to be, it is up to me."
You are responsible for your choices and actions. This includes food choices and your activites. It is up to you to eat from the vegetable tray and choose water with lemon. It is up to you to take the stairs instead of the elevator. No one else makes these choices for you, if you make choices which lead to an unhealthy life, you have no one to blame but yourself.

Doors open, when you work hard.

Film screenwriter, director and actor **Ben Affleck** and his childhood friend **Matt Damon** were struggling actors on the verge of being added to Hollywood's list of rejects. Bucking the system, they wrote their own screenplay, attracted their own financing, and produced and starred in their own movie. Within a year *Good Will Hunting* had become a financial success, earned several awards, and made Damon and Affleck stars.

downward facing dog pose

Kneel on hands and knees with the upper back relaxed. Exhale as you straighten your knees and push your back backwards from the pelvis, forming a line from your fingertips to lower back. Slowly press your heels to the floor as you bring your body into the shape of an inverted "V". With your head relaxed hanging down stretch out your arms and feel the stretch from two sides of the back–stretching from the pelvis and the arms.

Steps Walked:
Cardio Workout:
Strength Training:
Calories Consumed:
Calories Burned:
Difference:
Weight / Body fat:

DATE

Knowledge comes, but wisdom lingers.
–Lord Alfred Tennyson

Eating healthy tastes great!

Roasted Broccoli & Tomatoes

4 cups broccoli florets • 1 cup grape tomatoes • 1 tbs extra-virgin olive oil
3 tbs minced garlic
1/2 teaspoon freshly grated lemon zest
1 tablespoon lemon juice • 10 pitted black olives, sliced • 1 tsp dried oregano
Toss first five ingredients in large bowl. Spread evenly on a baking sheet and bake 10 to 13 minutes. Combine lemon zest and juice, olives and oregano in a large bowl. Add the roasted vegetables; stir to combine. Serve warm.

Read it, live it, love the results.

Eat plenty of cruciferous vegetables.

Studies show that cruciferous vegetables provide fiber and micronutrients which decrease LDL cholesterol and prevent hardening of arteries. They also contain indoles, a phytochemical which may protect against cancer. Some great choices of cruciferous vegetables include: broccoli, cauliflower, brussels sprouts and cabbage.

Write it down & get it done.

1
2
3
4
5
6
7
8
9
10

hands to feet pose

Stand in the Mountain Pose, then with palms facing raise arms straight overhead. Keeping your arms and legs straight, bend forward until your hands touch your feet. Then slowly bend a little further until your stomach touches your thighs and you are able to hold your toes or ankles. Hold for 10-15 counts.

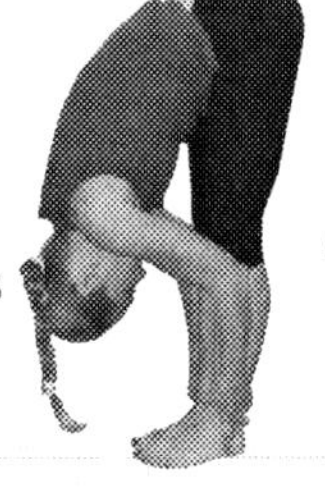

I am not rich, but I have what can make me rich: brains, education, and passion.
– author unknown

DATE

Steps Walked:
Cardio Workout:
Strength Training:
Calories Consumed:
Calories Burned:
Difference:
Weight / Body fat:

Write it down & get it done.

1
2
3
4
5
6
7
8
9
10

Read it, live it, love the results.

Close your kitchen.
More than likely, each time you enter the kitchen you will be tempted to grab something to eat. As soon as you finish with each meal, clean up the dishes and turn off the lights, then make a note to yourself that the kitchen is closed until the next meal.
There is plenty to do without spending your spare time snacking.

Doors open, when you work hard.

Walt Disney put his artistic ability to use at the age of sixteen, when he altered his birth certificate to show his year of birth as 1900—so he could enlist in the service and became a volunteer ambulance driver in World War I. Back home, in 1919, Walt left home and moved to Kansas City to begin his artistic career creating ads for newspapers, magazines, and movie theaters. From here he was motivated to go into business for himself.

We are insatiable beings and we always get our needs met. We will get these needs met in a healthy, conscious way, or we will get them met in an unhealthy, subconscious way.
– Sigmond Freud

sage twist
Sit on the floor with legs straight out, toes pointing to ceiling. Slowly bend your left knee bringing it to your chest. Rotate your body towards the knee, wrapping the right arm around it, positioning it in the crook of your right elbow. Holding here, clasp your hands together while keeping your back straight throughout the pose.

	DATE
Steps Walked:	
Cardio Workout:	
Strength Training:	
Calories Consumed:	
Calories Burned:	
Difference:	
Weight / Body fat:	

Eating healthy tastes great!

Apple Dip
8 oz package low fat cream cheese
1 cup Splenda®
1/4 cup Splenda® Brown Sugar Blend
1 tsp vanilla
4 apples, sliced

Combine all ingredients, except apples. Mix with a hand mixer until smooth. Chill, then serve with sliced apples.

Read it, live it, love the results.

Focus your thoughts on your desires.
Work smart towards your main desire by putting your subconscious mind to work for you. If you think about that which you desire, your mind will begin to devise ways to make your desire come true. It's at this point that you will experience sudden hunches, flashes of thought, inspiration and guidance, which will make your desire a reality.

Write it down & get it done.

1
2
3
4
5
6
7
8
9
10

leg pull

Lie on floor, face up with right knee bent, foot flat on the floor. Left leg extended out straight with hands at side palms face down. Slowly raise your left leg, holding it with both hands. If you cannot reach your ankle, hold your calf or thigh. Pressing your back into the floor, gently pull the leg toward you, as you flatten the shoulder blades and round your chest. Holding this position, extend your right leg out straight, then pull your left leg towards your chest. Continue pressing your back and shoulders into the floor so the shoulder blades flatten as you press both feet away from you, while continuing to gently pull the leg closer.

DATE

It is our attitude at the beginning of a difficult task which, more than anything else, will affect it s successful outcome. –William James

Steps Walked:
Cardio Workout:
Strength Training:
Calories Consumed:
Calories Burned:
Difference:
Weight / Body fat:

Write it down & get it done.

1
2
3
4
5
6
7
8
9
10

Read it, live it, love the results.

Choose fat free or low fat dairy products.
The American Dairy Council recommends consuming at least three cups of dairy products each day in order to reduce your risk of bone loss, which could lead to osteoporosis in later years.
By choosing fat free or low fat dairy products you can keep your saturated fat intake low, while meeting the daily recommendations.

Doors open, when you work hard.

Actor and cultural icon **Humphrey Bogart** was not a typical star. He was small, with weather beaten features, his face scarred and upper lip partially paralyzed from an injury he suffered during WWI, yet this did not stop him from reaching for the stars. He sought out rugged thrillers and action films, for which he was perfect, and as a result, became one of the number one movie legends of all time.

Whatever we plant in our subconscious mind and nourish with repetition and emotion will one day become a reality.
—Earl Nightengale

garland pose
With feet together squat down with hands resting near your feet. Stretch your arms forward, lengthening your back, letting your head hang down. Feel the stretch through your back as you lift your fingers from the ground.

	DATE
Steps Walked:	
Cardio Workout:	
Strength Training:	
Calories Consumed:	
Calories Burned:	
Difference:	
Weight / Body fat:	

Eating healthy tastes great!

Black Bean and Salsa Soup
2 cans black beans, drained
$1^1/_2$ cups vegetable broth
1 cup chunky salsa
1 tsp ground cumin
4 tbs sour cream
2 tbs thinly sliced green onion
Combine 1 can beans, broth, salsa, and cumin in blender. Heat the this bean mixture & add the other can of beans. Serve, topped with 1 tablespoon of the sour cream and $^1/_2$ tablespoon green onion.

Read it, live it, love the results.

Control your thoughts.
No thought, whether positive or negative, can enter into your subconscious mind without you allowing it to do so. Unfortunately, we often do not exercise control—which explains why so many of us end up overweight and unhealthy. If you feed your mind with thoughts of how wonderful fresh vegetables and fruits taste, you will then crave them. Try it, you'll be amazed.

Write it down & get it done.

1
2
3
4
5
6
7
8
9
10

seated reach

Sit on floor with legs stretched out, toes pointed upwards and arms stretched straight above your head with palms facing. Looking straight ahead, lengthen your back and slowly bend forward without moving your legs. Keeping your shoulders down, drop your hands to your lower legs, ankles or feet, then lightly pull and stretch. Move your breath through the entire length of your spinal column. With each exhale stretch your arms forward and bend even closer to your legs without losing the length in your back.

DATE

As we advance in life it becomes more and more difficult, but in fighting the difficulties the inmost strength of the heart is developed. – Vincent Van Gogh

Steps Walked:

Cardio Workout:

Strength Training:

Calories Consumed:

Calories Burned:

Difference:

Weight / Body fat:

Write it down & get it done.

1
2
3
4
5
6
7
8
9
10

Read it, live it, love the results.

Do the research then set goals. Knowledge is power, but only when organized into a definite action plan, with a beginning and end. If it's a healthy lifestyle you desire, research websites, magazines and medical journals. Learn all you can and fill your mind with health related information. Then, set a specific goal and write down the action plan necessary to reach that goal.

Success is the reward of hard work.

One of the all-time greatest female athletes **Jackie Joyner-Kersee** was inspired to compete in multi-disciplinary track and field events after seeing a 1975 made-for-TV movie about Babe Didrikson Zaharias. Ironically, Didrikson was chosen the *"Greatest Female Athlete of the First Half of the 20th Century."* Fifty years later, *"Sports Illustrated for Women"* magazine voted Joyner-Kersee *"The Greatest Female Athlete of All Time"*.

We have no more right to consume happinss without producing it than to consume wealth without producing it.
—George Berneard Shaw

bridge pose
Lie on the floor, face up with your knees bent, feet together, flat on the floor. Keeping your arms at your side with palms on the floor, lift your hips towards the ceiling, while keeping your feet and palms flat on the floor. Maintaining this position, place your arms behind your head. Hold this stretch for 30 to 60 counts.

Steps Walked:
Cardio Workout:
Strength Training:
Calories Consumed:
Calories Burned:
Difference:
Weight / Body fat:

DATE

Eating healthy tastes great!

Crab Cake Burgers
1 lb crabmeat • 1 egg, lightly beaten
1/2 cup panko breadcrumbs
1/4 cup light mayo • 2 tbs minced chives
1 tbs Dijon mustard
1 tbs lemon juice • 1 tsp celery seed
1 tsp onion powder
2 tsp unsalted light butter
hot sauce and pepper to taste
Mix all ingredients, form into patties. Heat 1 tbs olive oil and 2 tsp butter in skillet over medium heat until the butter stops foaming. Cook until golden brown.

Read it, live it, love the results.

Combat dry skin with fluids.
Studies show that increasing your fluid intake is essential for combating dry, aging skin. This includes drinking water and eating fruits and vegetables which contain a high water content such as celery, tomatoes, oranges, and watermelon. Decreasing your consumption of caffeine and alcohol may also help avoid dehydration of your skin, which may reduce wrinkles.

Write it down & get it done.

1
2
3
4
5
6
7
8
9
10

Leg reclining lunge
Lie face up on the floor, with legs extended out flat, your arms flat on floor near your sides, with palms down. Slowly bend your right leg, bringing the knee into your chest, then holding the sole of your foot with both hands. Move the knee to the side of your chest, positioning the right heel directly above the right knee, then pulling downward with your hands, attempting to touch the right knee to the floor. Keep your back and left leg flat on the floor.

Our plans miscarry because they have no aim. When a man does not know what harbor he is making for, no wind is the right wind.
– Seneca

DATE

Steps Walked:
Cardio Workout:
Strength Training:
Calories Consumed:
Calories Burned:
Difference:
Weight / Body fat:

Write it down & get it done.

1
2
3
4
5
6
7
8
9
10

Read it, live it, love the results.

Laugh more and enjoy life. When you take time to enjoy life and laugh on a daily basis, you will live a longer healthier life.

Your level of success is up to you.

Film director and producer **Steven Spielberg** applied to the film school at UCLA and University of Southern California's School of Cinema-TV, on three separate occasions, but was denied each time due to his C grade average. However, he never gave up on becoming a filmmaker. Today he is listed as *The Most Powerful and Influential Figure* in The Motion Picture Industry and as one of the *100 Greatest People of the Century.*

Little problems are big problems for little minds.
– Tom Zimmerman

Many feel the sole purpose to work the abdominal muscles is to achieve a great looking mid-section. However, even more important is that;

- A strong core provides stability for your entire body.
- Without a strong core, easy tasks will become more and more difficult.
- Abdominal muscles support and protect your internal organs and aid in breathing.
- Studies show strong abdominals reduce back pain.

	DATE
Steps Walked:	
Cardio Workout:	
Strength Training:	
Calories Consumed:	
Calories Burned:	
Difference:	
Weight / Body fat:	

Eating healthy tastes great!

Honey Curry Baked Chicken
$^{2}/_{3}$ cup light butter, melted
1 cup honey
$^{1}/_{2}$ cup prepared mustard
2 tbs curry powder
4 chicken breasts

Preheat oven to 350°F. Combine first four ingredients in a baking dish. Place chicken in the dish meaty side down. Cover and bake 50-60 minutes, until no longer pink inside.

Read it, live it, love the results.

Make your thoughts count.
"There are no limitations to the mind except for those we acknowledge. Both poverty and riches are the offspring of thought." –*Napolean Hill*
Treat your subconscious mind like a fertile garden, sowing only the seeds of desireable plants. If you don't take the time to sow that which you desire, weeds will take over. It's up to you to sow and reap that which you desire.

Write it down & get it done.

1
2
3
4
5
6
7
8
9
10

If it's a six pack you desire I will tell you up front that doing each of these exercises every day all day long will not give you a visible six-pack if you eat unhealthy! There are plenty of people who have great abs, but they will never actually see them, due to the layer of body fat that covers them. Doing ab exercises will not remove fat from the abdonimal area, it will however build the muscle. In order to see the muscle you must remove the fat by working out your entire body and EATING HEALTHY!!

The body only profits a little from exercising but the spirit profits a lot.

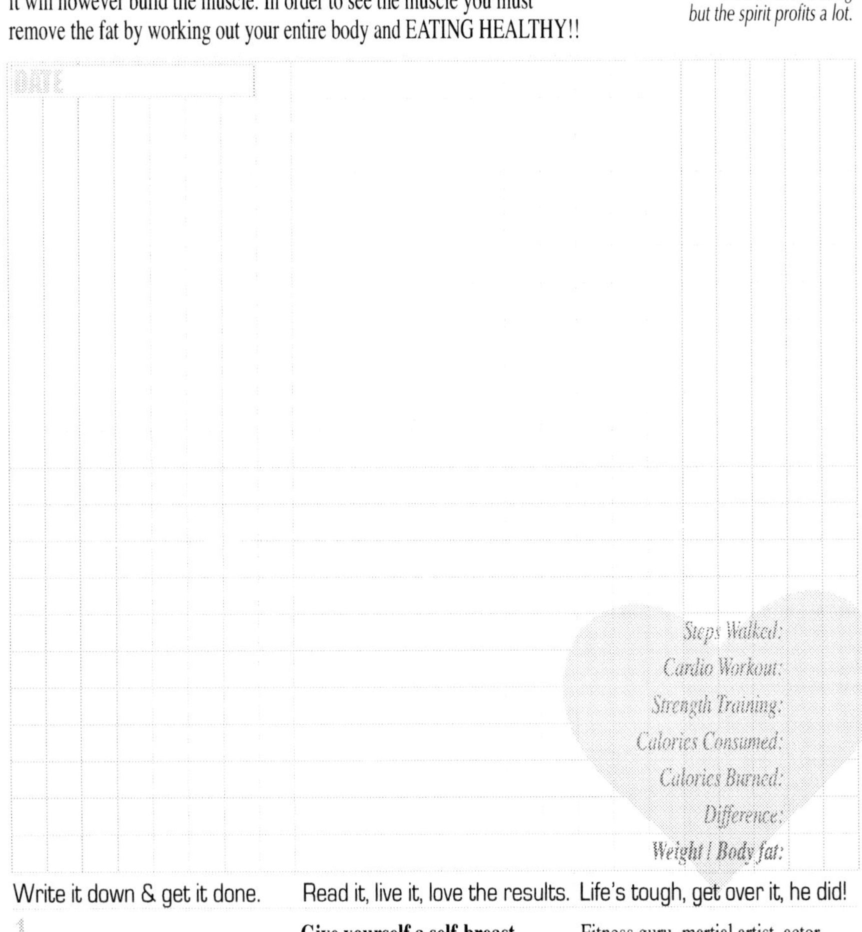

Write it down & get it done.

1
2
3
4
5
6
7
8
9
10

Read it, live it, love the results.

Give yourself a self-breast examination each month.
Over ninty-percent of breast cancers are found by women themselves. Though, since fewer than one-third of women perform regular breast self-examinations, these cancers are often found when they are over an inch in width. Generally, the smaller the lump, the better the chance of long-term survival. Note, men may also get breast cancer!

Life's tough, get over it, he did!

Fitness guru, martial artist, actor, and the inventor of the Tae Bo exercise program, **Billy Blanks** was born the fourth of fifteen children. His parents were hard working but poor. To make matters worse, Billy suffered from dyslexia and problems with his joints. However, this did not stop him from reaching for the stars. He became a great martial artist, film star, and one of the most sought after trainers and fitness consultants.

Plans are only good intentions unless they immediately degenerate into hard work. –Peter Drucker

dumbbell crunch

Lie flat on your back, knees bent with feet flat on the floor. Holding a dumbbell on your chest, cross your arms over the dumbbell. Contract you abs and curl up, lifting your body until your shoulder blades are 3-4 inches off the floor, hold for 2-3 counts, tightening the abdominal muscles, lower and repeat. Keep your chin pointed toward the ceiling, lower back and buns flat on the floor. Repeat 10-15 times.

Steps Walked:

Cardio Workout:

Strength Training:

Calories Consumed:

Calories Burned:

Difference:

Weight / Body fat:

DATE

Eating healthy tastes great!

Orange Chicken with Rosemary

4 chicken breasts
2 tsp paprika • 2 tsp pepper
12 oz frozen orange juice, thawed
2 tsp rosemary • 2 tsp thyme
2 tsp marjoram

Preheat oven to 350ºF. Place the chicken in a casserole dish, sprinkle with paprika and pepper. Mix together the remaining ingredients and pour over the chicken. Bake for about 1 hour, covered, until no longer pink inside.

Read it, live it, love the results.

Fill your mind with positive thoughts.

Do so and you will experience positive feelings. Individuals who lead a healthy life are generally happier than those who have an unhealthy lifestyle. If you truly love yourself you will find yourself focusing on creating the best life possible for yourself. High self-esteem and positive thoughts are essential for good health and a happy life.

Write it down & get it done.

1
2
3
4
5
6
7
8
9
10

reverse crunch

Lie face up on the floor with your hands at your sides, palms down and your knees bent with feet hovering 2-3 inches above the floor. Contract your abdominal muscles, lifting your pelvis up and bringing your knees up toward your chest. Hold for 2-3 counts, return to start position and repeat 10-15 times.

To truly laugh, you must be able to take your pain, and play with it!
– Charlie Chaplin

DATE

Steps Walked:
Cardio Workout:
Strength Training
Calories Consumed:
Calories Burned:
Difference:
Weight / Body fat:

Write it down & get it done.

1
2
3
4
5
6
7
8
9
10

Read it, live it, love the results.

Just as you learn from past failures, you should also learn from past successes.
Keep in mind those times you turned your dreams into reality. Reflect on what you did and how you felt when you achieved your goals. Know that you were able to achieve your dreams in the past and you will do it again in the present and future.

Without challenge, there is no change.

Actor and producer **Vince Vaughn**, moved to Hollywood where he struggled as an actor and faced many rejections. Though he held many smaller roles success, did not come until 1996 with his role in *Swingers* with Jon Favreau – from there his career took off. He has credited his mother as the inspiration behind his career, saying: “I saw her overcome stuff, and I thought if you worked hard at something you'd give yourself a chance.”

The thing always happens that you really believe in; and the belief in a thing makes it happen.
—Frank Lloyd Wright

side leg lifts

Lie on your right side with right hand supporting head, left hand flat on floor. Contract your obliques, as you lift both legs 8-12 inches off the floor. Tap toes together twice, then lower to the floor and repeat.If you would like to intensify this exercise, use ankle weights and/or don't let the feet touch the floor when returning to starting position. Repeat 15-20 times.

	DATE
Steps Walked:	
Cardio Workout:	
Strength Training:	
Calories Consumed:	
Calories Burned:	
Difference:	
Weight / Body fat:	

Eating healthy tastes great!

Peach Fizz Protein Shake
1 cup frozen peach slices
$^{1}/_{2}$ cup low fat vanilla yogurt
$^{1}/_{2}$ cup skim milk
2 scoops vanilla protein

Place all ingredients in blender and blend until smooth.
I recommend that women use soy protein and men use whey protein.

Read it, live it, love the results.

Use your imagination.
Don't have time for a healthy lunch? Enjoy a protein bar instead. No time for a workout? Do isometric exercises at your desk. Remember the words of the late Frank Lloyd Wright:
"The human race built most nobly when limitations were greatest and, therefore, when most was required of imagination in order to build at all."

Write it down & get it done.

1
2
3
4
5
6
7
8
9
10

middle "v" reach

Lie on the floor, face up with legs straight up, perpendicular to the floor, opened to form a "V". Keeping your chin pointing straight up to ceiling, contract your abdominals as you lift your shoulders, head and neck off the floor. Extend both arms and reach up through your legs. Hold here for 3-5 counts, then repeat 10-15 times.

I believe there's an inner power that makes winners or losers. And the winners are the ones who really listen to the truth of their hearts.
– Sylvester Stallone

DATE

Steps Walked:
Cardio Workout:
Strength Training:
Calories Consumed:
Calories Burned:
Difference:
Weight / Body fat:

Write it down & get it done. Read it, live it, love the results. Success is the reward of hard work.

1
2
3
4
5
6
7
8
9
10

Drinking green tea reduces your chances of cancer and stroke.
Green tea contains catechins, antioxidant compounds which protect against cancer by neutralizing free radicals. And, though other teas are good for you, studies show green tea to be stronger in blocking the growth of cancer cells. Catechins also prevent heart disease and stroke, primarily by defending against the harmful effects of artery-clogging LDL cholesterol.

Actor, director, producer and screenwriter, **Sylvester Stallone** was inspired to write, *"Rocky"*, after watching a 15 round boxing match between Mohammed Ali and an unknown. It took him just three days to write. Many film companies were interested, but Stallone insisted on being the star. Eventually he found a backer, and the oscar winning film was made on a very small budget in less than a month. Stallone became one of the biggest box office draws in the world.

A book is the only immortality.
–Rufus Choate

crunch with a punch

Sit on the floor with knees bent and heels on the floor. With a dumbbell in each hand, lean back slightly, engaging your abdominals. Twisting the upper body to the left, punch the right dumbbell to the outside of the left thigh. Complete 25-50 punches, then punch with the left to the right. You may also complete a set of alternating punches.

Steps Walked:
Cardio Workout:
Strength Training:
Calories Consumed:
Calories Burned:
Difference:
Weight / Body fat:

DATE

Eating healthy tastes great!

Parmesan Chicken

8 chicken breasts • ½ cup light butter, melted • 1 tsp Worchestershire sauce ½ tsp garlic powder • 1 cup bread crumbs 1 cup Parmesan cheese • 2 tbs parsley Preheat oven to 350ºF. Combine butter, Worchestershire, and garlic powder. In another bowl, combine the bread crumbs, Parmesan, and parsley. Dip breast into butter mixture, then into the crumb mixture. Place in baking pan and bake for 50-60 minute, until no longer pink inside.

Read it, live it, love the results.

Remove negative people from your life.

If you are in a relationship or surrounded by people who put you down and don't respect you, your subconscious mind will become cluttered with negatives. Staying in contact with negative people is similar to exposing yourself to carbon monoxide. It's a silent killer, and you're usually not aware of the danger until it's too late.

Write it down & get it done.

1
2
3
4
5
6
7
8
9
10

standing & twisting

Stand with feet slightly wider than shoulder-width apart, back straight, shoulders back and chest out with hands in beginner military press position. With dumbbells in hand, raise your right knee towards your left elbow, while simultaneously moving the left elbow towards the right knee. Your upper body should twist as you bring the two together. Return to starting position and repeat. Complete 10-15 repetitions on each leg.

Obstacles don't have to stop you. If you run into a wall, don't turn around and give up. Figure out how to climb it, go through it, or work around it.
—Michael Jordon

DATE

Steps Walked:
Cardio Workout:
Strength Training:
Calories Consumed:
Calories Burned:
Difference:
Weight / Body fat:

Write it down & get it done.

1
2
3
4
5
6
7
8
9
10

Read it, live it, love the results.

Drinking red tea may help in slowing the aging process and reducing your risk of cancer. Numerous studies have shown red tea to be a natural healing beverage. The tea, which contains anti-oxidants, Vitamin C, Calcium, Potassium, Magnesium, Iron, Zinc, Sodium, Copper, and Manganese, assists the immune system in fighting free radicals. It also works as an anti-inflammatory, anti-fungal and anti-allergen.

Success is the reward of hard work.

The founder of Mattel & creator of Barbie, **Ruth Handler**, started out in her garage in 1945. When she told her husband and his business partner of her idea to produce a plastic doll with an adult body they told her it wouldn't sell. She didn't let this discourage her. Instead, she created her doll, named it after her daughter, debuted it at the New York toy fair on March 9, 1959, and became an instant success.

Don't just learn the tricks of the trade. Learn the trade.
—James Bennis

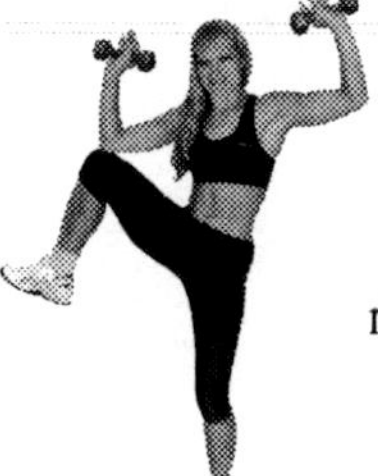

standing elbow to knee

Stand with feet slightly wider than shoulder-width apart, back straight, shoulders back and chest out with hands in military press position, holding dumbbells. Raise your right knee to your right elbow, touching or getting as close as possible. Return to the starting position and repeat. Complete 10-15 repetitions on each leg.

	DATE
Steps Walked:	
Cardio Workout:	
Strength Training:	
Calories Consumed:	
Calories Burned:	
Difference:	
Weight / Body fat:	

Eating healthy tastes great!

Red and Green Salad

1 large head romaine lettuce
3 cups tart red apples, diced
2 cups celery, diced
1/4 cup walnuts, chopped
1 oz blue cheese, crumbled
1 cup nonfat mayonnaise
1 cup nonfat yogurt
1/2 tsp black pepper

Combine torn lettuce, apples, celery, walnuts and blue cheese in a large bowl. In separate bowl whisk mayonnaise, yogurt and pepper, pour over salad and toss.

Read it, live it, love the results.

Learn all you can about that which you desire.

If it's a healthy lifestyle you desire, set aside a definite time every day for educating yourself. Whether it be twenty minutes of reading, taking special courses, or spending time at the library, *EDUCATE YOURSELF.* There is plenty of information out there, find it and use it, no one can do it for you...and no one can take it from you!

Write it down & get it done.

1
2
3
4
5
6
7
8
9
10

elbow to knee in pushup stance
On the floor, support yourself on hands and toes, in a full body pushup position. Curling the body, bring the right knee toward the left elbow. Hold for 2-3 counts then return to the extended position. Complete 10-15 repetitions on each leg.

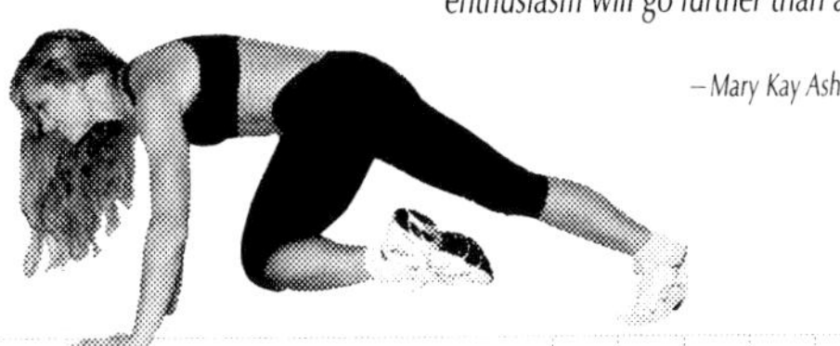

A mediocre idea that generates enthusiasm will go further than a

– Mary Kay Ash

DATE

Steps Walked:
Cardio Workout:
Strength Training:
Calories Consumed:
Calories Burned:
Difference:
Weight / Body fat:

Write it down & get it done.

1
2
3
4
5
6
7
8
9
10

Read it, live it, love the results.

Take a low dose aspirin each day. It has been public knowledge for some time that taking a low dose aspirin each day helps prevent heart attacks and strokes; now, according to an article in the British Journal of Cancer (Vol. 87:49-53), aspirin is reported to also cut lung cancer risks, especially in women. Though, this is not a license to smoke.

Life's tough, get over it, she did.

The founder of Mary Kay Cosmetics, **Mary Kay Ash**, started by working for Stanley Home Products. It wasn't until after retirement that she decided to live her dream by founding Mary Kay Cosmetics. Success did not come easy, but her philosophy endured, *"If you think you can, you can. And if you think you can't, you're right."* Her slogan *"God first, family second, career third"* expressed her insistence that the women in her company keep their lives in balance.

Yes, knowledge is power. But it's the ability to manipulate the knowledge, that sustains the power.
—aurthor unknown

single toe touch

Lie on the floor, face up with legs straight out, resting on the floor. Place right arm behind your head, the left arm resting at your side. (Holding a dumbbell is optional.) Simultaneously, raise your right arm and left leg off the floor, bringing your fingers and toes together above your chest. Hold together for 2-3 counts then slowly lower to starting position. Repeat 10-15 times, then complete a set on the opposite side.

	DATE
Steps Walked:	
Cardio Workout:	
Strength Training:	
Calories Consumed:	
Calories Burned:	
Difference:	
Weight / Body fat:	

Eating healthy tastes great!

Strawberry-Orange Shake
1 1/2 cups vanilla soymilk
2 cups ice
10 oz bag frozen strawberries
1 banana, cut into chunks
1/3 cup calcium-enriched OJ
1 banana, cut into chunks
1 scoop vanilla protein
Sweeten with honey, if desired.
Place all ingredients in blender and blend until smooth.
I recommend that women use soy protein and men use whey protein.

Read it, live it, love the results.

Organize and devise a plan of action with an end in mind.
If it's a healthy lifestyle you desire, research different exercises, learn about the foods you should be eating, then develop a plan and write it down. Don't leave anything to memory. In addition to the plan, record your workouts, the foods you eat, and the results of these actions as you progress towards your goals.

Write it down & get it done.

1
2
3
4
5
6
7
8
9
10

bent knee side leg raises

Lie on the floor, on your side. With both legs slightly bent prop yourself up on your elbow. Lifting your upper leg as high as you can, bring it into your chest, hold 2-3 counts, then return to the starting position.
Complete 10-15 repetitions on each leg.

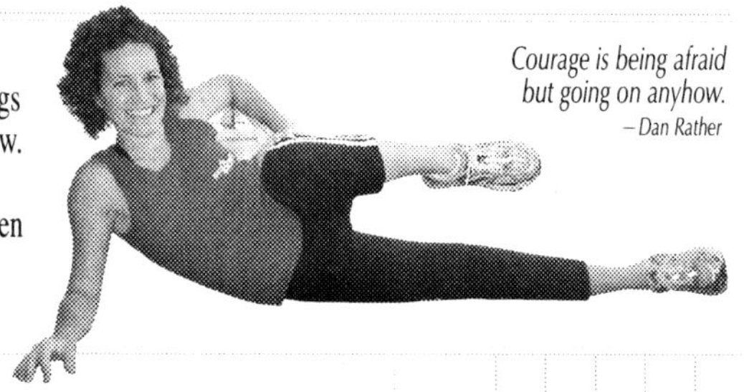

Courage is being afraid but going on anyhow.
– Dan Rather

DATE

Steps Walked:
Cardio Workout:
Strength Training:
Calories Consumed:
Calories Burned:
Difference:
Weight / Body fat:

Write it down & get it done.

1
2
3
4
5
6
7
8
9
10

Read it, live it, love the results.

Avoid consuming excessive amounts of alcohol.
Research shows that chronic heavy drinking is linked to an increased risk of cancer of the mouth, throat, esophagus, liver, pancreas and rectum. Consuming as little as three ounces of hard liquor every day for several years can cause major damage. Alcohol also reduces your metabolism, which leads to weight gain. It's better to keep it to a minimum.

Doors open when least expected.

News anchor **Dan Rather** from the CBS Evening News, had auditioned for the voice of cartoon character *Dudley Do-Right* in the 1960's. However, he was turned down by animator/director Jay Ward. In the long run, this worked out to his advantage. He anchored the CBS Evening News for 24 years, from March 9, 1981 to March 9, 2005, in addition to contributing to CBS' 60 Minutes. When one door closes, another always opens.

Try to realize it's all within yourself no one else can make you change.
– George Harrison

combined crunch

Lie face up on the floor, fingertips resting on your neck, with your knees directly over your hips at a 90-degree angle. Keeping your back pressed into the floor, tilt your pelvis up toward your chest in a small, controlled movement. With the pelvis lifted, bring your knees a few inches closer to your chest. At the same time, raise your torso. Contract the abdominals as you would in a standard crunch. Hold for 2-3 counts, repeat 10-15 times.

	DATE
Steps Walked:	
Cardio Workout:	
Strength Training:	
Calories Consumed:	
Calories Burned:	
Difference:	
Weight / Body fat:	

Eating healthy tastes great!

Hummus
1 can chick peas, drained
(Keep 1/3 cup liquid)
3 tbs lemon juice
1/3 cup sesame seed
2 tbs minced garlic
Chopped fresh parsley
Place beans, reserved bean liquid, lemon juice, sesame seed and garlic in blender and blend smooth.
Place in serving dish & sprinkle with parsley. Serve with pita bread wedges or raw vegetables.

Read it, live it, love the results.

Add onions and garlic to foods to help fight free radicals damage.
Research shows onions help clear waste materials from the body's cells. One of the most recognizable ways they do this is when they produce tears which wash the epithelial layers of the eyes. Garlic, also helps eliminate waste materials and dangerous free radicals from the body.

Write it down & get it done.

1
2
3
4
5
6
7
8
9
10

tilt back

Sit on the floor with knees bent, feet flat, arms straight out front. Keeping arms straight, lean back until you are 8-15 inches from the floor. Lift your feet and extend your legs until they are straight.Hold for 10-15 counts then lower and repeat 5-10 times.

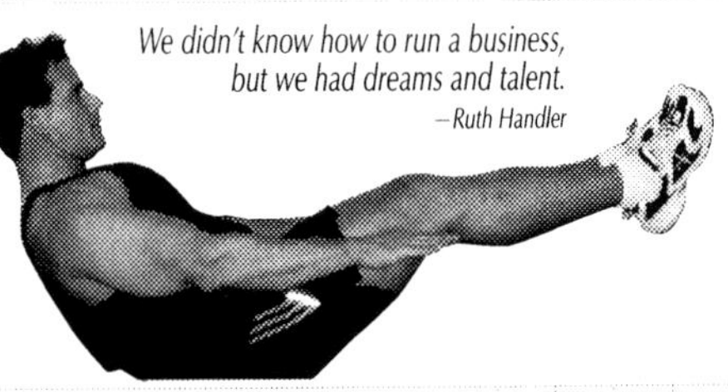

We didn't know how to run a business, but we had dreams and talent.
— Ruth Handler

DATE

Steps Walked:

Cardio Workout:

Strength Training:

Calories Consumed:

Calories Burned:

Difference:

Weight / Body fat:

Write it down & get it done.

1
2
3
4
5
6
7
8
9
10

Read it, live it, love the results.

Be self-motivated.
Without the power of self-motivation, the great leaders of business, industry and finance, along with the great artists, musicians, poets, and writers, would have been ordinary everyday people. These people became great because they were motivated to achieve that which they desired. Know what you desire and go for it.

Be the change you want to see.

Actor and film producer **Tom Selleck** lives on an avocado ranch. The following quote is from a Good Housekeeping interview titled *"Man of the House: Tom Selleck"*, *"So I like to get outside and work on the farm, from fixing roads to clearing brush. I hate going to the gym, so sweating outdoors sure beats sitting on a stationary bike staring at my navel. And I work cheaper than anyone I could hire to do it."*

A friend is one before whom I may think aloud.
– Ralph Waldo Emerson

oblique twist

Lie face up on the floor with legs up, knees bent at 90-degrees, fingertips resting on your neck. Keeping your elbows on the floor, twist from your waist, bringing your right elbow towards your left knee while extending your right leg out straight. The left elbow should remain on the floor. Complete 10-15 repetitions, then repeat on other side.

Steps Walked:
Cardio Workout:
Strength Training:
Calories Consumed:
Calories Burned:
Difference:
Weight / Body fat:

DATE

Eating healthy tastes great!

Pineapple Chicken
4 boneless skinless chicken breasts
14 oz unsweetened pineapple chunks, drained
1 tsp dried rosemary • pepper to taste
1/2 tsp paprika • 1/4 tsp ground ginger

Preheat the oven to 375°F.
Place breasts in a baking dish, and top with the pineapple chunks.
Combine other ingredients & sprinkle over the chicken. Cover and bake for one hour, until done.

Read it, live it, love the results.

Share your goals and ambitions with a supportive friend.
It's possible that you become successful without a friend at your side, but much of the real joy is lost if it cannot be shared.
If you've got at least one good friend you'll never be alone and you'll be more likely to succeed with his or her support.

Write it down & get it done.

1
2
3
4
5
6
7
8
9
10

cradle crunch

Lie on the floor, face up, with your knees bent at 90-degrees, feet elevated with ankles crossed. Rest fingertips on your neck, then contract your abdominals and crunch, lifting your shoulders, head and neck 3-4 inches off the floor. Hold for 3-5 counts, while pulling your knees in toward the chest. Return to start and repeat 10-15 times.

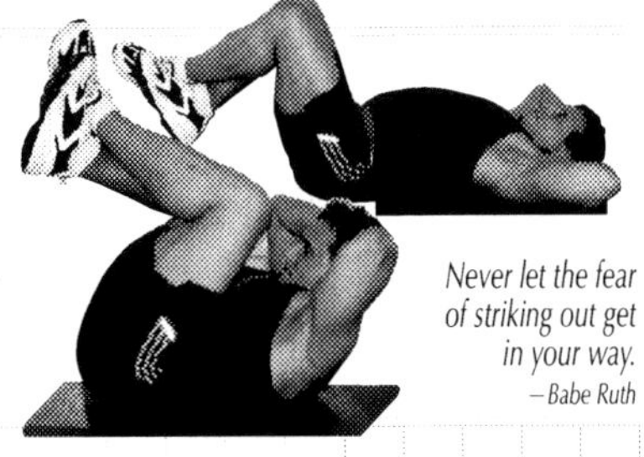

Never let the fear of striking out get in your way.
—Babe Ruth

DATE

Steps Walked:
Cardio Workout:
Strength Training
Calories Consumed:
Calories Burned:
Difference:
Weight / Body fat:

Write it down & get it done.

1
2
3
4
5
6
7
8
9
10

Read it, live it, love the results.

You determine how well you age. The fountain of youth does not reside in a magical pill, but in fruits and vegetables and in avoiding those things which expedite the aging process; such as smoking, excessive drinking, over-exposure to the sun, cold and stress. You are in control of your age, don't ever think differently or place the blame elsewhere.
One of the best things you can do is take responsibility for yourself.

Be the change you want to see.

Artist **Claude Monet** born into a wealthy family, had a love for art, not business. When young, Monet often drew caricatures of the locals, which got him into trouble at school. He was a rebel, and frequently disobeyed the rules. By the age of fifteen he was selling the caricatures. This did not set well with his parents, still he continued drawing and eventually began painting.

Many people fail in life, not for lack of ability or brains or even courage but simply because they have never organized their energies around a goal.
—Elbert Hubbard

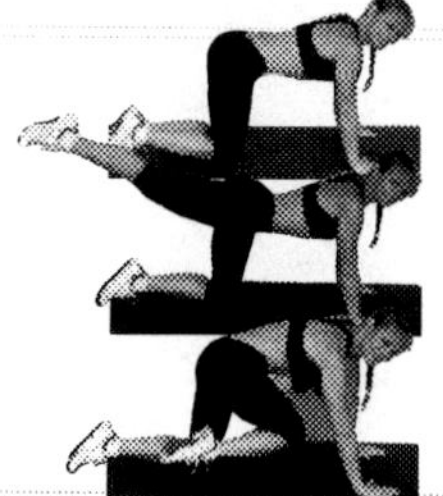

donkey kicks

On the floor support yourself with hands and knees. Extend the right leg straight up and back, hold here for 2-3 counts, then bring the knee to the left elbow, hold for 2-3 counts then return foot to extended position. Complete 10-15 repetitions on each leg.

	DATE
Steps Walked:	
Cardio Workout:	
Strength Training:	
Calories Consumed:	
Calories Burned:	
Difference:	
Weight / Body fat:	

Eating healthy tastes great!

Tuna Salad

12 oz can water-packed solid white tuna, drained
1/3 cup Fat Free plain yogurt
4 oz can crushed pineapple, drained
1/3 cup finely chopped celery
1/4 cup sweet pickle relish
1/4 cup chopped pecans
1 tsp yellow mustard
1/8 tsp ground cinnamon
Mix ingredients and serve with tomato or on low carb bread.

Read it, live it, love the results.

Focus on ways to reach your goals—on a daily basis.

Question yourself on a daily basis and push your mind to explore things you may not have considered. If it's a healthy lifestyle you desire, think of things you can do to get more exercise. Taking the stairs, walking the dog, playing with the kids, the list is endless.

Write it down & get it done.

1
2
3
4
5
6
7
8
9
10

weighted lower ab lifts

Lie on the floor face up with knees bent, holding a dumbbell between your feet. Extend legs straight up pressing your feet together tightly to hold the dumbbell in place. Contract your abdominals and lift your hips off the floor, raising the dumbbell toward the ceiling. Hold for 2-3 counts then slowly lower to the starting position. Repeat 10-15 times.

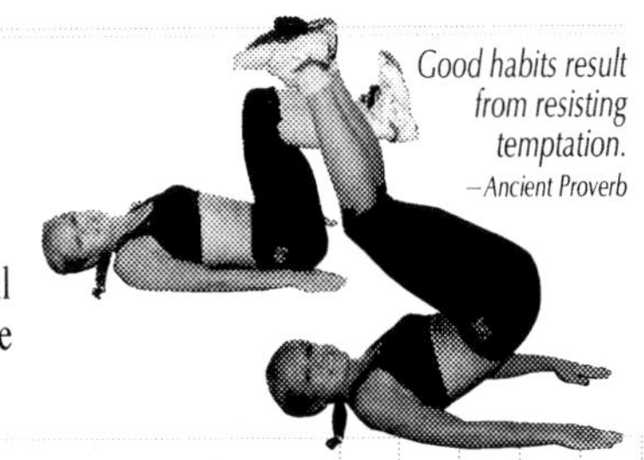

Good habits result from resisting temptation.
–Ancient Proverb

DATE

Steps Walked:
Cardio Workout:
Strength Training:
Calories Consumed:
Calories Burned:
Difference:
Weight / Body fat:

Write it down & get it done.

1
2
3
4
5
6
7
8
9
10

Read it, live it, love the results.

Don't get frustrated with your progress.
Losing fat is a long term goal, it doesn't happen overnight. Though it may seem that the unwanted pounds appeared overnight, it is more likely that it took several months or even years for them to appear. In contrast you should be able to take off two pounds a week, that's nearly ten pounds a month.

Life's tough, get over it, he did!

Seven-time winner of the Tour de France, **Lance Armstrong**, is also a cancer survivor. In 1996 Armstrong discovered that he had testicular cancer, which had spread to his brain and lungs. However, with surgery and heavy chemotherapy he beat the cancer and returned to his love of cycling. In 1999 he won his first Tour de France, and then repeated the victory the next five years in a row. He never gave up.

crunching leg drop

Lie on the floor, face up, with your fingertips resting on your neck and your legs extended straight up, with toes pointing toward the ceiling, feet slightly turned out. Lift your shoulders 2-3 inches off the floor and hold. Without arching your back, lower your legs to within 6-8 inches above the floor. Hold here for 3-5 counts, then return to the starting position. Complete 10-15 reps.

DATE

Steps Walked:
Cardio Workout:
Strength Training
Calories Consumed:
Calories Burned:
Difference:
Weight / Body fat:

Eating healthy tastes great!

Chocolate-Raspberry Shake
2 cups light chocolate soymilk
16 oz cup ice
1 cup raspberries, frozen or fresh
1/2 tsp vanilla
1 scoop chocolate protein

Place all ingredients in blender and blend until smooth.
I recommend that women use soy protein and men use whey protein.

Read it, live it, love the results.

Don't ever give up on yourself. Your success depends on you.
If you feel it is a lack of formal education that is keeping you from succeeding, keep in mind that Thomas A. Edison had only three months of *"schooling"* while Henry Ford made it only as far at sixth grade. Despite their lack of formal eduction, they were both extremely successful, moreso than many others who were more highly educated.

Write it down & get it done.

1
2
3
4
5
6
7
8
9
10

hip drop

Lie on the floor, on your side, supporting yourself with your left elbow and foot, with your right hand on your right hip. Lower your hip to the floor, then bring back to starting position. Hold here for 2-3 counts, before droppng to the floor again. Complete 10-15 repetitions on each side.

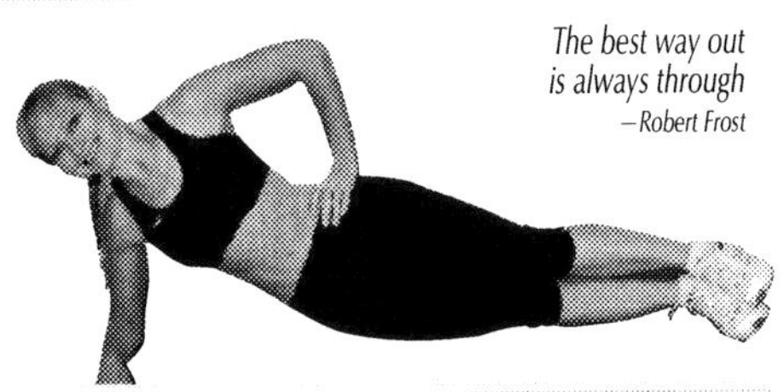

The best way out is always through
–Robert Frost

DATE

Steps Walked:
Cardio Workout:
Strength Training
Calories Consumed:
Calories Burned:
Difference:
Weight / Body fat:

Write it down & get it done.

1
2
3
4
5
6
7
8
9
10

Read it, live it, love the results.

Exercise on a regular basis.
Exercise releases endorphins, the feel good substances which reduce stress, depression, anxiety, irritability and anger.
When feeling overwhelmed or upset, take a walk or jog and you'll soon view things in a different light.

Life's tough, get over it, he did.

Four time Pulitzer Prize winning poet, **Robert Frost** attended Harvard but left without a degree, in order to support his family. Over the next ten years he wrote poetry, but was seldom published. He also operated a farm, given to him by his grandfather, and taught at Derry's Pinkerton Academy. At the age of 38, determined to become a successful writer, he sold the farm and moved to England. Here, he wrote some of his best work.

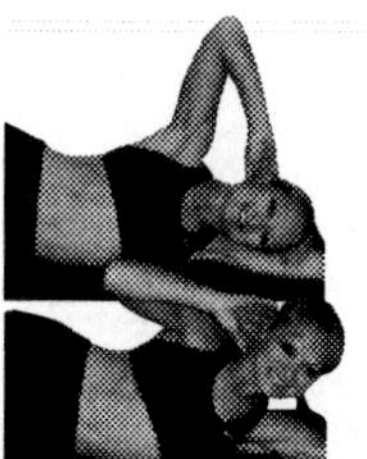

Ability is what you're capable of doing. Motivation determines what you do. Attitude determines how well you do it.
– Lou Holtz

side crunch

Lie on the floor, on your right side, with both legs slightly bent, with your left hand fingers resting on your neck. Concentrate on flexing your oblique abdominal muscles as you lift your upper body. Hold for 2-3 counts, return to the floor and repeat 10-15 times. Note, you won't be able to come up too high, this is a concentrated short movement.

	DATE
Steps Walked:	
Cardio Workout:	
Strength Training:	
Calories Consumed:	
Calories Burned:	
Difference:	
Weight / Body fat:	

Eating healthy tastes great!

Coconut Oven Fried Chicken
1/4 cup melted light butter
4 boneless, skinless chicken breasts
1/2 cup flaked unsweetened coconut
1/4 cup fine bread crumbs
Preheat oven to 350°F. Brush the chicken pieces with melted butter. Combine the coconut and the bread crumbs, then roll the chicken pieces in the coconut mixture. Place chicken in a baking pan and drizzle any remaining butter over the chicken. Bake for about an hour.

Read it, live it, love the results.

Let your imagination run wild.
Don't put limitations on what you can do. As stated by Earl Nightengale, "*Whatever the mind of man can conceive and believe, it can achieve.*" Realize that the only limitations you face, within reason, lie within your own imagination and motivation to take action. If you have a desire, you can do it.

Write it down & get it done.

1
2
3
4
5
6
7
8
9
10

toe reach

Lie on the floor, face up with legs straight up, perpendicular to the floor. Keeping your chin pointing straight up, contract your abdominals and crunch, lifting your shoulders, head and neck off the floor as you extend both arms and reach up to touch your toes. Alternate sides, reaching up first to your left foot, then to your right. Hold each reach for 2-3 counts. Repeat this alternating count 10-15 times.

Always bear in mind that your own resolution to succeed is more important than any other one thing.
– Abraham Lincoln

DATE

Steps Walked:
Cardio Workout:
Strength Training
Calories Consumed:
Calories Burned:
Difference:
Weight / Body fat:

Write it down & get it done.

1
2
3
4
5
6
7
8
9
10

Read it, live it, love the results.

Don't make the mistake of living the dreams of others. When setting goals, make sure they are your goals. If they're not, you won't have a real desire to make them a reality. This is your one and only life, you must embrace it and live it to the fullest. Letting others goals become your goals, living the dreams of others and/or focusing on empty goals will get you nowhere.

Doors open, when you work hard.

The sixteenth President of the United States, **Abraham Lincoln**, grew up in a wild region without much education. Instead, he learned all he could while working on a farm and at a store. Later he became a captain in the Black Hawk War, spent eight years in the Illinois legislature, and rode the circuit of courts for many years. His law partner said of him, *"His ambition was a little engine that knew no rest."*

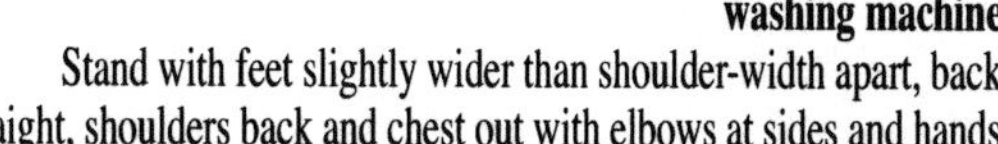

Ideas are the beginning point of all fortunes. Ideas are the products of the imagination.
—Napolean Hill

washing machine

Stand with feet slightly wider than shoulder-width apart, back straight, shoulders back and chest out with elbows at sides and hands pressed together in front of chest, holding dumbbells. Bend knees to squatting position. Then, without moving your hips or head, twist the body to the right for a 2-3 count hold, then to the left for a 2-3 count hold. Continue this alternating count 15-30 times.

DATE

Steps Walked:
Cardio Workout:
Strength Training:
Calories Consumed:
Calories Burned:
Difference:
Weight / Body fat:

Eating healthy tastes great!

Frozen Mango Pops

1 ripe mango, peeled and diced
1 cup vanilla yogurt
1/2 lime, juice plus a few scrapings zest
2 packets Splenda®
1/4 tsp vanilla

Blend all ingredients until smooth. Pour into popsicle molds and freeze.

Read it, live it, love the results.

Be creative when striving to reach your goals.

If you have tried unsuccessfully in the past to create a healthy lifestyle, determine why you failed, then use your imagination to change your approach. When you use your imagination and think *"outside of the box"* you will be amazed at the solutions which arise.

Write it down & get it done.

1
2
3
4
5
6
7
8
9
10

kneeling elbow to knee

On floor, support yourself on hands and knees. (Using a dumbbell is optional.) Extend the right arm straight out front, the left leg straight out back and hold for 2-3 counts. Curling the body, bring the right elbow to the left knee, and hold for another 2-3 counts. Return to extended position, repeat 10-15 times, then complete a set on the opposite side.

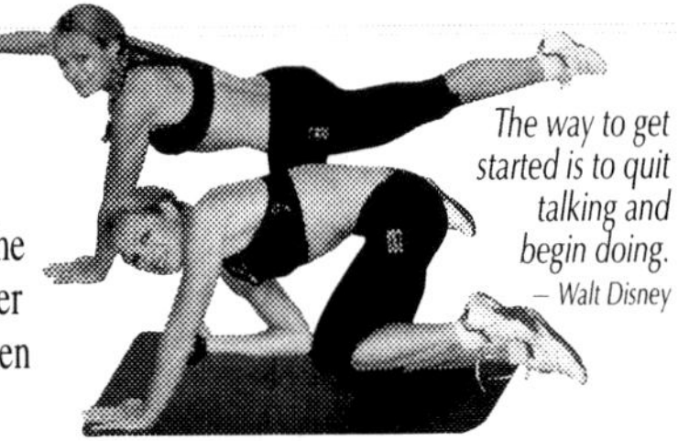

The way to get started is to quit talking and begin doing.
– Walt Disney

DATE

Steps Walked:
Cardio Workout:
Strength Training
Calories Consumed:
Calories Burned:
Difference:
Weight / Body fat:

Write it down & get it done.

1
2
3
4
5
6
7
8
9
10

Read it, live it, love the results.

Don't be pessimistic.
In a study published in the August 2002 issue of *Mayo Clinic Proceedings*, it was found that people who expect misfortune and see only the darker side of life don't live as long as those with a more optimistic view.
No matter what happens to you there is always a brighter side.
Be creative, find the brighter side and enjoy a longer, happier, healthier life.

Be the change you want to see.

St. Louis Cardinal superstar **Albert Pujols** was raised in the Dominican Republic by his grandmother. Then, in 1996 they immigrated to the U.S.—he became a citizen in 2007, scoring a perfect 100 on his citizenship test!
Not only is he admired by many for his incredible baseball talent, he is also hailed a hero due to his dedication to *"the love, care and development of people with Down syndrome and their families."*
His foundation has helped many.
www.pujolsfamilyfoundation.org

Success is the progressive realization of a worthy goal or ideal. –Earl Nightengale

knee raise lying and twisting

Lie on the floor, face up with legs exended straight out, flat on the floor. Place fingertips on your neck with elbows out. Contract your abdominals and crunch, lifting your shoulders, head and neck 3-4 inches off floor. Twisting your upper body, bring the right elbow to meet the left knee. Hold 2-3 counts, then return to starting position, keeping the left leg slightly suspended above the floor. Repeat 10-15 times, then complete a set on the opposite side.

	DATE
Steps Walked:	
Cardio Workout:	
Strength Training	
Calories Consumed:	
Calories Burned:	
Difference:	
Weight / Body fat:	

Eating healthy tastes great!

Chicken and Summer Squash

4 chicken breast • 1 tomato, diced
$^{3}/_{4}$ pound yellow squash, sliced
$^{3}/_{4}$ pound zucchinis, sliced
pepper to taste • olive oil

Sauté chicken in olive oil. Remove, then sauté vegetables for about 3 minutes. Reduce heat, and return chicken to skillet. Cover partially, and cook until squash is soft, serve hot.

Read it, live it, love the results.

Develop an organized plan.
With the help of those who support you in achieving your desire, develop a plan to accomplish your goals, and write it down. If you are working toward a healthier lifestyle you may want to work with a personal trainer or dietician. You may also refer to the library or internet, each is a great source of information. *Knowledge is power.*

Write it down & get it done.

1
2
3
4
5
6
7
8
9
10

the plank
Lie on the floor, face down with elbows resting on floor next to your chest. Push your body off the floor in a push-up position, supporting yourself on your elbows and toes. Contract your abs, keeping your body in a straight line from head to toes. Hold for 30-60 counts. Repeat 1-5 times.

side plank on step Lie on the floor, on your side with elbows resting on floor, toes on step. Push your body off the floor in a push-up position, then rotate to the right, supporting yourself on your right elbow and foot.Hold for 30-60 counts.Repeat 2-5 times, then complete a set on theother side.

DATE

Tomorrow hopes that we have learned something from yesterday. –John Wayne

Steps Walked:
Cardio Workout:
Strength Training:
Calories Consumed:
Calories Burned:
Difference:
Weight / Body fat:

Write it down & get it done.

1
2
3
4
5
6
7
8
9
10

Read it, live it, love the results.

Enjoy an optimistic outlook.
In the November 2004 issue of the *Archives of General Psychiatry*, it was noted that your mental health can influence your physical health. And, that certain personality traits such as optimism or pessimism, can influence how well and how long you live. Needless to say, it is the optimist who lives a long happy life. So, remove all negative thoughts and enjoy a long, happy optimistic life.

Doors open when least expected.

Academy Award and Golden Globe Award-winning actor **John Wayne** entered the film business while working as a laborer on the Fox lot during summer vacations. His first big movie was a major flop, but he never gave up. Eventually, he became one of the most popular leading men in Hollywood history. He was honored by the film community, the U.S. Congress, and the American people unlike any actor before or since.

but they will never forget how you made them feel.
—Carl W. Buechner

plank with leg extension

While in the plank position, contract your abs, keeping your body in a straight line from head to toes, then raise your right foot 10-12 inches from the floor. Hold for 30-60 counts. Repeat lift with left leg.

plank with rotation

While in the plank position, contract your abs and drop your heels to the right, hold here for 2-3 counts then rotate to the left. Complete 10-15 reps.

DATE

Steps Walked:
Cardio Workout:
Strength Training:
Calories Consumed:
Calories Burned:
Difference:
Weight / Body fat:

Eating healthy tastes great!

Cheesy Baked Fish

1 lb fish fillets • 1 tsp lemon juice
1/2 cup light cheddar cheese, grated
2/3 cup wheat bread crumbs
1/2 tsp dried basil • 1/4 tsp nutmeg
Salt and pepper to taste

Preheat oven to 450ºF. Combine first six ingredients, then spread half of the mixture in a greased baking dish. Place the fish on top of the crumbs. Sprinkle the lemon juice over the fish.Sprinkle remaining crumbs over the fish. Bake about 10-12 minutes until fish flakes easily.

Read it, live it, love the results.

Give your brain a boost with fish.

Fish, which is rich in omega 3 fatty acids, is essential for brain function and development. The healthy fats have actually been found to have many benefits including; lower dementia and stroke risks; slower mental decline; and may play a vital role in enhancing memory, especially as we age.

It's recommended that you eat two servings of fish weekly.

Write it down & get it done.

1
2
3
4
5
6
7
8
9
10

pikes

Lie on the floor, face up with legs flat on the floor, straight out and arms outstretched behind head. Simultaneously, raise your shoulders and legs off the floor, bringing your fingers and toes together in the middle. Hold here for 2-3 counts then slowly lower your hands and feet to starting position, without touching the floor. Repeat 10-15 times.

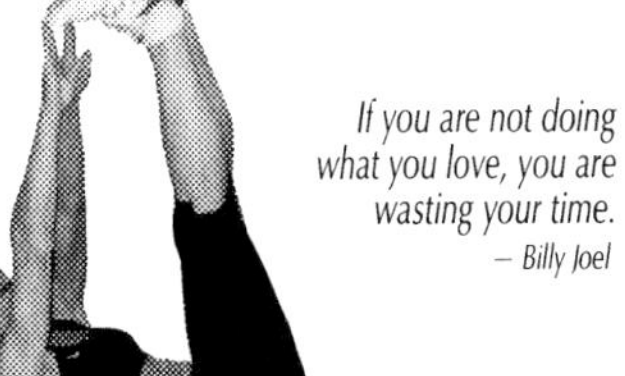

If you are not doing what you love, you are wasting your time.
– Billy Joel

DATE

Steps Walked:
Cardio Workout:
Strength Training:
Calories Consumed:
Calories Burned:
Difference:
Weight / Body fat:

Write it down & get it done.

1
2
3
4
5
6
7
8
9
10

Read it, live it, love the results.

Play well with others.
Your ability to get along with others is critical to achieving those things you desire. Treat people as you would like to be treated, even when they do things you object to, after all, we are all mere humans. In life's lessons we learn you cannot change others—however we can change ourselves. Focus your energy on becoming all you can be.

Life's tough, get over it, he did!

Six-time Grammy Award winner pianist and singer-songwriter, **Billy Joel** had an intense interest in music at a young age, so his mother pushed him into piano lessons. Unfortunately, his interest in music, instead of sports, was the source of teasing and bullying from classmates. However, instead of giving up music he took up boxing to defend himself.

Planning is bringing the future into the present so that you can do something about it now.
–Alan Lakein

side elbow to knee

Lie face down on the floor then push yourself up into a plank position on elbows and toes. Slowly turn your body to the right into a t-stand. Place fingertips on your neck with elbow extended out. Supporting your body with the lower left leg, bring the right knee up to the right elbow, hold here for 2-3 counts, then extend leg back out straight, keeping it suspended inches above the floor. Repeat 10-15 times, then complete a set on the opposite side.

DATE

Steps Walked:
Cardio Workout:
Strength Training
Calories Consumed:
Calories Burned:
Difference:
Weight / Body fat:

Eating healthy tastes great!

Garlic and Balsamic Chicken

4 chicken breasts • 2 tbs minced garlic
2 tbs olive oil • 1 cup apple juice
1 tsp oregano • pepper to taste
1/4 cup Parmesan cheese
3 tbs balsamic vinegar

Preheat oven to 450°F. Combine all ingredients, except balsamic vinegar. Place breasts in a baking dish and pour mixture over them. Bake for 45 to 60 minutes, until no longer pink inside. Pour the balsamic vinegar over the breasts and serve.

Read it, live it, love the results.

Create a roadmap for success and write it down.

Don't create the *"perfect plan"* in your head. Use this journal and record each and every step necessary to reach your ultimate goal. Know what you will be doing each day in order to reach your destination. Without a map to your destination you may end up sitting at too many rest stops and never getting anywhere.

Write it down & get it done.

1
2
3
4
5
6
7
8
9
10

t-stand with elbow support

You must pay the price if you wish to secure the blessing.
—Andrew Jackson

Lie face down on the floor then push yourself up into a plank position on elbows and toes. Slowly turn your body to the right in a plank position, lifting the right hand straight up toward the ceiling. Hold here 10-20 counts, lower and repeat 2-5 times. Complete a set on each side. If too difficult, drop to your knees for this exercise.

DATE

Steps Walked:
Cardio Workout:
Strength Training
Calories Consumed:
Calories Burned:
Difference:
Weight / Body fat:

Write it down & get it done.

1
2
3
4
5
6
7
8
9
10

Read it, live it, love the results.

Don't make excuses to skip your workouts.
You may think you are far to busy to workout, that your job is much more important than spending 30-minutes a day to improve your health. However, the real truth is that life is far more precious than any amount of money. Even the heftiest bank account may not be able to save your life when you ignore your health.

Life's tough, get over it, he did!

The seventh President of the United States, **Andrew Jackson** was born in the backwoods of the Carolinas, and orphaned at age 14 when his entire immediate family died from war-related hardships. Jackson received only sporadic education, including a scanty legal education, though he knew enough to practice law on the frontier. Since he was not from a distinguished family, he had to make his career by his own merit and determination, which he did.

*Life is what happens to us,
while we are making other plans.*
—author unknown

t-stand

Lie face down on the floor then push yourself up into a push-up position on hands and toes. Slowly turn your body, lifting the right hand straight up. Hold here for 10-30 counts, lower and repeat 2-5 times. Complete a set on each side.

	DATE						
Steps Walked:							
Cardio Workout:							
Strength Training							
Calories Consumed:							
Calories Burned:							
Difference:							
Weight / Body fat:							

Eating healthy tastes great!

Peach Jello Salad

2 small boxes peach gelatin
1 1/2 cups boiling water
20 oz can crushed pineapple
14 oz can sweetened condensed milk
8 oz container light sour cream
1 cup chopped pecans

Dissolve gelatin in boiling water. Stir in remaining ingredients. Pour into 13 x 9-inch pan. Chill.

Read it, live it, love the results.

Make realistic plans and don't ever give up on them.

In order to succeed you must make realistic plans. This is not to say that your plans won't fail, however, if they do fail, remember this is only a temporary defeat, it is not permanent failure.
Don't ever give up, simply make needed adjustments to your plans and get started again. Only those who give up become failures.

Write it down & get it done.

1
2
3
4
5
6
7
8
9
10

I've heard many confess they refuse to wear shorts or skirts due to their "cottage cheese" thighs, and though this is a great reason to keep/get your legs in shape, it's not the only reason. The muscles in the legs are the most powerful as well as the largest in our bodies. They are used for everyday activities such as walking, sitting, standing, driving, climbing stairs, running, and the list goes on. In addition to developing strength and endurance and enhancing the appearance, leg exercises also improve balance and stability.

If you don't have time to do it right, When will you have time to do it over?
– John Wooden

DATE

Steps Walked:
Cardio Workout:
Strength Training:
Calories Consumed:
Calories Burned:
Difference:
Weight / Body fat:

Write it down & get it done.

1
2
3
4
5
6
7
8
9
10

Read it, live it, love the results.

Don't rely on good luck to get you to the top.
Winners know that it takes more than good luck to succeed. They know that they must take responsibility for themselves in order to achieve those things they desire. They take responsibility for the thoughts they think, the words they speak and the actions they take.

Life's tough, get over it, he did!

Actor, model, businessman, and politician, **Arnold Schwarzenegger**, grew up in Austria in a strict Roman Catholic household. He remembers; *"Back then in Austria it was a very different world, if we did something bad or we disobeyed our parents, the rod was not spared."* His father had *"no patience for listening or understanding your problems..."* The household also had money problems. Schwarzenegger recalled the highlight of his family purchasing their first refrigerator.

Our thoughts create our reality—where we put our focus is the direction we tend to go.
—Peter McWilliams

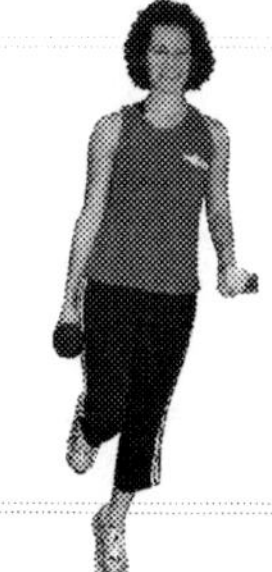

single leg calf raise
Using a chair for balance, stand tall with back straight, shoulders back and chest out. Place your right foot behind your left calf, then raise up on the toes of your left foot and hold for 2-3 counts. Lower to floor, then raise again. Repeat 10-15 times on each leg.

	DATE
Steps Walked:	
Cardio Workout:	
Strength Training	
Calories Consumed:	
Calories Burned:	
Difference:	
Weight / Body fat:	

Eating healthy tastes great!

Whole-Grain Snack Mix
2 cups Fiber One® bran cereal
2 cups Fiber One® Honey Clusters®
2 cups Honey Nut Cheerios®
1 cup raisins
1 cup peanuts

Mix ingredients and serve.

Read it, live it, love the results.

Eat legumes and/or other whole grains on a daily basis.
Studies show that eating two to three servings of legumes and/or whole grains on a daily basis can improve your blood sugar levels and lower your bad, LDL cholesterol. Beans, peanuts and whole wheat bread are among the best choices to fulfill this recommendation. Add them to your grocery list today and you may add years to your life.

Write it down & get it done.

1
2
3
4
5
6
7
8
9
10

squats

Stand with feet shoulder-width apart, back straight, shoulders back and chest out, with toes pointed straight ahead or slightly outward. Focus your vision straight ahead. Keeping your heels planted firmly on the floor, squat down and back, as if you are sitting in a chair. Keep your knees behind your toes as you squat down, stop when your thighs are parallel with the floor. Hold for 2-3 counts, then return to starting position. Repeat 10-15 times. *Hold dumbbells to intensify.*

Success seems to be largely a matter of hanging on after others have let go.
—William Feather

DATE

Steps Walked:
Cardio Workout:
Strength Training:
Calories Consumed:
Calories Burned:
Difference:
Weight / Body fat:

Write it down & get it done.

1
2
3
4
5
6
7
8
9
10

Read it, live it, love the results.

Have your bone density tested. It's estimated that there are an overwhleming 300,000 plus, hip fractures every year. And unfortunately, after six months of painful recovery only fifteen percent of patients can walk across a room unaided; another twenty five percent will require long-term care and may become disabled. Fortunately, there are steps you can take to build strong bones and prevent such fractures.

Doors open, when you work hard.

Actress, singer, record producer, dancer, fashion designer and television producer, **Jennifer Lopez** didn't just get "lucky". At 19, she financed singing and dancing lessons for herself. She divided her time between working in a legal office, dance classes and dance performances in New York clubs. After months of auditioning and rejections, she gained her first regular job for the comedy program *"In Living Color"*. Hardwork and desire brought her success.

narrow squats

Stand with feet inches apart, toes pointing straight ahead or slightly outward. Holding a dumbbell in each hand, focus your vision straight ahead. Keeping your heels planted firmly on the floor, inhale and move your buns back and downward, as if you are sitting in a chair. Keeping your knees behind your toes, stop when your thighs are parallel to the floor. Hold for 2-3 counts, then return to starting position and repeat 10-15 times.

The greatest barrier to success is the fear of failure.
–Sven Goran Eriksson

Steps Walked:

Cardio Workout:

Strength Training:

Calories Consumed:

Calories Burned:

Difference:

Weight / Body fat:

DATE

Eating healthy tastes great!

Red Onion and Pepper Fish

1 lb fish fillets • 1 tbs olive oil
1 sweet red pepper, cut in thin strips
1 red onion, cut in thin slices
1 tbs minced garlic • 1/2 tsp oregano
1 tsp parsley • pepper to taste

Sauté peppers, onion, garlic and oregano in olive oil. In another skillet, cook fish until it flakes easily. Sprinkle with parsley and season with pepper to taste. Spoon the red pepper mixture over the fish and serve immediately.

Read it, live it, love the results.

Never stop learning.

Those who are not successful usually make the mistake of believing knowledge is only acquired in schools. Spend time each day learning everything you can about that which you desire. If it's a healthy lifestyle you desire read all you can on the subject and talk to others who have made lifestyle changes. This is the knowledge you need succeed.

Write it down & get it done.

1
2
3
4
5
6
7
8
9
10

leg extension with dumbbell

Sit tall, abs in, shoulders back and chest out with hands in lap or holding sides of a chair. With a dumbbell between your feet, raise legs straight out front. Hold for 2-3 counts, then lower and repeat 10-15 times.

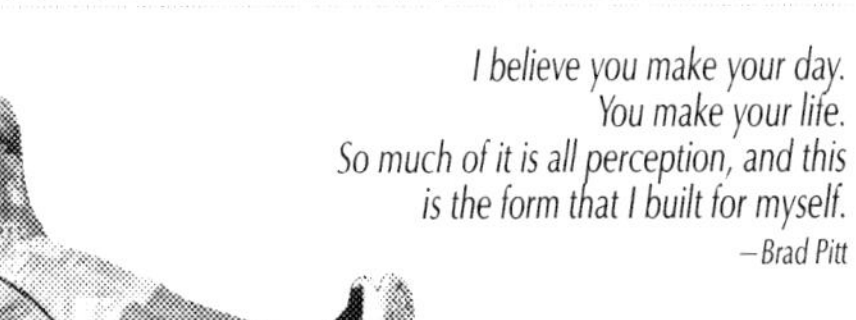

*I believe you make your day.
You make your life.
So much of it is all perception, and this
is the form that I built for myself.*
–Brad Pitt

DATE

Steps Walked:
Cardio Workout:
Resistance Workout:
Calories Consumed:
Calories Burned:
Difference:
Weight / Body fat:

Write it down & get it done.

1
2
3
4
5
6
7
8
9
10

Read it, live it, love the results.

"But I don't care how poor you are – you can turn off the television set during the week." *–Barrack Obama*

Turning off the television is perhaps one of the best things you can do for yourself. When doing anything at all, you need to ask yourself; *"Is this taking me closer to my goals or further from them?"* 99% of the time, TV is taking you AWAY from your goals. So, get up off the couch and MOVE. Stop watching others live there lives, and start living yours!

Life's tough, get over it, he did!

Actor and film producer, **Brad Pitt** did not always have it so easy. Before becoming successful, he supported himself by driving a limo, moving refrigerators and dressing as a giant chicken while working for the restaurant El Pollo Loco. He knew these were not the jobs that would define him, they were simply stepping stones, taking him closer to his real desire.

front kicks

Stand with feet shoulder-width apart, back straight, shoulders back and chest out with hands clinched in fists, positioned at your chest or holding dumbbells at your sides. Keeping the left knee slightly bent, raise the right leg straight out front as high as possible, then lower to starting position. Keep the movement controlled as you repeat 25-50 kicks. Repeat the same number of kicks with the left leg.

There is only one good, knowledge, and one evil, ignorance.
—Socrates

DATE

Steps Walked:
Cardio Workout:
Strength Training
Calories Consumed:
Calories Burned:
Difference:
Weight / Body fat:

Eating healthy tastes great!

Rootbeer Float Protein Shake
1 tsp rootbeer extract
16 oz cup of ice
$^{1}/_{2}$ cup low fat yogurt
2 scoops vanilla protein
Place all ingredients in blender and blend until smooth.

I recommend that women use soy protein and men use whey protein. Be sure to read the lables when purchasing protien, all are not created equal.

Read it, live it, love the results.

Focus your thoughts on being healthy and fit.
You become that which you focus your thoughts on. Think about being healthy and you'll find it easier to stick with your workouts and eat healthy. When you envision yourself as an eighty-year old man or woman, do you see yourself in a wheelchair or golf cart? Envision the golf cart and your subconscious will steer you in making healthy decisions.

Write it down & get it done.

1
2
3
4
5
6
7
8
9
10

tiptoe squat

With a pair of dumbbells positioned in front of you, stand with feet shoulder-width apart, toes pointed straight ahead or slightly outward. Bend down, placing hands on weights, as you bring yourself up on tiptoes. Holding this position, drop your buns down as far as possible, then lift again. Repeat 10-15 times.

All my life I have tried to pluck a thistle and plant a flower wherever the flower would grow in thought and mind.
–Abraham Lincoln

DATE

Steps Walked:
Cardio Workout:
Strength Training:
Calories Consumed:
Calories Burned:
Difference:
Weight / Body fat:

Write it down & get it done.

1
2
3
4
5
6
7
8
9
10

Read it, live it, love the results.

Get off the couch and move!

In a study performed at the University of Illinois, researchers found that sedentary individuals who took up a walking program of just forty-five minutes, three times a week, improved their scores on tests of mental sharpness by up to twenty percent.

As these individuals become more fit, the circuits that support their cognition and perception became more efficient.

Success is the reward of hard work.

Actor, comedian, singer, musician, songwriter, screenwriter, and film producer, **Adam Sandler**, found he was a natural comic while in high school. He nurtured this talent while at New York University by performing regularly in clubs and on campuses. Later in his career, he drew on these earliest experiences to become the star he is today.

I believe that one of life's greatest risks is never daring to risk. –Oprah Winfrey

toe touch squat

Stand with feet together, toes pointed straight ahead or slightly outward. Keeping your knees as straight as possible, bend at the waist and place hands on top of feet. Hold this position, then drop your buns down as far as possible, hold for 2-3 counts, then return to starting position. Repeat 10-15 times.

Steps Walked:	DATE
Cardio Workout:	
Strength Training:	
Calories Consumed:	
Calories Burned:	
Difference:	
Weight / Body fat:	

Eating healthy tastes great!

Zesty Bean Dip and Chips

1/4 cup fat free canned refried beans
1 tbs salsa
1 1/2 tsp fresh cilantro, chopped
1 scallion, minced

Combine all ingredients.
Serve with baked tortilla chips.

Read it, live it, love the results.

Find a good support partner.
You've heard it before, *"behind every great man is a great woman."* This is not far from the truth, as even the strongest individuals need a little help every now and then. Someone who will support you and renew your enthusiasm when you are ready to throw in the towel. With a good support partner you are more likely to maintain a healthy lifestyle.

Write it down & get it done.

1
2
3
4
5
6
7
8
9
10

fire hydrants
On floor, position yourself on hands and knees. With your right leg remaining bent at the 90-degree angle, slowly lift it out to the side, until it is parallel to the floor, hold here for 2-3 counts, then lower to starting position. Complete10-15 repetitions, then complete a set on the opposite side. To intensify, place a dumbbell behind your knee.

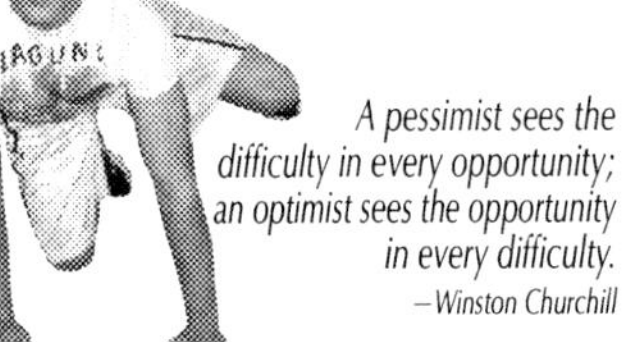

A pessimist sees the difficulty in every opportunity; an optimist sees the opportunity in every difficulty.
—Winston Churchill

DATE

Steps Walked:
Cardio Workout:
Strength Training:
Calories Consumed:
Calories Burned:
Difference:
Weight / Body fat:

Write it down & get it done.

1
2
3
4
5
6
7
8
9
10

Read it, live it, love the results.

Keep your mind in motion. According to research, performed at the Saint Louis University School of Medicine, if you challenge your brain to take on new tasks, it has the ability to rewire itself. This study indicated that people who spend most of their time participating in mentally stimulating activities such as reading, playing games, or doing puzzles, may be cutting their risk of dementia in half.

Life's tough, get over it, he did!

One of the most important leaders in world history, **Winston Churchhill**, served as Prime Minister of the United Kingdom. He was a noted statesman and orator, an officer in the British Army, a historian, a Nobel Prize-winning writer, and an artist. Unfortunately, his childhood was not so great. He spent much of it at boarding schools, sending letters begging his mother to either come to visit him, or let him come home, yet he rarely saw her or his father.

Slow down and enjoy life. It's not only the scenery you miss by going too fast—you also miss the sense of where you are going and why.
—Eddie Cantor

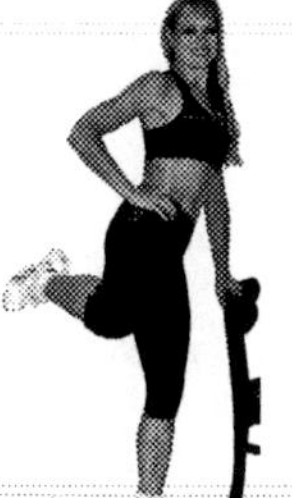

standing fire hydrants

Standing on your left foot, bend your right knee to a 90-degree angle. Slowly lift this bent leg out to the side, until it is parallel to the floor, hold here for 2-3 counts, then lower to starting position. Complete 10-15 repetitions, then complete a set on the opposite side. *To intensify, place a dumbbell behind your knee.*

	DATE
Steps Walked:	
Cardio Workout:	
Strength Training:	
Calories Consumed:	
Calories Burned:	
Difference:	
Weight / Body fat:	

Eating healthy tastes great!

Not "Just" Oatmeal
1 cup skim milk
$^{1}/_{2}$ cup oatmeal
1 tbs vanilla
$^{1}/_{4}$ tbs cinnamon
2 packets Splenda®

Mix all ingredients and microwave on high for two minutes, stirring twice during cooking.

Read it, live it, love the results.

Add cinnamon and honey to your diet.
In a recent study, arthritis patients were given a half teaspoon of cinnamon powder with one tablespoon of honey every morning before breakfast.
The result was a significant relief in arthritis pain after one week and they could walk without pain within one month.

Write it down & get it done.

1
2
3
4
5
6
7
8
9
10

lying hamstring curl

Lie on the floor, face down, legs extended out flat, with a dumbbell locked between your feet. Rest your head on your folded arms. Keeping the glutes tight, slowly bend your knees bringing the dumbbell up toward your glutes. Hold for 2-3 counts then return to starting position, stopping within inches of the floor. Repeat this curling motion 10-15 times.

The greatest glory in living lies not in never falling, but in rising every time we fall.
– Nelson Mandela

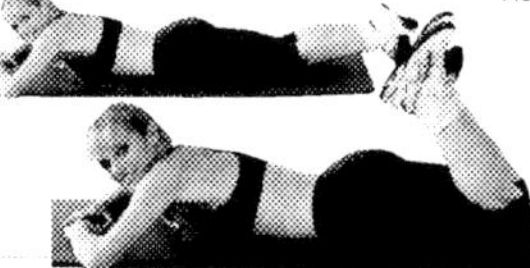

DATE

Steps Walked:
Cardio Workout:
Strength Training:
Calories Consumed:
Calories Burned:
Difference:
Weight / Body fat:

Write it down & get it done.

1
2
3
4
5
6
7
8
9
10

Read it, live it, love the results.

Learn from the past and others. No need to make your own mistakes when you can learn from the mistakes of others.
Read biographies and autobiographies, they are a great insight to the experiences of those who have come through hard times and succeeded. And yes, everyone goes through hard times!

Life's tough, get over it, he did!

Former President of South Africa **Nelson Mandela**, was one of the chief anti-apartheid activists, anti-apartheid saboteur and guerrilla leader. As a result, he spent 27 years in prison for crimes. Upon release his policy became one of reconciliation and negotiation as he helped lead the transition to multi-racial democracy in South Africa. He's now widely praised, and has received hundreds of awards, including the 1993 Nobel Peace Prize.

The thing always happens that you really believe in; and the belief in a thing makes it happen.
– Frank Lloyd Wright

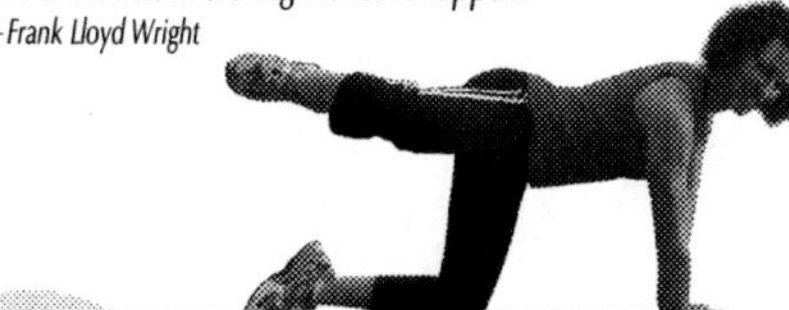

side leg curls

On the floor, position yourself on hands and knees. Extend your right leg straight out to the right side, 8-10 inches off the floor. Hold here as you curl the foot back toward your glutes, holding here for 2-3 counts, then extending out straight. Repeat 10-15 times, then complete a set with the left leg.

	DATE
Steps Walked:	
Cardio Workout:	
Strength Training:	
Calories Consumed:	
Calories Burned:	
Difference:	
Weight / Body fat:	

Eating healthy tastes great!

Greek Salmon
1 lb salmon fillets • 1 tbs olive oil
1 tbs lemon juice • 1 tsp oregano
1/2 tsp basil • 1/2 tsp pepper
1/2 cup sliced black olives
2 tomatoes and 1 red onion, sliced
1/2 cup light feta cheese, crumbed
2 tbs fresh parsley
Preheat oven to 400°F. Place Salmon in greased glass baking dish. Place all ingredients on fish. Cover with foil. Bake for 15 minutes. Remove foil, bake another 10 more minutes.

Read it, live it, love the results.

Keep your memory sharp by feeding your brain great foods such as salmon and beans.
Studies indicate that older individuals who have low levels of vitamins B12 and/or B9,have more trouble recalling certain words, then those who don't. Studies show that getting a total of 700 micrograms of foliate per day in food and supplements can help sharpen your memory.

Write it down & get it done.

1
2
3
4
5
6
7
8
9
10

step-ups

Stand facing a step with a dumbbell in each hand, arms hanging at sides. Step up first with the left foot, planting it flat on the step. Then keeping your shoulders back, chest out and abs in, step up with the right. Once the right foot is flat on the step, step back down with the left foot, then the right. Complete 10-15 step-ups leading with the left foot, then complete a set leading with the right foot.

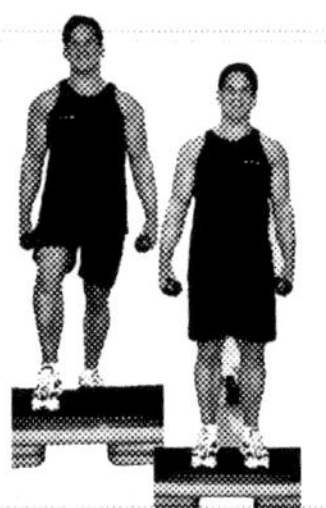

Open your eyes, look within. Are you satisfied with the life you're living?
— Bob Marley

DATE

Steps Walked:

Cardio Workout:

Strength Training:

Calories Consumed:

Calories Burned:

Difference:

Weight / Body fat:

Write it down & get it done.

1
2
3
4
5
6
7
8
9
10

Read it, live it, love the results.

Stay calm.
Although lung function naturally declines with age, recent research suggests it may decline faster in those with bad tempers. The next time you are upset, close your eyes, relax your muscles, and imagine yourself far away from that which is making you angry, breath deeply and place yourself in a positive state of mind. Good emotional health and well-being also helps you look and feel many years younger.

Life's tough, get over it, he did!

Singer, guitarist and songwriter **Bob Marley**, was from the ghettos of Jamaica. He was born to a black mother and a white father. Due to the white upper classes' disdain for the mixed affair Marley never got the opportunity to know his father. Perhaps this is why much of his work delt with the struggles of the impoverished and/or powerless. He used his experiences to become the best-selling reggae artist ever.

Four steps to achievement:
Plan purposefully.
Prepare prayerfully.
Proceed positively.
Pursue persistently.
—William A. Ward

dumbbell squat sprints

Stand with feet shoulder-width apart, toes pointed straight ahead or slightly outward. Holding a dumbbell in each hand, focus your vision straight ahead. Keeping your heels planted firmly on the floor, inhale and move your buns back and downward, as if you are sitting in a chair. Keep knees behind toes. When the thighs are parallel with the floor, rise up 2-3 inches then go back down immediately, repeat this short up and down motion quickly 10-15 times before returning to the upright starting position.

	DATE
Steps Walked:	
Cardio Workout:	
Strength Training:	
Calories Consumed:	
Calories Burned:	
Difference:	
Weight / Body fat:	

Eating healthy tastes great!

Pina Colada Salad

3/4 cup crushed pineapple, drained
2 tbs lemon juice
1/3 cup granulated sugar
1 cup light cream cheese
2 cups chilled cooked brown rice
1/2 cup coconut, shredded
Combine pineapple, lemon juice, sugar and salt. Fold mixture into whipped cream. Fold in chilled rice, then shredded coconut. Chill, then serve over fresh pineapple.

Read it, live it, love the results.

Develop a plan and organize.

Setting out to reach your final desination without a specific plan is like taking a roadtrip without a map. You will unevitably end up somewhere other than where you want to be. Without a plan the probability of failure is greatly increased— don't set yourself up for failure. Know where you want to be, and the steps you will take to get there.

Write it down & get it done.

1
2
3
4
5
6
7
8
9
10

squat and hop

Stand with feet slightly wider than shoulder-width apart, toes pointing straight ahead. Holding a dumbbell in each hand, position hands in front of your chest. Keeping your heels planted firmly on the floor, squat down slightly, then hop as far to the right as possible, then without pause hop back to the left. Repeat this hop 10 to 15 times, while keeping your body in a squatting position with the glutes tightened.

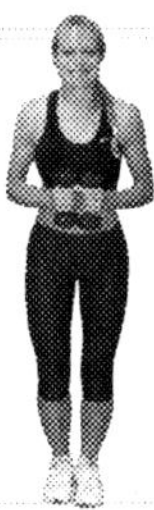

Begin with the end in mind.
–Steven Covey

DATE

Steps Walked:
Cardio Workout:
Strength Training:
Calories Consumed:
Calories Burned:
Difference:
Weight / Body fat:

Write it down & get it done.

1
2
3
4
5
6
7
8
9
10

Read it, live it, love the results.

Exercise daily to slow aging.
As your body ages it produces fewer potent white blood cells, making you more vulnerable to viruses, bacteria, carcinogens, and other disease-causing organisms. Vaccinations, such as flu shots, seem to become less effective and wounds take longer to heal. Regular exercise can greatly slow this decline of white blood cells and prevent the age-related decline in your immune system's antibody response.

Be the change you want to see.

Grammy Award-winner musician, **Ozzy Osbourne**, actually began his career as a burgler, though not a good one. He wore gloves during the burgleries, however they were fingerless and he left fingerprints. He was soon arrested and sentenced to six weeks at Winson Green Prison, here he used his time to think about different career choices. As a musician he has sold millions of albums and was inducted into the US Rock and Roll Hall of Fame.

The difference between a successful person and others is not alack of strength, not a lack of knowledge, but rather in a lack of will.
– Vincent T. Lombardi

plié squat

Stand with feet wider than shoulder-width apart, toes pointing out at a comfortable angle, shoulders back, chest out, abs and back tight and straight. Hold dumbbells in front of your chest. Bending your knees, slowly lower your body until your thighs are parallel with the floor, hold for 2-3 counts then keeping your knees in line with your toes, push your weight into your heels as you return to starting position. Repeat 10-15 times.

	DATE
Steps Walked:	
Cardio Workout:	
Strength Training:	
Calories Consumed:	
Calories Burned:	
Difference:	
Weight / Body fat:	

Eating healthy tastes great!

Grilled Lime Chicken

2 chicken breasts
1/2 cup lime juice
1/4 cup cilantro, chopped
1 tsp olive oil
pepper to taste

Mix lime juice, cilantro, salt and black pepper. Rub chicken with oil then coat with lime mixture. Refrigerate 2 hours. Grill chicken 10-15 minutes per side or until juices run clear.

Read it, live it, love the results.

Get motivated.

Motivation, is the most important part of your workout. You can't buy it, borrow it, rent it, lease it—nor can you do without it. To keep yourself motivated you must focus on the positives and discard the negatives. Get rid of thoughts of procrastination and set realistic goals you can and will achieve.

Write it down & get it done.

1
2
3
4
5
6
7
8
9
10

lunges with dumbbells

Stand with feet shoulder-width apart, arms at sides with palms facing in, holding dumbbells. Keeping shoulders back and abs in, step forward about two feet with your right foot. As you plant your right foot bend the right knee to about 90-degrees. Your left knee will bend automatically and should come within an inch of the floor. Hold for 2-5 counts, then push off with your right foot to return to starting position. Complete 10-15 repetitions, then perform the exercise, leading with the left foot.

I want to get old gracefully. I want to have good posture, I want to be healthy and be an example to my children.
– Sting

DATE

Steps Walked:
Cardio Workout:
Strength Training:
Calories Consumed:
Calories Burned:
Difference:
Weight / Body fat:

Write it down & get it done.

1
2
3
4
5
6
7
8
9
10

Read it, live it, love the results.

Look and feel better when you avoid sugar.

Sugar is not your friend, it causes skin to wrinkle, impairs immune function, and causes hormone imbalances, particularly insulin and cortisol. When your insulin levels go up, your body's metabolism slows, inflammation increases and chronic pain conditions worsen. In raising the cortisol levels, memory loss is accelerated, stress is harder to adapt to, and clinical depression may be induced.

Life's tough, get over it, he did!

Musician and former member of *The Police*, **Sting**, worked as a ditch digger and an English teacher before he became famous. His first music gigs were with local jazz bands, playing wherever they could. Despite rough times, he knew what he wanted and he never gave up on reaching his goals. With *The Police* he sold more than fifty million albums worldwide. The *Rolling Stone* ranked them 70, on their list of the *100 Greatest Artists of All Time*.

Most of the important things in the world have been accomplished by people who have kept on trying when there seemed to be no hope at all.
—Dale Carnegie

lunge with lateral raise

Stand with feet shoulder-width apart, arms hanging straight down with a dumbbell in each hand, palms facing the body. Step forward with the right leg, bending the knee to a 90-degree angle. As you step, lift the dumbbells straight out to the sides. Hold this position for 2-3 counts, then pushing with the right leg, return to starting position. Complete 10-15 repetitions, then perform this exercise on the opposite side.

DATE

Steps Walked:
Cardio Workout:
Strength Training:
Calories Consumed:
Calories Burned:
Difference:
Weight / Body fat:

Eating healthy tastes great!

Cedar-Barbecued Salmon

boneless salmon fillets • cedar plank
olive oil • soy sauce
barbecue spice • lemon slices

Soak cedar plank in water for 15 minutes and place on preheated grill. Coat salmon with olive oil and soy sauce then place on plank. Sprinkle with barbecue spice and top with thin slices of lemon. Barbecue for about 15 or 20 minutes, until the fish flakes easily with a fork.

Read it, live it, love the results.

You must be persistent.

Persistence is the quality you need to get you through the tough times—and there will be tough times. Presistence has often been the difference between the individual who succeeds and another who fails. Combine your desire with willpower and you will become a truly persistant individual who will succeed. You are priceless, don't ever give up on yourself.

Write it down & get it done.

1
2
3
4
5
6
7
8
9
10

step with a twist
Holding a dumbbell in each hand, stand with your back to a step. Place the left foot on the step, then keeping your torso straight, bend the right knee 90-degrees, keeping knee aligned with ankle. Turn the upper body to the right , bringing the dumbbells over the right thigh, hold for 2-3 counts, then return to starting position.

I have been impressed with the urgency of doing. Knowing is not enough; we must apply. Being willing is not enough; we must do.
– Leonardo da Vinci

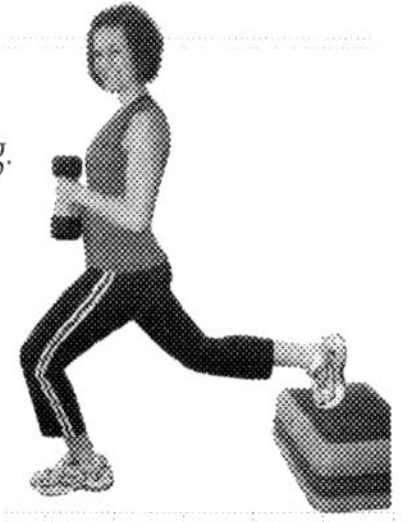

DATE

Steps Walked:
Cardio Workout:
Strength Training:
Calories Consumed:
Calories Burned:
Difference:
Weight / Body fat:

Write it down & get it done.

1
2
3
4
5
6
7
8
9
10

Read it, live it, love the results.

Let go of past failures.
It doesn't matter how many times you fail at something, what's important is that you never give up trying!
Past failures should stay in the past. Learn from your failures, but don't use them as an excuse for not being successful today. You can do anything you put your mind to—the only way to fail is to give up.

Your level of success is up to you.

One of the true innovators in the retail industry, **Maxine Clark**, founded her first Build-A-Bear Workshop® in 1997 at the St. Louis Gallaria—she now has 400 stores worldwide! Clark attributes this great success to her 35 years of experience in the areas of marketing, merchandising, store operations, digital technology, entertainment, strategic planning, and real estate along with her service on the Board of Directors of The JCPenney Company.

You have no control over what the other guy does. You only have control over what you do. – A. J. Kitt

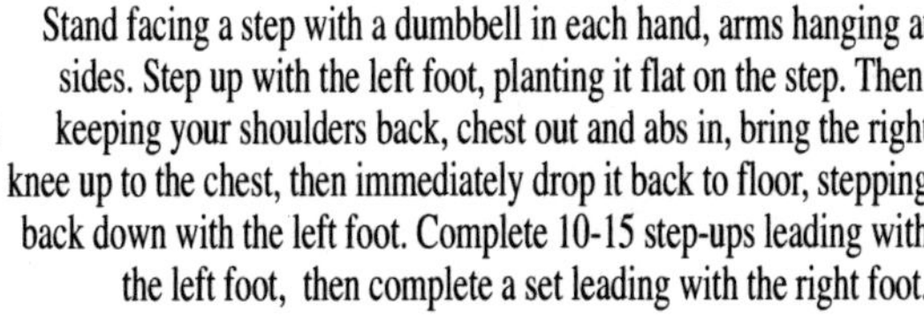

step-up with knee lift

Stand facing a step with a dumbbell in each hand, arms hanging at sides. Step up with the left foot, planting it flat on the step. Then, keeping your shoulders back, chest out and abs in, bring the right knee up to the chest, then immediately drop it back to floor, stepping back down with the left foot. Complete 10-15 step-ups leading with the left foot, then complete a set leading with the right foot.

DATE

Steps Walked:
Cardio Workout:
Strength Training:
Calories Consumed:
Calories Burned:
Difference:
Weight / Body fat:

Eating healthy tastes great!

Chicken and Green Bean Soup

1 chicken breast, cooked
1 can low sodium chicken broth
1 can green beans, drained
1 onion, diced
1 tsp light butter
hot sauce and pepper to taste

Combine all ingredients and cook until onions are tender.

Read it, live it, love the results.

Don't be guilty of *"folding when the going gets tough."*

It's the lack of persistence, more than any other quality, that keeps the majority of people from accomplishing great things. Don't let yourself fall into this category, you are capable of great things. Develop the habit of being persistent and never giving up. With this habit you are sure to succeed in whatever it is you desire to accomplish.

Write it down & get it done.

1
2
3
4
5
6
7
8
9
10

single leg squat off step

Stand on step with feet shoulder-width apart, hands at chest with a dumbbell in each hand, palms facing. Step forward off the step with the right leg, bending the left knee as you step down. Keeping the right leg extended, lower your body until the right thigh is parallel to the floor. Repeat this single leg squat 10-15 times, then complete a set with the left leg extended. When performing this exercise keep the knee behind your toes.

In wisdom gathered over time I have found that every experience is a form of exploration.
–Ansel Adams

DATE

Steps Walked:
Cardio Workout:
Strength Training:
Calories Consumed:
Calories Burned:
Difference:
Weight / Body fat:

Write it down & get it done.

1
2
3
4
5
6
7
8
9
10

Read it, live it, love the results.

Get blood tests and have your blood pressure checked yearly. Studies show that heart disease is the number one killer of American women. One in three will die of heart disease each year. When you know your risk for developing heart disease, you may be able to ward off disaster. Checking your blood pressure and having blood tests done at least once a year, could result in saving your life.

Doors open, when you work hard.

One of the most recognizable photographers in the world, **Ansel Adams**, worked as a commercial photographer to pay his bills. And though he had written many technical works and encouraged museums and colleges to add photography departments, he did not actually achieve financial success for his art until late in his life. Today his photographs are often reproduced on calendars, posters, and in books.

Gifts make slaves.
– Levi Strauss

press and lunge

Stand with feet shoulder-width apart, arms at sides with palms facing body, holding dumbbells. Lift dumbbells out to side and overhead. Then lift the right leg straight out until it' s parallel to the floor. Hold for 2-3 counts, then drop the foot into a front lunge, hold for 2-3 counts, then return to starting position and repeat . Complete 10-15 repetitions, then perfom exercise lunging with the left leg. This also works the shoulders.

	DATE
Steps Walked:	
Cardio Workout:	
Strength Training:	
Calories Consumed:	
Calories Burned:	
Difference:	
Weight / Body fat:	

Eating healthy tastes great!

Waldorf Salad
3 apples, peeled and diced
1 cup concord seedless grapes
1 1/2 cups miniature marshmallows
1 cup celery, diced
1 cup nuts, chopped
1 1/2 cups Fat Free Miracle Whip®
Splenda® to taste
Mix first five ingredients together. Stir in Miracle Whip®, Splenda® and salt. Refrigerate to chill.

Read it, live it, love the results.

Be persistent for success.
As Earl Nightengale stated;
"It will seem as though there's no longer any reason to continue. Everything in you will tell you to give up, to quit trying. It is right here that if you'll go that extra mile and keep going, the skies will clear and you'll begin to see the first signs of the abundance that is to be yours because you had the courage to persist."

Write it down & get it done.

1
2
3
4
5
6
7
8
9
10

side toe tap

Stand sideways on a step with feet together, arms hanging straight down with a dumbbell in each hand, palms facing the body. Step off the step with the right leg, bending the left knee as you step down. Tap the right toe on the floor, then quickly return the foot to the step, tapping the step, then returning again to the floor. Repeat this right toe tap 20-30 times, then complete a set with the left toe tapping.

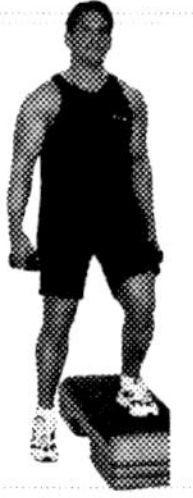

Out of clutter, find simplicity. From discord, find harmony. In the middle of difficulty lies opportunity.
Albert Einstein's three rules of work.

DATE

Steps Walked:
Cardio Workout:
Strength Training:
Calories Consumed:
Calories Burned:
Difference:
Weight / Body fat:

Write it down & get it done.

1
2
3
4
5
6
7
8
9
10

Read it, live it, love the results.

Eat plenty of beans.
Studies show that beans provide fiber, which in turn reduces your level of LDL cholesterol, the *"bad cholesterol."* Additionally, if you eat beans as a substitute for meat, you will reduce the amount of saturated fat in your diet, which also decreases LDL cholesterol and prevents hardening of arteries. The best bean choices are black beans, pinto beans, lentils, and soy products such as tofu or soyburgers.

Doors open, when you work hard.

When genius, **Albert Einstein**, was a child, some thought he was *"retarded."* Einstein claimed that he didn't begin speaking until the age of three and only then hesitantly, even beyond the age of nine. It was due to this late speech development and his tendency to ignore any subject in school which bored him, that brought about this belief. Today he is best known for his theory of relativity. He also received the 1921 Nobel Prize in Physics.

You can make more friends in two months by becoming interested in other people than you can in two years by trying to get other people interested in you.
– Dale Carnegie

reverse toe tap

Stand on a step with feet together, arms hanging straight down with a dumbbell in each hand, palms facing your body.Step off the back of the step with the right leg, bending the left knee as you step down. Tap the right toe on the floor, then quickly return the foot to the step, tapping the step. Repeat this quick right toe tap 20-30 times, then complete a set with the left toe tapping.

DATE

Steps Walked:

Cardio Workout:

Strength Training:

Calories Consumed:

Calories Burned:

Difference:

Weight / Body fat:

Eating healthy tastes great!

Cinnamon Ricotta Crème
1 cup light ricotta cheese
1 tsp vanilla extract
1 tsp cinnamon
2 packets Splenda®

Combine all ingredients in blender. Blend until smooth. Refrigerate to chill.

Read it, live it, love the results.

Discuss your idea with others.
Many great ideas have been born as a result of having talked with others. Always be open to talking and listening to those who have knowledge that will help you reach your goals. There are many great ideas that would have never been "born" without group discussion. Promotion and advertising agencies use this brainstorming tactic on a regular basis.

Write it down & get it done.

1
2
3
4
5
6
7
8
9
10

plié sprint

Stand with feet wider than shoulder-width apart, toes pointing out at a comfortable angle, shoulders back, chest out, abs in and back straight. Hold a dumbbell with both hands, allowing it to hang straight down. Bending your knees, slowly lower your body until the thighs are parallel with the floor, hold here, then rise up 2-3 inches and go back down immediately. Repeat this short up and down

As we advance in life it becomes more and more difficult, but in fightingthe difficulties the in most strength of the heart is developed.

DATE

Steps Walked:
Cardio Workout:
Strength Training:
Calories Consumed:
Calories Burned:
Difference:
Weight / Body fat:

Write it down & get it done.

1
2
3
4
5
6
7
8
9
10

Read it, live it, love the results.

SLEEP!!

Lack of sleep can cause many problems. It can affect your mood, productivity, immune function, and cognitive ability. It's also connected to many health issues including; tooth decay, wrinkles, muscle pain, slower recovery time, depression and mental disorders. Increase your sleeping time and you may improve the quality of your life.

Be the change you want to see.

One of the world's best known, most popular and most expensive artists,**Vincent William van Gogh**, sold only one painting during his entire life. Still this did not stop him from continuing to paint, he had a dream and he never gave up. As a result, he produced more than 2,000 works, which included aproximately 900 paintings and 1,100 drawings and sketches, during the last ten years of his life. Most of his best-known works were produced in the final two years of his life.

You must have long term goals to keep you from being frustrated by short term failures.
– Charles C. Noble

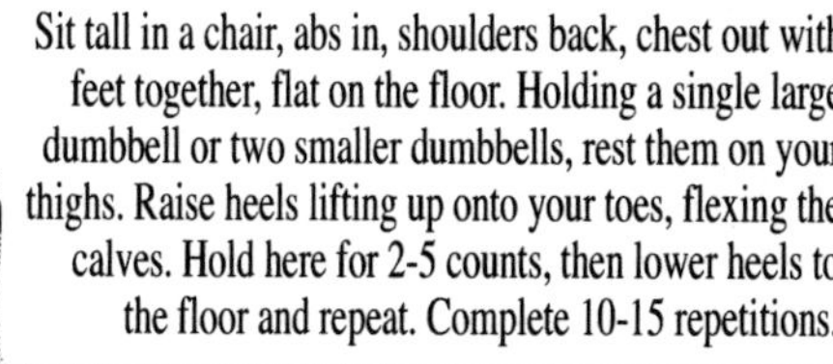

seated calf raise

Sit tall in a chair, abs in, shoulders back, chest out with feet together, flat on the floor. Holding a single large dumbbell or two smaller dumbbells, rest them on your thighs. Raise heels lifting up onto your toes, flexing the calves. Hold here for 2-5 counts, then lower heels to the floor and repeat. Complete 10-15 repetitions.

	DATE
Steps Walked:	
Cardio Workout:	
Strength Training:	
Calories Consumed:	
Calories Burned:	
Difference:	
Weight / Body fat:	

Eating healthy tastes great!

Tuna Celery Crunch
14 oz light tuna, drained
3 tbs light butter • 3 cups celery, diced
3 tbs wheat flour • pepper to taste
2 cups skim milk • 1 cup light cheese
In saucepan, melt butter, add celery and sauté until bright green but still crisp. Add flour and salt then gradually stir in the milk. Cook over medium heat, stirring, until the sauce comes to a boil and thickens.
Add the cheese and tuna, stirring until heated through.

Read it, live it, love the results.

Talk and listen to those who have knowledge that will help you reach your goals.
This doesn't mean you should let others do your thinking for you, far from it. It's a tactic meant to stimulate your own thinking through the association with other minds. No one knows everything. Learn from the experience and knowledge of others, and you'll reach your ultimate goal faster than ever.

Write it down & get it done.

1
2
3
4
5
6
7
8
9
10

wall squats
Stand two to three feet from a wall with your feet shoulder-width apart. Sit back into a squatting position, with the thighs parallel to the floor, pressing your back against the wall, with hands resting on your thighs. Make sure your knees are behind your toes. Hold this position for 30 to 60 counts.
Repeat 2-5 times.

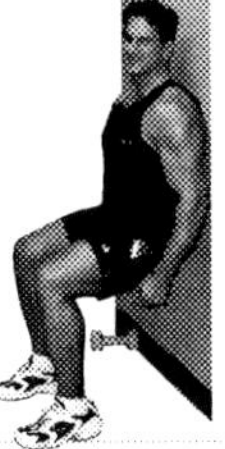

The only failure is not to try.
– George Clooney

DATE

Steps Walked:
Cardio Workout:
Strength Training:
Calories Consumed:
Calories Burned:
Difference:
Weight / Body fat:

Write it down & get it done.

1
2
3
4
5
6
7
8
9
10

Read it, live it, love the results. Your level of success is up to you.

Dream BIG!
This is your life, no one can make your dreams come true except for you. You are limited only by the extent of your thoughts and dreams. When you dream big you can accomplish great things. Become excited about your future and all of which it holds for you. When you do this you will ultimately do everything in your power to make this dream a reality.

Academy Award and Golden Globe award winning actor, director, producer, and screenwriter, **George Clooney**, spent his first ten years of acting as an unknown. Yet he never gave up. It was his role on *"E.R."* that turned things around for him, making him TV's hottest heartthrob. He left *"E.R."* five years later and led an even more successful career in films as an actor.

The truth of the matter is that you always know the right thing to do. The hard part is doing it.
—General H. Norman Schwarzkopf

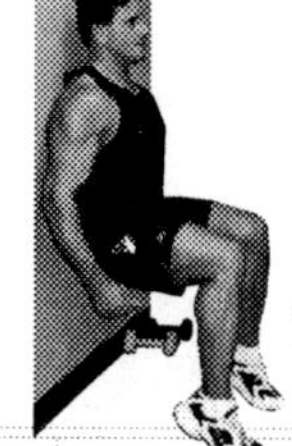

wall squat calf raise

Stand two to three feet from a wall with your feet shoulder-width apart. Sitting back into a squatting position, with the thighs parallel to the floor, press your back against the wall. Make sure your knees are behind your toes. Holding this position, raise up on your toes and hold for 2-3 counts, completing 15-25 repetitions.

DATE

Steps Walked:

Cardio Workout:

Strength Training:

Calories Consumed:

Calories Burned:

Difference:

Weight / Body fat:

Eating healthy tastes great!

BIG Breakfast Cookie

1/3 cup oatmeal • 1 tbs wheat flour
1/3 cup fat free dry milk
1/4 cup unsweetened applesauce
1/4 tsp cinnamon
1/4 tsp baking powder
1 packet Splenda®

Preheat oven to 350°F. Mix all ingredients and place in pam coated cookie sheet. Bake for 15-20 minutes, until golden brown on edges.

Read it, live it, love the results.

Know who you want to become, what you stand for and what you consider to be important.
Choose two people you admire, then list what it is you like about them. Creating this list of qualities targets the qualities you would most like to see in yourself. When you know what you want to become it is much easier to become that person. Remember, it is never to late to become the person you thought you could be.

Write it down & get it done.

1
2
3
4
5
6
7
8
9
10

big circles

Lie on your side with your bottom leg slightly bent to support your body. Keeping the upper leg straight, lift it in a controlled movement, "drawing" a big circle with your foot. Complete 10-15 circles clockwise, then complete a set counter clockwise. To intensify, wear an ankle weight.

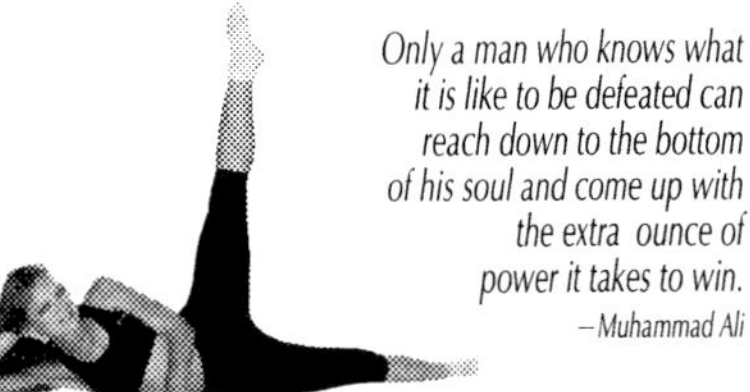

Only a man who knows what it is like to be defeated can reach down to the bottom of his soul and come up with the extra ounce of power it takes to win.
– Muhammad Ali

DATE

Steps Walked:

Cardio Workout:

Strength Training:

Calories Consumed:

Calories Burned:

Difference:

Weight / Body fat:

Write it down & get it done.

1
2
3
4
5
6
7
8
9
10

Read it, live it, love the results.

Don't put off until tomorrow what you can do today.

If you had began working out and eating healthy this time last year, losing just a pound a week, you could now be up to fifty-two pounds lighter AND much healthier. Imagine where you will be next year when you get started NOW!

Be the change you want to see.

Football superstar **Brett Favre's** father passed away one day before the Monday Night game against the Raiders. Favre passed for four touchdowns in the first half and 399 total yards in a 41–7 victory on international television. Afterwards, he said, *"I knew that my dad would have wanted me to play. I love him so much and I love this game. It's meant a great deal to me, to my dad, to my family, and I didn't expect this kind of performance. But I know he was watching tonight."*

What the mind can conceive and believe, it can achieve.
—Napoleon Hill

hip adduction

Lie on the floor, on your right side, balancing your body with your elbow and bottom leg slightly bent for support. Keeping the left leg straight, lift it as high as you can, then hold in this position. Next, raise the right foot to touch the left foot. Hold for 2-3 counts, then lower to starting position, keeping the left leg up in the same positon. Repeat 10-15 times, then complete a set on the opposite side.

	DATE
Steps Walked:	
Cardio Workout:	
Strength Training:	
Calories Consumed:	
Calories Burned:	
Difference:	
Weight / Body fat:	

Eating healthy tastes great!

Salmon Patties

12 oz canned salmon • 2 eggs
1 cup whole wheat bread crumbs
½ cup corn • ¼ cup red onion, diced
2 tbs cornmeal • 2 tsp olive oil
pepper to taste

Mix salmon, eggs, ½ cup bread crumbs, corn, onion, cornmeal, salt and pepper. Form patties, then coat with remaining bread crumbs.
In skillet, cook a few minutes on each side, until browned.

Read it, live it, love the results.

See yourself already having accomplished your goals.

The subconscious mind is best developed when you know what you want, define it clearly, and then stamp it into your mind.
Do this often and your subconscious will lead you towards your goals.
Make it a regular habit to see yourself as having accomplished your goals, and you will be amazed at how easy your life will become.

Write it down & get it done.

1
2
3
4
5
6
7
8
9
10

Nearly everyone desires great looking buns—though your glutes do have a purpose other than filling out a pair of jeans. As many, with desk jobs, soon discover, sitting for long periods of time, not using the glutes and putting constant pressure on them, can cause atrophy. Studies show this may also be associated with lower back pain and difficulty with movements which require the glute muscles—such as standing from a seated position and climbing stairs. Athletes rely upon strong glutes to help them run faster, jump higher and last longer than the competition. Whatever your reason may be, the exercises in this section will help you develop great glutes.

DATE

Steps Walked:
Cardio Workout:
Strength Training:
Calories Consumed:
Calories Burned:
Difference:
Weight / Body fat:

Write it down & get it done.

1
2
3
4
5
6
7
8
9
10

Read it, live it, love the results.

Know what you desire and picture yourself as having achieved it.
If you have the desire to lose twenty pounds—envision yourself twenty pounds thinner. You must establish this vision firmly in your mind. There are times when you will become overwhelmed and side tracked—that is why you must read your desire statement on a daily basis. The key is to never give up.

Doors open, when you work hard.

Musician **Marc Anthony** has been dubbed the *"Reigning King of Salsa"* by the *New York Times.* Ironically, his career began as a writer for other club performers. Then, in 1991 he released his own Latin album— the Latin listeners loved him. In 1999 he made his English-language debut and went platinum in just six weeks. He also won a 1999 Gammy for *Best Tropical Latin Performance.*

Knowledge of what is possible is the beginning of happiness.
–George Santayana

butt blaster

On the floor support yourself on elbows and knees with a dumbbell tucked tightly behind your right knee or an ankle weight on the ankle. Keeping your knee bent at 90-degrees, raise your leg until the thigh is parallel to the floor. *DO NOT lift too high as it may cause back injury.* Tighten your glutes, squeezing for 2-3 counts before returning to the start position. Repeat 10-15 times, then complete a set with the left leg.

	DATE
Steps Walked:	
Cardio Workout:	
Strength Training:	
Calories Consumed:	
Calories Burned:	
Difference:	
Weight / Body fat:	

Eating healthy tastes great!

Parmesan Spinach Cakes

12 oz fresh spinach
$^1/_2$ cup low fat cottage cheese
$^1/_2$ cup Parmesan cheese
2 large eggs • 2 tbs minced garlic
pepper to taste
Preheat oven to 400 F. Finely chop spinach in food processor, combine with other ingredients. Place mixture in greased 8 cup muffin pan. Bake 18-20 minutes. Let stand for 5 minutes, remove from pan and sprinkle with more Parmesan.

Read it, live it, love the results.

Follow in the footsteps of Popeye.
Popeye was on track with his can of spinach. Studies show that spinach is perhaps one of the healthiest foods you can eat. It's a powerhouse loaded with vitamins, antioxidants and essential nutrients. Eating just $^1/_2$ cup of cooked spinach can give you 100% of your daily requirement for vitamins A and K.

Write it down & get it done.

1
2
3
4
5
6
7
8
9
10

butt blaster crossover

On the floor, position yourself on elbows and knees with a dumbbell tucked tightly behind your right knee or an ankle weight on the ankle. Keeping the knee bent at a 90-degree angle, raise leg up until your thigh is parallel to the floor. DO NOT lift too high as it may cause back injury. Drop the leg down, crossing over the left leg, then return to the up position, hold for 2-3 counts. Repeat10-15 times, then complete a set with the left leg.

This is one small step for a man, one giant leap for mankind.
— Neil Armstrong

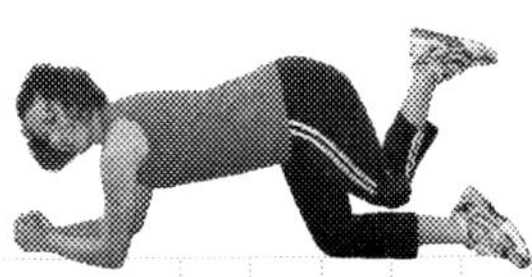

DATE

Steps Walked:
Cardio Workout:
Strength Training:
Calories Consumed:
Calories Burned:
Difference:
Weight / Body fat:

Write it down & get it done.

1
2
3
4
5
6
7
8
9
10

Read it, live it, love the results.

Prepare your own meals.
In today's busy society many opt for the so-called *"healthy"* or *"lean"* microwavable meals. Although they may be low in carbs and calories, these quick fixes are often high in sodium, and contain many preservatives, unhealthy oils and fats. Instead, prepare large meals and freeze portions which you can later thaw and microwave when you need a *"quick fix"*.

Success is the reward of hard work.

Former American Astronaut **Neil Armstrong**, the first human being to set foot on the moon, worked hard to receive this honor. As a Navy fighter pilot he flew 78 combat missions over Korea then joined NASA as a civilian test pilot. He was accepted into the astronaut corps in 1962, became the pilot of the Gemini 8 mission, launched 16 March 1966, and was then named commander for the Apollo 11 mission of 1969, which allowed him to walk on the moon.

butt blaster combo

On the floor, support yourself on elbows and knees with a dumbbell tucked tightly behind your right knee or an ankle weight on the ankle. Keeping your knee bent at a 90-degree angle, raise leg up until thigh is parallel to floor. DO NOT lift too high as it may cause back injury. Drop your leg straight down, bring back up to parallel position then drop again crossing over the left leg as you lower. Return to starting position hold for 2-3 counts, then repeat the combination move. Perform 10-15 repetitions, then complete a set with the left leg.

	DATE
Steps Walked:	
Cardio Workout:	
Strength Training:	
Calories Consumed:	
Calories Burned:	
Difference:	
Weight / Body fat:	

There is one quality that one must possess to win, and that is definiteness of purpose, the knowledge of what one wants, and a burning desire to possess it. –Napoleon Hill

Eating healthy tastes great!

Chocolate Mint Protein Shake
1 tsp mint extract
16 oz cup of ice
1/2 cup low fat vanilla yogurt
2 scoops chocolate protein

Place all ingredients in blender and blend until smooth.
I recommend that women use soy protein and men use whey protein. Be sure to read the lables when purchasing protien, all are not created equal.

Read it, live it, love the results.

Make it a passion.
Although you know working out and eating healthy is the right thing to do, you won't stick with it unless you make it your passion. You must have the desire to care for yourself as you would an expensive car or home. Often we take better care of material items then we do ourselves, these are replaceable, you are not.

Write it down & get it done.

1
2
3
4
5
6
7
8
9
10

standing butt blaster

With a dumbbell placed snuggly behind your knee, brace yourself using a chair or the wall. Curl the leg back toward your buttocks as close as possible. Get a peak contraction at the top, then lower the dumbbell to the starting position. Complete 10-15 repetitions, then complete a set with the other leg.

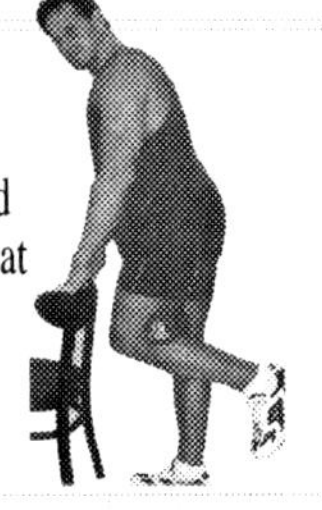

People who are unable to motivate themselves must be content with mediocrity, no matter how impressive their other talents.
– Andrew Carnegie

DATE

Steps Walked:
Cardio Workout:
Strength Training:
Calories Consumed:
Calories Burned:
Difference:
Weight / Body fat:

Write it down & get it done.

1
2
3
4
5
6
7
8
9
10

Read it, live it, love the results.

Repeat only those habits which are good.
There are habits which destroy our lives and habits which improve our lives. Determine the habits in your life that need to be changed or improved upon, then begin today in making those changes. Creating a healthy lifestyle requires repeating those habits which are good and getting rid of those which are not.

Doors open, when you work hard.

One of the 20th century's most famous philanthropists, **Andrew Carnegie**, has an incredible rags-to-riches story. He was born in Scotland, then as a teenager, moved to Pennsylvania with his family, where he began working in factories. His hard work and wise investments led to early success in the railroad business. He then founded the *Carnegie Steel Company* where he made his fortune.

straight leg lift

On the floor, support yourself on elbows and knees with your right leg extended straight out behind you. Slowly lift the right leg high enough to feel the hamstrings working, yet not so high that you arch your back, as this may cause injury. Hold for 2-3 counts then lower to within inches of the floor. Complete 10-15 repetitions on each leg.

All great achievements require time.
–David Joseph Schwartz

DATE

Steps Walked:
Cardio Workout:
Strength Training:
Calories Consumed:
Calories Burned:
Difference:
Weight / Body fat:

Eating healthy tastes great!

Crockpot Salsa Chicken
4 chicken breasts
1 cup salsa
4 tbs yellow mustard
red pepper and hot sauce to taste

Mix salsa and mustard and layer between chicken breasts placed in crock pot. Cook on low until done. Wrap in whole wheat tortilla, with lettuce and tomatoes.

Read it, live it, love the results.

Control your thoughts.
You have control over the thoughts which reach your subconscious mind. It is the consciously thinking mind which controls those thoughts that are fed into the subconscious.
If it is fried foods you crave, tell yourself repeatedly that fried foods make you ill, that you can taste more of the grease than the food. You will be surprised at how your tastes will change.

Write it down & get it done.

1
2
3
4
5
6
7
8
9
10

side kick

Stand with feet shoulder-width apart, back straight, shoulders back and chest out with hands clinched in fists, positioned in front of your chest. Keeping the left knee slightly bent, kick the right leg straight out to the side as high as possible, then lower to starting position, keeping the movement controlled. Repeat 25-50 kicks then repeat with left leg.

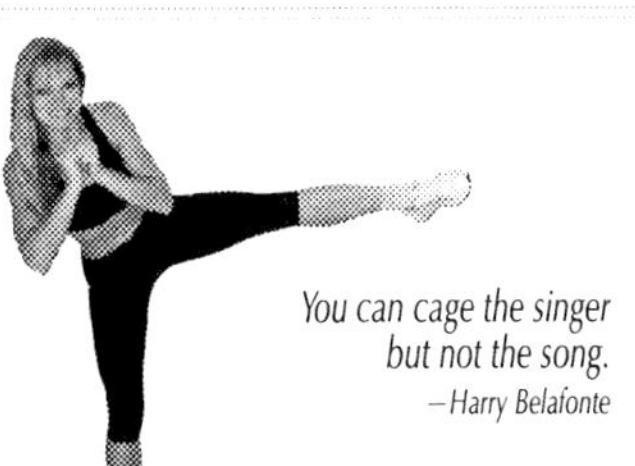

You can cage the singer but not the song.
– Harry Belafonte

DATE

Steps Walked:
Cardio Workout:
Strength Training:
Calories Consumed:
Calories Burned:
Difference:
Weight / Body fat:

Write it down & get it done.

1
2
3
4
5
6
7
8
9
10

Read it, live it, love the results.

Keep your body fat at twenty-four percent or less.
Fat cells produce hormones which raise your risk of type 2 diabetes. They also make substances called cytokines, causing inflammation and stiffening the arteries. In addition, carrying excess fat also raises your risk of cancer. Studies show that those under the age of seventy-five can cut their chances of premature death in half, by keeping their body fat in a healthy range.

Doors open, when you work hard.

Musician, actor and social activist, **Harry Belafonte**, one of the first African-American producers in television, grew up in both Jamaica and Harlem in New York City. It was in New York that he started his career in music as a club singer, to pay for his acting classes. Upon earning a recording contract he brought Jamaica's calypso beat to mainstream audiences he also starred in several films. Once famous he used his fame to fight against racial and social inequality.

Fill your world with excellence in each thought and in each endeavor for universal benefit.
– Vashi Chandiramani

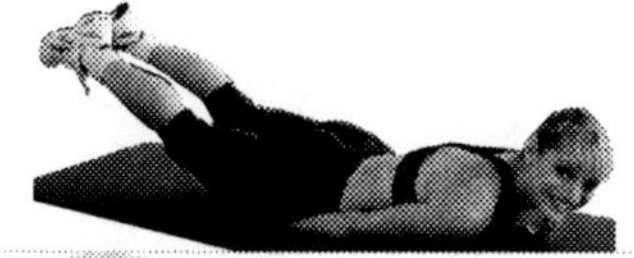

prone glute squeeze
Lie on the floor, face down with hands under your thighs. Raise your legs off the floor as high as you can, keeping your feet pressed together with your heels pointing towards the ceiling. Hold this position for 7-10 counts then slowly lower and repeat 10-15 times.

	DATE
Steps Walked:	
Cardio Workout:	
Strength Training:	
Calories Consumed:	
Calories Burned:	
Difference:	
Weight / Body fat:	

Eating healthy tastes great!

Black Bean Salad
1/2 cup onion, minced
3 tbs minced garlic
15 oz can black beans, drained
1 cup frozen corn, thawed
8 cherry tomatoes, quartered
1/2 cup red bell pepper, diced
2 tbs pumpkin seeds, chopped
1/4 cup fresh cilantro, chopped
2 tbs olive oil • pepper to taste
3 tbs fresh lemon juice
Combine ingredients then chill.

Read it, live it, love the results.

You are in charge of your thoughts.
If negative thoughts fill your mind, get rid of them. Replace them with positive thoughts. If something bad happens look for the silver lining and I guarantee you will find it. It's not what happens to you that determines your future, it's how you respond to that which happens. The next time a negative thought enters your mind, strike it out immediately.

Write it down & get it done.

1
2
3
4
5
6
7
8
9
10

hack squat
Stand with feet 2-4 inches apart, heels on a board or book one inch thick. With your back straight, shoulders back and chest out, with toes pointed straight ahead or slightly outward, focus your vision straight ahead. Keeping your heels planted firmly on the floor, squat down and back, as if you are sitting in a chair. Keeping your knees behind your toes, stop when your thighs are parallel with the floor. Hold for 2-3 counts, then return to the starting position.

This search for what you want is like tracking something that doesn't want to be tracked. It takes time to get a dance right, to create something memorable.
— Fred Astaire

DATE

Steps Walked:
Cardio Workout:
Strength Training:
Calories Consumed:
Calories Burned:
Difference:
Weight / Body fat:

Write it down & get it done.

1
2
3
4
5
6
7
8
9
10

Read it, live it, love the results.

Feel great with Ginger Tea.
Ginger tea is known as a remedy for nausea, especially for pregnant women suffering from morning sickness. It can also be helpful if you get the flu. Additionally, ginger tea may alleviate the symptoms of a cold or cough, as it helps clear your lungs and sinuses. Some have also found it beneficial to combat acid reflux and heartburn.

Your level of success is up to you.

Academy Award-winning film and Broadway stage dancer, choreographer, singer and actor, **Fred Astaire**, whose routines were a staple of movie highlight reels, was a huge star in the thirties and fourties. Despite his lack of typical movie star good looks he became a popular romantic lead. It was his mix of elegance and nice-guy charm which landed him this title. He was named the fifth *Greatest Male Star of All Time* by the *American Film Institute*.

Our business in life is not to get ahead of others, but to get ahead of ourselves—to break our own records, to outstrip our yesterday by our today.
—Stewart B. Johnson

reverse lunge

Stand with feet shoulder-width apart, arms at sides with palms facing in, holding dumbbells. Keeping shoulders up and abs in, step backwards about two feet with your right foot, dropping down to within an inch of the floor. Hold for 2-5 counts, then push off and return to starting position. Complete 10-15 repetitions, then perform the exercise using the left leg.

Steps Walked:
Cardio Workout:
Strength Training:
Calories Consumed:
Calories Burned:
Difference:
Weight / Body fat:

DATE

Eating healthy tastes great!

Maple Pork Chops
6 thick pork chops
1/2 cup chopped onion
1/2 cup maple syrup
2 tbs cider vinegar
2 tbs Worchestershire sauce
1 tsp chili powder • pepper to taste

Preheat oven to 350°F. Place pork chops in baking dish. Combine the remaining ingredients and pour over pork chops. Bake for 50-60 minutes until no longer pink inside.

Read it, live it, love the results.

Don't dwell on yesterdays.
Yesterday doesn't matter. If you have not been able to stick to a healthy lifestyle in the past don't dwell on it. Make today, and every day, a brand-new start. Forget the past, discard the thoughts of what you could have/should have done. Yesterdays are gone forever—focus on today and how you can make the present and your future the best it can possibly be.

Write it down & get it done.

1
2
3
4
5
6
7
8
9
10

side lunge
Stand with feet together, arms at sides with palms facing in, holding dumbbells. Keeping shoulders back and abs in, step to the right as far as possible with your right foot, dropping down into a side lunge position. Hold for 2-5 counts, then push off and return to starting position. Complete 10-15 repetitions, then perform exercise using the left leg.

I don't know anybody's road who's been paved perfectly for them, there are no manuals, you don't know what life has in store for you.
–Drew Barrymore

DATE

Steps Walked:
Cardio Workout:
Strength Training:
Calories Consumed:
Calories Burned:
Difference:
Weight / Body fat:

Write it down & get it done.

1
2
3
4
5
6
7
8
9
10

Read it, live it, love the results.

Stay active to stay young.
With age, blood vessel walls tend to stiffen, similar to old tires; this is the reason two-thirds of people older than 60 have high blood pressure. The good news is that exercise can help keep the vessels pliable. Exercise also reduces the risk of many other diseases, including diabetes, certain cancers, depression, aging of the skin, and dementia.

Life's tough, get over it, she did!

Actor and film producer, **Drew Barrymore**, best known for her start in E.T. the Extra-Terrestrial and Charlie's Angels, began her career headed for trouble. By age 10 she was using alcohol and marijuana, at 13 she was in rehab, and at 17 posed nude for Interview magazine. Despite her downward spiral, she turned it around and became a prolific and respected actress when she reached her twenties.

We can let circumstances rule us, or we can take charge and rule our lives from within.
– Earl Nightengale

reverse step up

Stand directly in front of a step with a dumbbell in each hand, arms hanging at sides. Step up first with the left foot, planting it flat on the step, then keeping your shoulders back, chest out and abs in, step up with the right. Step back down with the left then the right. Complete 10-15 reverse step-ups leading with the left foot, then complete a set leading with the right foot.

DATE

Steps Walked:
Cardio Workout:
Strength Training:
Calories Consumed:
Calories Burned:
Difference:
Weight / Body fat:

Eating healthy tastes great!

Cajun-Style Baked Fish
1 lb fish fillets • 4 tsp olive oil
1 tbs paprika • 2 tsp thyme leaves
1 tsp onion powder
2 tbs minced garlic
red pepper to taste

Preheat oven to 400°F. Combine oil with spices. Spread mixture evenly on one side of each fillet. Place fillets on a lightly oiled baking pan, seasoning side up. Bake until fish flakes easily– 8 to 10 minutes.

Read it, live it, love the results.

Begin each day with a to-do list that will take you closer to your ultimate goal.
If you are trying to create a healthy lifestyle your list may look like this;
1) Bike to work.
2) Workout at gym 45 minutes.
3) Stop by farmer's market for fresh produce.
4) Walk dog for 20 minutes.
A life without goals is like taking a road trip without a map.

Write it down & get it done.

1
2
3
4
5
6
7
8
9
10

basic bridge

Lie on the floor, face up with knees bent, feet on the floor hip-width apart, arms at sides with palms facing down. Pressing into your heels, lift your hips toward the ceiling. Hold for 10 counts, then slowly lower your hips to the floor. Repeat 5-10 times.

It's amazing how much you can learn, if your intentions are truly earnest. – Chuck Berry

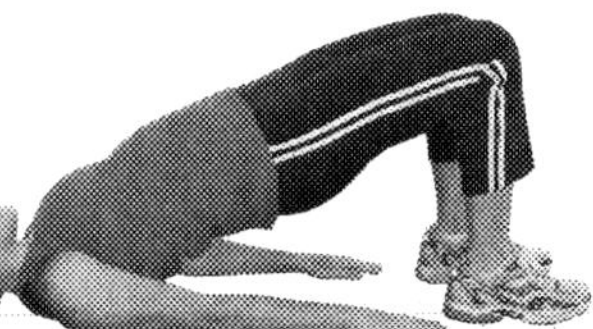

DATE

Steps Walked:
Cardio Workout:
Strength Training:
Calories Consumed:
Calories Burned:
Difference:
Weight / Body fat:

Write it down & get it done.

1
2
3
4
5
6
7
8
9
10

Read it, live it, love the results.

Stay active.
Researchers reported on a study that looked at the effect of fitness training on the physical condition and cognitive abilities of thirty-seven male sailors in the Norwegian navy.
This study revealed that when individuals did not workout for four weeks they had lower aerobic fitness, lower heart rate variability, and lower scores on tests of executive function.

Life's tough, get over it, he did!

Rock legend, **Chuck Berry** was sent to prison for three years in the early 60's. At this point he felt his best years were behind him. Fortunately, he re-entered the scene with new recordings and performances, creating even bigger hits then before. He still earns respect to this day as he truly is an incredible entertainer. He is also known as "The Father of Rock & Roll".

The great oak sleeps in the acorn.
The birds waits in the egg ,
and the highest vision of the
soul, a waking angel stirs.
Dreams are the
seedlings of reality.
–Napoleoan Hill.

bridge with single leg lift

Lie on floor face up in bridge position, arms extended at sides with palms down or locked together under buttocks. Plant the right foot flat on the floor or step, extend the left leg out straight. Pressing through your right heel lift your hips toward the ceiling. Hold this position as you raise and lower your left leg. Complete a set of 10-15 repetitions with each leg.

Steps Walked:

Cardio Workout:

Strength Training:

Calories Consumed:

Calories Burned:

Difference:

Weight / Body fat:

DATE

Eating healthy tastes great!

Fruit Kebabs and Dipping Sauce

16 oz can unsweetened pineapple
1 papaya • 1 banana • 16 grapes
2 mangoes • Juice of 1 lime
2 cups lowfat plain yogurt
1/2 cup honey
2 tsp orange zest, minced fine
1/2 tsp vanilla extract

Cut fruit into small pieces and place on skewer. Sprinkle with the lime juice, Made dip by mixing the honey, zest, vanilla and yogurt. Chill each.

Read it, live it, love the results.

Set realistic goals and clarify what it is you really want.

For example; "I want to quit taking my blood pressure medication by July." "I want to lose ten pounds by June 20th." Set realistic goals and get started in acheiving them. Set unrealistic goals and you will become frustrated, unsuccessful and probably back to your old habits. Don't set yourself up for failure.

Write it down & get it done.

1
2
3
4
5
6
7
8
9
10

bridge with a step

An alternative to the basic bridge. Lie on floor, face up with heels, shoulder-width apart, positioned on a step. Arms extended at sides with palms down or locked together under buttocks. Pressing your heels into the step lift your hips toward the ceiling. Hold for 5 counts, then slowly lower and repeat. Complete 10-15 repetitions.

We all do 'do, re, mi,' but you have got to find the other notes yourself.
—Louis Armstrong

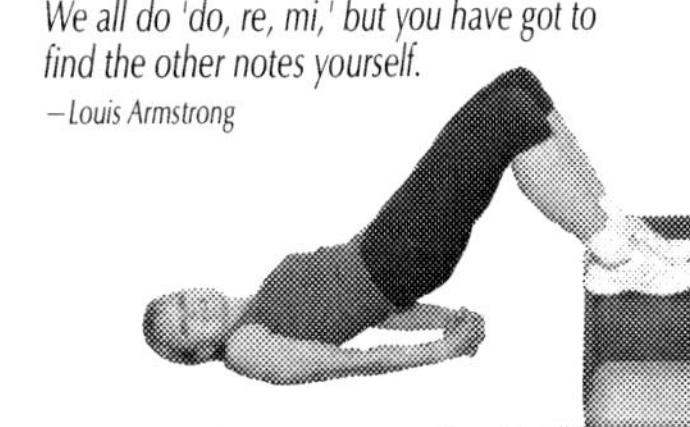

DATE

Steps Walked:
Cardio Workout:
Strength Training:
Calories Consumed:
Calories Burned:
Difference:
Weight / Body fat:

Write it down & get it done.

1
2
3
4
5
6
7
8
9
10

Read it, live it, love the results.

Get seven to eight hours of sleep each night.
Researchers have discovered that sleep-deprived individuals have high levels of hunger-stimulating ghrelin and lower levels of leptin, the appetite-regulating hormone. Study participants also reported stronger cravings for sweet, fatty and salty foods.
Get your sleep and you may avoid overeating throughout the day.

Success is the reward of hard work.

Radio host and author **Laura Ingraham,** who is ranked eighth among most-listened-to talk radio programs, is a woman with drive. When attending Dartmouth College she became the first female editor of the school's newspaper. Received a law degree from the University of Virginia School of Law. Worked as a speechwriter in the Ronald Reagan administration. Became a CBS commentator and hosted the MSNBC program Watch It! Then in 2001 launched The Laura Ingraham Show.

A change in scenery doesn't always improve the view. –author unknown

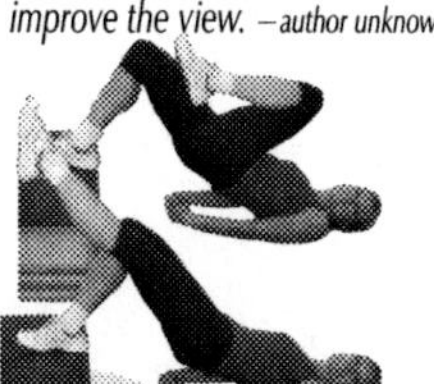

bridge with kickout

Lie on floor face up in bridge position, arms extended at sides with palms down or locked together under buttocks. Plant the right foot flat on the floor or step, bring the left knee into your chest, then pressing through your right heel lift your hips toward the ceiling. Hold this position as you kick the left leg out, then bring back into chest. Perform 10-15 kicks, then complete a set of kicks with the right leg.

DATE

Steps Walked:

Cardio Workout:

Strength Training:

Calories Consumed:

Calories Burned:

Difference:

Weight / Body fat:

Eating healthy tastes great!

"Cocoa-Nut" Bananas

4 tsp cocoa powder
4 tsp toasted unsweetened coconut
2 bananas, sliced on the bias

Place cocoa and coconut on separate plates. Roll each banana slice in the cocoa, shake off the excess, then dip in the coconut.

Read it, live it, love the results.

Say no to projects that won't fit into your schedule.

Often when you try to fit too much into your life you compromise your health. Taking on too much can cut into your sleep and workouts. There is no one more important in this world then you, and if you don't take care of yourself, no one else will.

Write it down & get it done.

1
2
3
4
5
6
7
8
9
10

bridge march

Lie on floor, face up with heels, shoulder-width apart, positioned on a step. Arms extended at sides with palms down or locked together under buttocks. Pressing your heels into the step lift the right foot 6-10 inches from the step, return and then lift the left. Complete this "marching" movement for 10-15 repetitions.

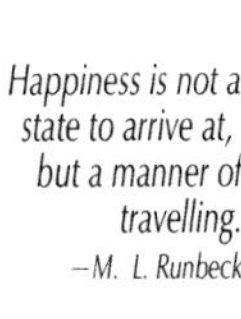

Happiness is not a state to arrive at, but a manner of travelling.
—M. L. Runbeck

DATE

Steps Walked:
Cardio Workout:
Strength Training:
Calories Consumed:
Calories Burned:
Difference:
Weight / Body fat:

Write it down & get it done.

1
2
3
4
5
6
7
8
9
10

Read it, live it, love the results.

Don't forget to read your desire statement daily.
Teachers often encourage students with test anxiety to tell themselves *"I will ace this test"* — repeating it, until they really believe they can do it. And, as a result, they generally do much better. If you work hard and tell yourself you will be successful, you will be. Of course it's not all magic, you must put effort towards that which you desire.

Success is the reward of hard work.

Fashion designer and business executive **Liz Claiborne** quit high school to study art in Europe. From here she went to New York, where she worked as a designer for twenty-five years before starting her own business. Ultimately, her hard work and creativity built a billion dollar business, which became the first company founded by a woman to make the Fortune 500.

Winners have simply formed the habit of doing things losers don't like to do.
—Albert Gray

kickback

Stand with legs 2-4 inches apart, with an ankle weight on the right leg *(weight optional)*, balance by holding onto a wall. Leaning slightly forward so your entire body is in a straight line, shift your weight to the left leg. With the right knee slightly bent, move the leg up and back as far as you can, without arching your back, feeling the contraction in your glutes. Hold here for 2-3 counts, then lower to starting position. Repeat 10-15 times, then complete a set with the

DATE

Steps Walked:
Cardio Workout:
Strength Training:
Calories Consumed:
Calories Burned:
Difference:
Weight / Body fat:

Eating healthy tastes great!

Fish Puffs
4 fish fillets • 1 egg white
$^1/_4$ tsp dill • $^1/_4$ tsp onion juice
$^1/_4$ cup fat free mayonnaise
pepper to taste
Preheat oven to 425°F. Place fish in greased baking dish, season with salt and pepper. Add $^1/_8$ tsp salt to egg white and whip until stiff, fold in mayonnaise, dill and onion juice. Spoon over fillets. Bake about 12 minutes or until top is puffed and brown.

Read it, live it, love the results.

Read autobiographies and biographies of successful individuals.
Whether people are successful at losing weight or becoming millionaires, understand they all went through difficulties in achieving their goals. Life is not easy for anyone, everyone has problems, it's how we choose to deal with those problems that sets the winners apart from the losers. It's your choice to be a winner.

Write it down & get it done.

1
2
3
4
5
6
7
8
9
10

deadlifts with dumbbells

Stand with feet shoulder-width apart, back straight, shoulders back and chest out. With a dumbbell in each hand, arms hang in front with the dumbbells resting on your thighs. Keeping dumbbells pressed against your legs, bend forward, until your upper body is parallel with the floor. Hold here briefly, then slowly return to the starting position, pulling your shoulders back and arching your lower back for a complete lower back contraction. Complete 10-15 repetitions.

Life is not certain, life is not easy. It is up to you, and only you, to make the best of it.
–author unknown

DATE

Steps Walked:
Cardio Workout:
Strength Training:
Calories Consumed:
Calories Burned:
Difference:
Weight / Body fat:

Write it down & get it done.

1
2
3
4
5
6
7
8
9
10

Read it, live it, love the results.

Control your weight.
Obesity is a chronic disease that accelerates aging, a disease of which you have control. Obesity is a result of eating too much, eating the wrong foods and not getting enough physical activity. If you want to hold on to your youth choose your foods wisely and stay active.

Your level of success is up to you.

One of the best-selling authors in the United States, **Tom Clancy**, began his career as an insurance broker. Most brokers are not known for entertaining conversation, though Clancy broke this mold. Many of his books have also become commercially successful films. He also founded Red Storm Entertainment, a multimedia company specializing in computer games.

one-legged deadlifts

Stand with feet shoulder-width apart with the left leg shifted back about two feet. Keeping the right foot planted on floor, lift the left foot, balancing on your toe if needed. With shoulders back, chest out and abs in, hold dumbbells close to your thighs, palms facing your body. Bend at the hips, dropping the dumbbells down, keeping them close to your leg. Hold for 2-3 counts, then contract your glutes and hamstrings as you return to the starting position. Repeat 10-15 times, then complete a set with the left leg.

Steps Walked:

Cardio Workout:

Strength Training:

Calories Consumed:

Calories Burned:

Difference:

Weight / Body fat:

DATE

If you do not hope, you will not find what is beyond your hopes. –St. Clement of Alexandra

Eating healthy tastes great!

Codfish Cakes

1 lb cooked cod • 1 onion, diced
8 parsley sprigs, chopped
2 cups potatoes, boiled and cubed
2 hardboiled eggs, chopped
3 tbs melted light butter
pepper to taste • olive oil
Seasoned wheat bread crumbs
Cut cod into pieces, mix with other ingredients and chill for one hour. Shape into 10 round, flat cakes, coat with seasoned bread crumbs, then pan fry in olive oil.

Read it, live it, love the results.

Use the internet to help develop a well-executed plan for reaching your objective.

With the internet you have access to unlimited information. You can research the experiences of others, educate yourself and explore endless possibilities to achieving that which you desire. The web also has a great selection of websites that allow you to track your meals, with calorie, fat and carb information and more.

Write it down & get it done.

1
2
3
4
5
6
7
8
9
10

plié squat with flye

Stand sideways in front of stairs, holding dumbbells in front of pelvic area, with elbows slightly bent. Keeping the feet spread wide and toes turned out, place the right foot on the step, the left foot on the floor. Lower your body into a plié squat. Bring dumbbells out to side, keeping elbows slightly bent, while lowering hips. Hold for 2-3 counts, then slowly return to starting position. Repeat 10-15 times on each side.

This became a credo of mine... attempt the impossible in order to improve your work.
– Bette Davis

DATE

Steps Walked:
Cardio Workout:
Strength Training:
Calories Consumed:
Calories Burned:
Difference:
Weight / Body fat:

Write it down & get it done.

1
2
3
4
5
6
7
8
9
10

Read it, live it, love the results.

Stay active, stay healthy.
One of the most comprehensive Alzheimer's studies, being performed in Sweden, follows everyone over the age of 75 living on one of the islands of greater Stockholm. This study indicates that leisure activities of almost any kind seem to be protective against Alzheimer's. So whether it's riding your bike, walking your dog, or pulling weeds, the important thing is to stay active!

Life's tough, get over it, she did!

Academy award-winning actress **Bette Davis** had a rough start, beginning with her arrival in Hollywood. Davis and her mother were stranded at the train station. The studio employee sent to pick her up left because he didn't see anyone who *"looked like an actress."* This *"unlikely actress,"* was the first to receive ten *Academy Award* nominations and the first woman to receive a *Lifetime Achievement Award*.

God doesn't want to deliver you from difficulty, he wants to take you through it... it's the only way to grow and learn.
–author unknown

duke curtsey

Stand with heels touching, toes turned out, shoulders back, chest out, abs in and hands on your waist. You may need to hold a chair back for balance. Once balanced, put the left foot behind the right, then bend both knees into a curtsy while keeping the back straight. Hold the pose 2-3 counts then return to starting position. Complete 10-15 repetitions, then perfom with the right foot behind the left.

DATE

Steps Walked:
Cardio Workout:
Strength Training:
Calories Consumed:
Calories Burned:
Difference:
Weight / Body fat:

Eating healthy tastes great!

Bloody Mary Salmon
1 lb salmon fillets
pepper to taste
1 cup spicy Bloody Mary mix
Preheat the broiler.
Place salt & peppered salmon fillets in baking dish. Pour spicy Bloody Mary mix over the fillets. Cover, and refrigerate at least 30 minutes. Broil 7-9 minutes, until fish is easily flaked with a fork and surface is lightly browned.

Read it, live it, love the results.

Don't eat too much red meat if you want to avoid heart disease.
Though you don't have to give up steak completely, eating too much red meat has been linked to heart disease and colon, breast, pancreatic and prostate cancers. On the other hand, fish, such as salmon, sardines, and mackerel, is rich in omega-3 fatty acids which have been shown to lower your risk of heart disease and cancers.

Write it down & get it done.

1
2
3
4
5
6
7
8
9
10

walking lunges

Stand with feet shoulder-width apart, arms resting at sides with palms facing in, holding dumbbells. Keeping shoulders back and abs in, step forward about two feet with your right foot. As you plant your right foot bend the right knee to about 90-degrees. Your left knee will bend automatically and should come within an inch of the floor. Tighten your glutes as you return to standing position. Next step forward with the left foot. Continue stepping and walking 10-15 steps.

DATE
Life is not a spectator sport. If you're going to spend your whole life in the grandstand just watching what goes on, in my opinion you're wasting your life. –Jackie Robinson
Steps Walked:
Cardio Workout:
Strength Training:
Calories Consumed:
Calories Burned:
Difference:
Weight / Body fat:

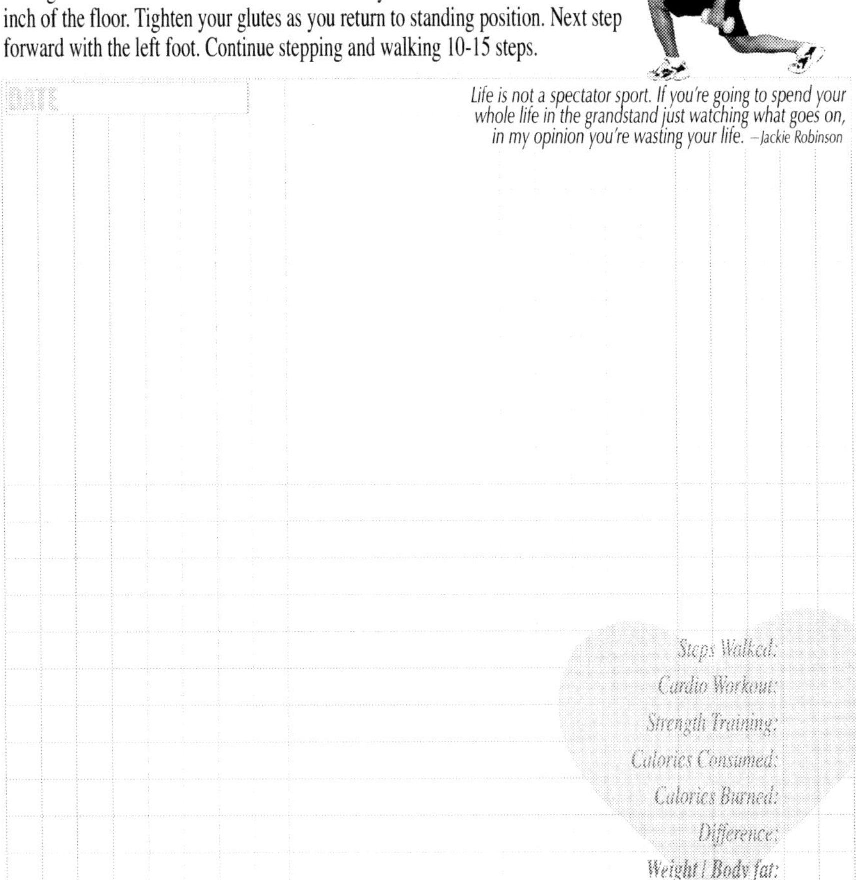

Write it down & get it done.

1
2
3
4
5
6
7
8
9
10

Read it, live it, love the results.

Think positive thoughts.
The dominating thoughts of your mind will eventually become a reality. Promise yourself that you will focus on positive self-improving thoughts for at least thirty minutes a day, creating in your mind a clear mental picture of what you will become—whether it be one hundred pounds lighter or simply leading a healthier, happier life. You become what you think.

Your level of success is up to you.

The first African-American Major League player, **Jackie Robinson,** had once been a gang member, fortunately a friend convinced him to abandon this life. His older brother, Matthew, then inspired him to pursue his talent and love for athletics. Due to these influences and his wise decisions Jackie became a huge success. He's now in the *Baseball Hall of Fame* and has won numerous awards for his baseball talent.

When solving problems, dig at the roots instead of just hacking at the leaves.
–Anthony J. D'Angelo

lunge and lift

An addition to the walking lunge. Step forward about two feet with your right foot. As you plant your right foot bend the right knee to about 90-degrees. Your left knee will bend automatically and should come within an inch of the floor. Tighten your glutes as stand, bringing the left foot up and forward, raising it to your chest before planting it on the floor next to the right foot. Continue stepping with the right foot leading, 10-15 steps. Then complete a set with the left foot leading.

Steps Walked:
Cardio Workout:
Strength Training:
Calories Consumed:
Calories Burned:
Difference:
Weight / Body fat:

DATE

Eating healthy tastes great!

Mexican Skillet Supper
1 lb chicken, diced
1 cup onion, diced
14 oz can tomatoes, not drained
1 tbs chili powder
$1^1/_2$ cups brown rice, cooked
1 cup lettuce, shredded
1 cup light cheese, shredded
Brown chicken and onion in a skillet. Add tomatoes, chili powder and rice. Simmer until any liquid is absorbed. Serve over lettuce, top with cheese.

Read it, live it, love the results.

Reward yourself each time you reach a benchmark or successfully change a habit.
For example, if you skip the cheesecake at the dinner party, reward yourself with a manicure, pedicure or a long relaxing bath. The reward needn't be expensive, just make sure it's something you truly enjoy.

Write it down & get it done.

1
2
3
4
5
6
7
8
9
10

single dumbbell squat

Stand with feet shoulder-width apart, back straight, shoulders back and chest out, with toes pointed straight ahead or slightly outward. Holding a dumbbell with both hands, let it hang straight down, as you focus your vision straight ahead. Keeping your heels planted firmly on the floor, squat down and back, as if you are sitting in a chair. Keeping your knees behind your toes, stop when your thighs are parallel with the floor. Hold for 2-3 counts, then return to starting position. Repeat 10-15 times, focus on using the glutes to execute the move.

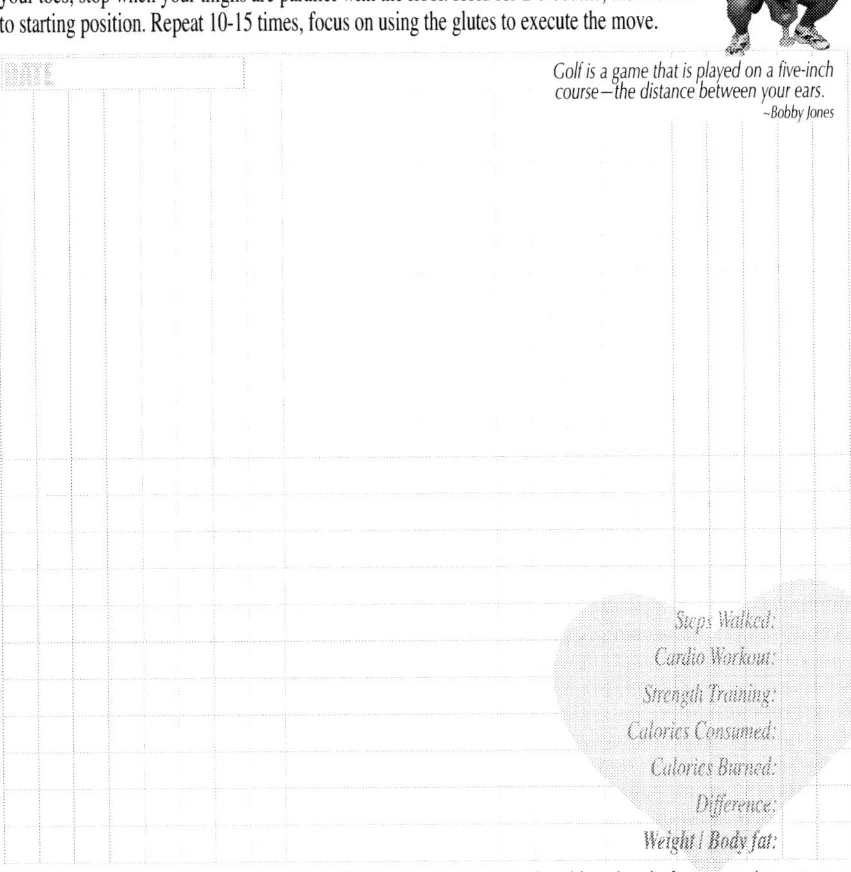

Write it down & get it done.

1
2
3
4
5
6
7
8
9
10

Read it, live it, love the results.

Get whole grains in your diet. Research performed at Wake Forest University, revealed that people who eat two and a half servings of whole grains each day, are about one-fifth less likely to have heart disease than those who skimp on whole grains. Whole grains are a good source of B vitamins, Vitamin E, magnesium, iron and fiber, as well as other valuable antioxidants not found in some fruits and vegetables.

Your level of success is up to you.

Golfer **John Daly** became a favorite when he came out of nowhere to win the *1991 PGA Championship* and *Rookie of the Year.* However, his temper, drinking and gambling nearly brought an end to the dream. Through the years his play has gone up and down. Despite the challenges he has never given up. He remains one of the most popular and intriguing figures on *The Tour.*

plié with a twist

Stand with feet slightly wider than shoulder-width apart, toes pointing out at a comfortable angle, shoulders back, chest out, abs in and back straight. Holding dumbbells in a military press position, bend your knees and slowly lower your body until the thighs are parallel with the floor. Hold here for 2-3 counts then rotate your entire body 90-degrees to the left, holding here for 2-3 counts. Return to the center then the starting position. Repeat 10-15 repetitions on each side.

Steps Walked:

Cardio Workout:

Strength Training:

Calories Consumed:

Calories Burned:

Difference:

Weight / Body fat:

DATE

Success is simple. Do what's right, the right way, at the right time. – Arnold H. Glasow

Eating healthy tastes great!

Honey Fish

4 fish fillets • 1/4 cup honey
1/4 cup Dijon mustard
2 tbs lemon juice
1 tsp curry powder

Mix honey with spices, then coat the fillets. Cover and refrigerate for 15 minutes. Place fillets on a lightly greased rack in a roasting pan. Broil 10 to 12 minutes, about 4 inches from heat, basting occasionally with reserved marinade.

Read it, live it, love the results.

Do what's right.

Often we know the answers, however, *"we can't handle the truth."* Bottom line, there are no magic pills. If there were, all doctors and nurses would be fit and trim. The magic to being healthy is eating right, staying active, drinking water and sleeping seven to eight hours a night. You know what you should do, so stop making excuses and simply do what's right!

Write it down & get it done.

1
2
3
4
5
6
7
8
9
10

monster march

Stand with feet shoulder-width apart, toes pointing straight ahead or slightly outward. Holding a dumbbell in each hand, squat down, keeping your heels planted firmly on the floor and your knees behind your toes. Stop when your thighs are parallel with the floor, then lift your right foot 8-10 inches from the floor, hold for 2 counts return to floor and lift your left foot and hold for 2 counts. Complete 10-15 alternating steps.

I told my psychiatrist that everyone hates me. He said I was being ridiculous— everyone hasn't met me yet.
–Rodney Dangerfield

DATE

Steps Walked:

Cardio Workout:

Strength Training:

Calories Consumed:

Calories Burned:

Difference:

Weight / Body fat:

Write it down & get it done.

1
2
3
4
5
6
7
8
9
10

Read it, live it, love the results.

Practice good posture.
An Australian study revealed that good posture works your abdominal muscles and helps flatten your stomach. Experts observed twenty participants as they sat slumped in chairs and stood with their backs arched and bellies pooched out, and then again when they sat and stood erect. They found that when using good posture participants muscles were engaged and working, which is essential to building strong muscles.

Doors open when least expected.

Comedian **Rodney Dangerfield** made a very successful career out of telling audiences *"I don't get no respect."* However, he nearly missed "his calling" when he quit comedy for more than a decade to live the "normal" life in sales. It was after his divorce that he returned to stand-up. Fate intervened one Sunday night in New York, when *The Ed Sullivan Show* needed a replacement for another act. Dangerfield became a surprise hit.

Success is the prize for those who stand true to their ideas!
– Josh S. Hinds

squat with kicks

Stand with feet shoulder- width apart, toes pointing straight ahead or slightly outward. Holding a dumbbell in each hand, focus your vision straight ahead. Keeping your heels planted firmly on the floor and your knees behind toes, move your buns back and downward, as if you are sitting in a chair. Hold here 2-3 counts then return to the standing position, kicking your right foot to side. Complete another squat, kicking out your left foot. Complete10-15 kicks on each leg.

DATE

Steps Walked:
Cardio Workout:
Strength Training:
Calories Consumed:
Calories Burned:
Difference:
Weight / Body fat:

Eating healthy tastes great!

Chunky Salsa
1/2 white onion
2 stalks celery • 1 mango
red, yellow, orange and green peppers
12 cherry tomatoes
1 bunch cilantro • cumin
2 1/2 cups salsa

Dice all ingredients, add Cilantro and Cumin to taste, then combine with salsa. Chill and serve.

Read it, live it, love the results.

Add cilantro to your recipes for the health of it!
Researchers have discovered many benefits of organic cilantro including just a few listed here;
- Reduces arthritis pain
- Relieves stomach gas
- Wards off urinary tract infections
- Eases hormonal mood swings
- Reduces menstrual cramping
- Reduces minor swelling
- Helps detoxify the body
- Helpful in fighting anemia

Write it down & get it done.

1
2
3
4
5
6
7
8
9
10

squat with toe tap
Stand with feet shoulder-width apart, toes pointing straight ahead or slightly outward. Holding a dumbbell in each hand, keeping your heels planted firmly on the floor and knees behind your toes, squat down. When your thighs are parallel with the floor, shift your weight to the right foot and extend your left foot straight out to the side. Tap your toe on the floor then return to the upright starting position. Complete 10 to 15 taps with each leg.

I don't spend a lot of time thinking about regrets because there's nothing I can do.
– Sheryl Crow

DATE

Steps Walked:
Cardio Workout:
Strength Training:
Calories Consumed:
Calories Burned:
Difference:
Weight / Body fat:

Write it down & get it done.

1
2
3
4
5
6
7
8
9
10

Read it, live it, love the results.

Once you have decided what it is you desire, stick with it, despite what others say.
Many people who fail in reaching their goals, do so because they are influenced by the opinions of others. In Napolean Hill's analysis of several hundred millionaires, he discovered that the majority of them would reach decisions promptly and change these decisions slowly, if in fact they were ever changed.

Your level of success is up to you.

Singer, songwriter and breast cancer survivor, **Sheryl Crow**, worked as a backup and studio session singer until her platinum solo album, *"Tuesday Night Music Club"* was released. This album went on to sell more than seven million copies in the US and UK during the 1990's, and won three Grammy Awards for Crow.
Due to her determination, she become extremely successful– she never gave up.

Create a vision and never let the environment, other people's beliefs, or the limits of what has been done in the past shape your decisions. Ignore conventional wisdom.
—Anthony Robbins

step overs

Stand on a step with a dumbbell in each hand, arms hanging at sides. Keeping your shoulders back, chest out, abs in and the right foot stationary, step forward with the left foot, placing the entire foot on the ground, then quickly picking the foot back up and placing it behind the bench, again, putting the entire foot on the ground. Continue this back and forth motion without stopping for 10-15 steps, then complete a set with the right foot stepping.

	DATE
Steps Walked:	
Cardio Workout:	
Strength Training:	
Calories Consumed:	
Calories Burned:	
Difference:	
Weight / Body fat:	

Eating healthy tastes great!

Miso Soup

1 tsp sesame oil • 1 cup onion, diced
1 large carrot, thinly sliced
3 cups water • 2 tbs miso
1 tbs soy sauce • 3 green onions, sliced
$^1/_2$ cup firm tofu, diced

Sauté onion and carrot. Add the water and bring to a boil. Reduce heat and simmer for a few minutes. Remove from heat. Add the miso soy sauce, green onions and tofu. Stir until miso is dissolved.

Read it, live it, love the results.

Remember your successes and reflect upon them.

Remember the times you've turned your dreams into reality and know that you are capable of doing it over and over again. Often we spend too much time reflecting on the things we didn't accomplish, and thinking less of ourselves for not getting them done. Never let yesterdays ruin your todays, remember the good times!

Write it down & get it done.

1
2
3
4
5
6
7
8
9
10

toe tap

Lie on floor face up, with legs up, knees bent at 90-degrees with calves parallel to the floor. Keeping your back pressed into the floor, slowly lower your right foot touching your toe to the floor, then slowly return it to the starting position. If your back starts to arch, stop at that point. As your abs get stronger, you'll be able to get closer to the floor. Complete 10-12 repetitions with each leg and then do both legs at the same time.

It's through curiosity and looking at opportunities in new ways that we've always mapped our path at Dell. There's always an opportunity to make a difference.
– Michael Dell

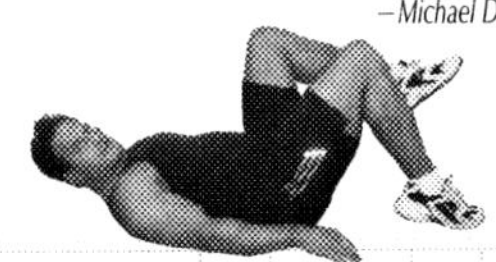

DATE

Steps Walked:
Cardio Workout:
Strength Training:
Calories Consumed:
Calories Burned:
Difference:
Weight / Body fat:

Write it down & get it done.

1
2
3
4
5
6
7
8
9
10

Read it, live it, love the results.

If a robber asks for your wallet and/or purse, DON'T hand it to him or her.
Instead toss it away from you—far away from you.
Chances are that he/she is more interested in your wallet and/or purse than you, and will instinctively run for your money leaving you alone to run like crazy in the other direction!

Doors open, when you work hard.

The founder of Dell Computer Corp., **Michael Dell**, began by selling computers out of his dorm room at the University of Texas. He sold computers directly to consumers, built to their specifications, without the cost of the "middle man." Following this dream made him a huge success. He became *"Entrepreneur of the Year"* from Inc. magazine; *"Man of the Year"*, PC Magazine; *"Top CEO in American Business"*, Worth Magazine.

Strong back muscles are essential, as they involve nearly every movement and activity in which you participate. The back serves as the structural support for the lumbar spine, supports and holds the weight of your body when you stand, acts as a hinge between the upper and lower body, allows you to bend or rotate at the waist and protects the spinal cord and nerves as they enter and leave the spinal column. Unfortunately, many people suffer from lower back pain due to overuse and muscle strain or injury. This is one of the primary reasons it's important to perform back exercises. Studies show that exercise may not only help decrease lower back pain, but it may also aide in faster injury recovery, injury prevention, and reduce the risk of disability from back pain.

Steps Walked:

Cardio Workout:

Strength Training:

Calories Consumed:

Calories Burned:

Difference:

Weight / Body fat:

DATE

The quality of your life will never exceed the quality of your thoughts. Change one and you'll change the other.
— Vic Johnson

Eating healthy tastes great!

Fresh Veggie Delight
1 cup each diced;
zucchini, green pepper, eggplant, onion and tomatoes
16 oz can white beans
3 tbs minced garlic • 2 tbs olive oil
1/2 cup Parmesan cheese
Place veggies in baking dish with 2 tbs olive oil, mix well and broil for 5 minutes. Remove from oven, cool and mix in remaining ingredients. Chill and serve.

Read it, live it, love the results.

Don't ever put limits on yourself.
The only limitations you have are those you place upon yourself, you can do anything you put your mind to. When you open your mind and think big, you will become more successful than you ever thought possible.
By limiting your thoughts, you hold youself back from achieving those things you may think are impossible.

Write it down & get it done.

1
2
3
4
5
6
7
8
9
10

straight leg wide decline row

Stand with feet 8-10 inches apart, legs straight, holding dumbbells with an overhand grip. Bend at your waist with arms extended down, slightly wider than shoulder-width apart. Keeping your body stationary and your hands out wide, sowly lift the dumbbells to chest level, hold 2-3 counts, then lower to the start position. Repeat10-15 times.

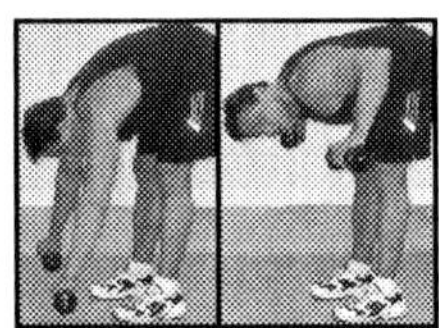

Always do right. This will gratify some people and astonish all others.
—Mark Twain

DATE

Steps Walked:
Cardio Workout:
Strength Training:
Calories Consumed:
Calories Burned:
Difference:
Weight / Body fat:

Write it down & get it done.

1
2
3
4
5
6
7
8
9
10

Read it, live it, love the results.

Respect yourself as you respect others.

If Mark Twain were to visit your home for dinner, you would not serve fast food or unhealthy choices.You would serve a healthy home cooked meal. You are the most important person in the world. Treat yourself even better than those individuals you respect the most!

Your level of success is up to you.

Humorist, satirist, lecturer and writer, **Samuel Clemens**, known as **Mark Twain** had originally gone west to became a miner—though failed to strike it rich. He then went to work for a newspaper in Virginia City, where he adopted the pen name *"Mark Twain."* Today he is most noted for *The Adventures of Tom Sawyer* and *Adventures of Huckleberry Finn,* which has since been called the *Great American Novel.*

Our attitude toward life determines life's attitude towards us.
– Earl Nightengale

goodmornings
Stand with feet shoulder-width apart, dumbbells resting on your shoulders. Keep your back straight with knees locked. Bend forward from the waist until your upper body is nearly parallel to the floor. Make sure your head is up during this movement. Hold for 2-3 counts, then return to the starting position. Repeat 10-15 times.

	DATE
Steps Walked:	
Cardio Workout:	
Strength Training:	
Calories Consumed:	
Calories Burned:	
Difference:	
Weight / Body fat:	

Eating healthy tastes great!

Cabbage Salad Recipe
1/3 cup fat free mayonnaise
1 tsp cider vinegar
2 large carrots, grated
2 cups cabbage, grated
1/2 cup cucumber, diced
1/4 cup pine nuts
Combine the mayonnaise and the cider vinegar. Add the carrots, cabbage, cucumber and pine nuts. Stir well. Serve chilled.

Read it, live it, love the results.

Eat brightly colored vegetables.
Spinach, romaine lettuce, winter squash, carrots, bell peppers, and tomatoes are all fiber rich vegetables which aid in digestion. They also contain phytochemicals such as beta-carotene and lutein which may protect against heart disease, abnormal blood clotting, and macular degeneration, an eye disease that can cause blindness.

Write it down & get it done.

1
2
3
4
5
6
7
8
9
10

straight arm pullovers

Lie on the floor, face up, holding a large dumbbell straight above your chest, using both hands to clasp the ends. Knees should be bent at 90-degrees with your ankles crossed. Keeping your arms as straight as possible, lower the dumbbell behind your head, stopping when it's 1-2 inches above the floor. Hold for 2-3 counts, then return to the starting position. Focusing on your back muscles, repeat the exercise 10-15 times.

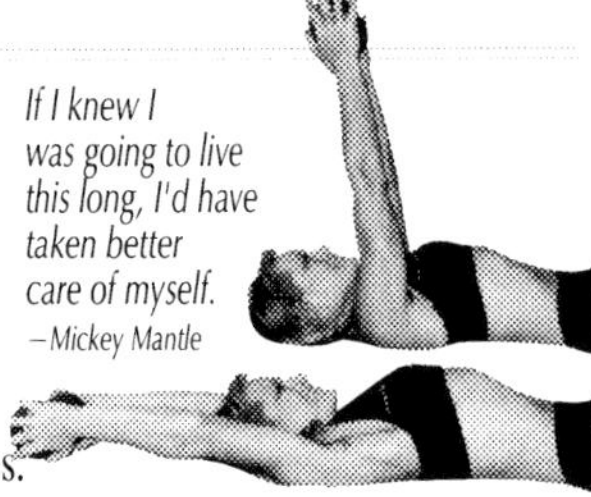

If I knew I was going to live this long, I'd have taken better care of myself.
–Mickey Mantle

DATE

Steps Walked:

Cardio Workout:

Strength Training:

Calories Consumed:

Calories Burned:

Difference:

Weight / Body fat:

Write it down & get it done.

1

2

3

4

5

6

7

8

9

10

Read it, live it, love the results.

Avoid Alzheimer's.

Studies indicate you may be able to reduce your risk of Alzheimer's by following these *"rules"*;

- Don't smoke
- Don't carry excessive body fat
- Avoid becoming diabetic
- Avoid being chronically stressed
- Get plenty of exercise
- Eat a brain-healthy diet
- Drink coffee
- Keep your mind active
- Sleep regularly and restfully

Life's tough, get over it, he did!

National radio and television host, **Glenn Beck**, began his radio career when he won a local radio contest and was granted a part-time job. He then hosted Christian radio on Saturday, rock on Sunday and country on weeknights. His personal life was also difficult. His mother and brother commited suicide, another brother died, and he fought with drugs and alcohol. Despite all of the negatives, he never gave up.

Your world is a living expression of how you are using and have used your mind.
—Earl Nightengale

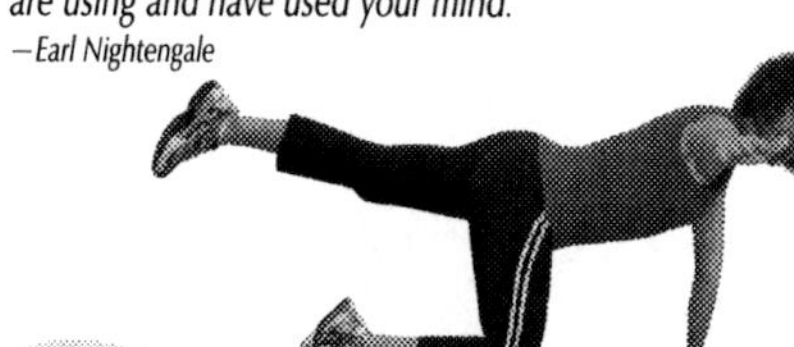

airplane

On the floor support yourself on your hands and knees. *(Using dumbbells with this exercise is optional.)* Extend your right arm straight out to the right side, the left leg straight out back, hold for 10 counts. Return to the starting position and repeat 2-5 times on each side.

	DATE
Steps Walked:	
Cardio Workout:	
Strength Training:	
Calories Consumed:	
Calories Burned:	
Difference:	
Weight / Body fat:	

Eating healthy tastes great!

Apple Pie Oatmeal

1 cup water
$^1/_2$ cup old-fashioned oats
2 tsp Splenda® brown sugar blend
1 tbs chopped apple
1 dash apple pie spice

Cook oatmeal as specified on box. Blend, chopped apple and spice with cooked oatmeal then top with Splenda® Brown Sugar.

Read it, live it, love the results.

Don't focus on limitations.

When your focus is placed on limitations, successes are limited. You are capable of being successful at anything you desire. Looking for a healthier body? Then focus your thoughts on what you need to do to achieve a healthy lifestyle and your body and attitude will follow. Forget about limitations and your mind and body will forget them also.

Write it down & get it done.

1
2
3
4
5
6
7
8
9
10

seated bent over row
Sit in a chair with feet together, then bend over bringing your chest, as close as possible to your knees. With a dumbbell in each hand, extend arms straight down, with palms facing forward. Using your back muscles, lift the dumbbells up to the side of your chest, rotating hands to face your sides. Squeeze your elbows together behind you and hold for 2-3 counts, lower and repeat 10-15 times.

I am selfish, impatient and a little insecure, I make mistakes... out of control at times, hard to handle but, if you can't handle me at my worst, you sure don't deserve me at my best.
–Marilyn Monroe

DATE

Steps Walked:
Cardio Workout:
Strength Training:
Calories Consumed:
Calories Burned:
Difference:
Weight / Body fat:

Write it down & get it done.

1
2
3
4
5
6
7
8
9
10

Read it, live it, love the results.

If you are ever thrown into the trunk of a car, kick out the back tail lights.
Once the light is kicked out, stick your arm out of the hole and start waving like crazy. The driver won't see you, but everybody else will. This has saved lives... perhaps yours will be one of them.

Life's tough, get over it, she did!

Actress, singer, model and film producer, **Marilyn Monroe** had a rough childhood. She never knew her father, and her mother was committed to a mental institution. She then spent most of her childhood in foster homes and orphanages. At 16 she married, however it was short lived, she had a bigger dream. She began a modeling career which soon led to acting. In 1999, she was ranked the sixth greatest female star of all time.

My interest is in the future, because I'm going to be spending the rest of my life there.
—Charles Kettering

lower back extensions

Lie on the floor, face down, arms extended straight out in front with legs flat on the floor extended out back. Keeping your head in line with your spine, lift your right leg and left arm off the floor. Contracting the muscles in your back, hold for 2-3 counts, then lower to the floor, repeating the lift using the left leg and right arm. Complete10-15 repetitions. You may use 3-5 lb dumbbells with this exercise.

	DATE
Steps Walked:	
Cardio Workout:	
Strength Training:	
Calories Consumed:	
Calories Burned:	
Difference:	
Weight / Body fat:	

Eating healthy tastes great!

Shrimp and Mango Salad
1 lb cooked shrimp • 1 red onion, sliced
1/4 cup olive oil • 3 tbs rice vinegar
1 tsp sesame oil • pepper to taste
3 ripe mangoes, diced
3 ripe avocados, diced
3 green onions, thinly sliced
In a large bowl, mix the olive oil, rice vinegar, sesame oil, salt and pepper. Whisk until well mixed. Add remaining ingredients. Mix well and serve chilled.

Read it, live it, love the results.

At times individuals get into their cars and just sit—doing their checkbook, making a list, etc. Don't do this!
A predator may be watching you, and this is the perfect opportunity for them to get in on the passenger side, put a gun to your head, and tell you where to go.
Instead, get in, lock the doors and go to your destination.

Write it down & get it done.

1
2
3
4
5
6
7
8
9
10

Character, not circumstances, makes the man. – Booker T. Washington

lying pull up
Place a bar between two sturdy chairs, then lie on the floor face up, under the bar. Hold the bar with an underhand grip with hands shoulder width apart. Slowly pull yourself up, keeping your body perfectly straight throughout the movement. Bring your chin up to touch the bar, holding here for 2-3 counts. Then, slowly lower to the starting position and repeat 10-15 times.

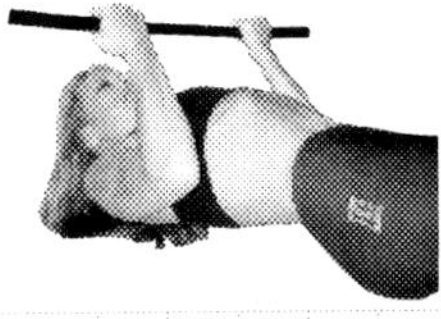

DATE

Steps Walked:
Cardio Workout:
Strength Training:
Calories Consumed:
Calories Burned:
Difference:
Weight / Body fat:

Write it down & get it done.

1
2
3
4
5
6
7
8
9
10

Read it, live it, love the results.

Look younger with Vitamin C. Vitamin C is an antioxidant which helps defend your skin from the free radicals that age it. Vitamin C also affects your skin's collagen, the elasticity, by ensuring normal formation, maintenance and structural stability—this can make you look years younger.

Your level of success is up to you.

American educator and author, **Booker T. Washigton** was born a slave. Still, he remained tolerant and open minded at all times—a dreamer, without limitations. As a result he was appointed to lead a teachers' college for blacks. He then rose into a nationally prominent role as spokesman for African-Americans. Although his non-confrontational approach was criticized by some blacks, he became very successful.

lying close grip pullup

Place a bar between two sturdy chairs, then lie on the floor face up, under the bar. Hold the bar with an underhand grip with hands at center, pinky fingers touching. Slowly pull yourself up, keeping your body perfectly straight throughout the movement. Bring your chin up to touch the bar, holding here for 2-3 counts before lowering to the starting position. Repeat 10-15 times.

Effort only fully releases its reward after a person refuses to quit.
–Napolean Hill

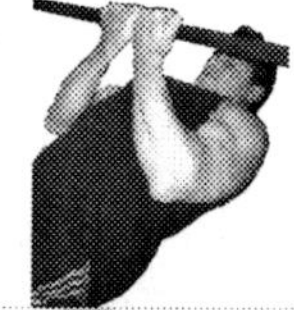

Steps Walked:

Cardio Workout:

Strength Training:

Calories Consumed:

Calories Burned:

Difference:

Weight / Body fat:

Eating healthy tastes great!

Tuna Ball

1 large can tuna, drained well
8 oz fat free cream cheese
1/4 cup onion, minced
1/4 tsp chili powder
pepper, parsley and paprika to taste
Mix all ingredients and roll into a ball. Sprinkle with paprika, served chilled.

Read it, live it, love the results.

Don't ever quit.

Leading a healthy lifestyle is not easy, if it were everyone would be doing it. It's unfortunate that most people will never stick with it long enough to experience the "success high" gotten from creating a healthy body. There is something grand about refusing to quit and creating a body that feels great mentally and physically. Everyone has the ability to do this, don't ever think differently.

Write it down & get it done.

1
2
3
4
5
6
7
8
9
10

superman/woman

Lie on the floor, face down with arms extended straight out in front with legs flat on floor extended out back. Raise your arms, chest and legs off the floor, squeeze, and hold for 10-15 counts. It's as if you are flying through the air. Lower and repeat 2-5 times.

Patience and perseverance have a magical effect before which difficulties disappear and obstacles vanish.
–John Quincy Adams

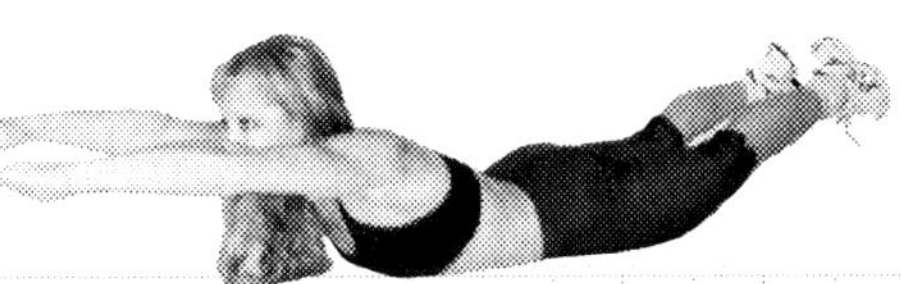

DATE

Steps Walked:
Cardio Workout:
Strength Training:
Calories Consumed:
Calories Burned:
Difference:
Weight / Body fat:

Write it down & get it done.

1
2
3
4
5
6
7
8
9
10

Read it, live it, love the results.

Exercise to avoid osteoporosis. Osteoporosis is a major cause of disability in older women, however, with exercise you may be able to avoid its destruction. Exercise increases your muscle strength, improves balance and and may keep your bone density high and your bones strong. You are in charge of your future, why not make it enjoyable?

Success is the reward of hard work.

Businessman, **Levi Straus** was only 18 when he moved from Germany to New York City to join his brothers in their dry goods business. Then, in the 1850's he moved to San Francisco to sell canvas for tents and wagons during the gold rush. Seeing a need to protect the minor's clothing, he made overalls out of the canvas. In the early 1860's he replaced the canvas with a softer material, denim, which he later dyed with indigo blue to minimize soil stains. Levi's jeans were born.

Patience, persistence and perspiration make an unbeatable combination for success.
– Napolean Hill

bent-arm pullovers

Place a large dumbbell on the floor at the head of a flat bench, then lie on the bench face up. Reaching back, grab the dumbbell. Keeping your arms bent, raise the dumbbell over your head to your chest. Then, slowly lower the dumbbell to the starting position without touching the floor. Make sure you stretch your chest and back muscles to their fullest on the way down. Complete 10-15 repetitions.

DATE

Steps Walked:
Cardio Workout:
Strength Training:
Calories Consumed:
Calories Burned:
Difference:
Weight / Body fat:

Eating healthy tastes great!

Baked Chicken Fingers
2lbs chicken breast, cut in 1" strips
1 cup wheat bread crumbs
1 cup crushed corn flakes
2 tbs brown sugar • 2 tbs olive oil
1/2 cup wheat flour • 3 eggs, beaten
pepper to taste
Preheat oven to 375^{0} F. Mix first four ingredients, place in bowl. Put flour and eggs in seperate bowls. Dip chicken in flour, then eggs, then breading. Place on cookie sheet & bake 15 minutes.

Read it, live it, love the results.

Be patient and persistent when working to achieve your desires.
All to often people start a workout routine, only to give up within a couple of weeks when they have not gotten the expected results. Those who have patience, persistence and perspiration are guaranteed success. Only when you give up can you become a failure. Realize that success does not come easy, if it did, everyone would be successful.

Write it down & get it done.

1
2
3
4
5
6
7
8
9
10

lying shrug

Lie on the bench, face down, with your chin over the edge. Straddle your legs on either side of the bench with your feet resting on the floor. With a dumbbell in each hand, let arms hang straight down with palms facing. Keeping your arms straight, pull the dumbbells up, squeezing your shoulder blades together. Hold for 2-3 counts, lower to the starting position, and repeat 10-15 times.

The truth will make you odd.
– Judy Blume

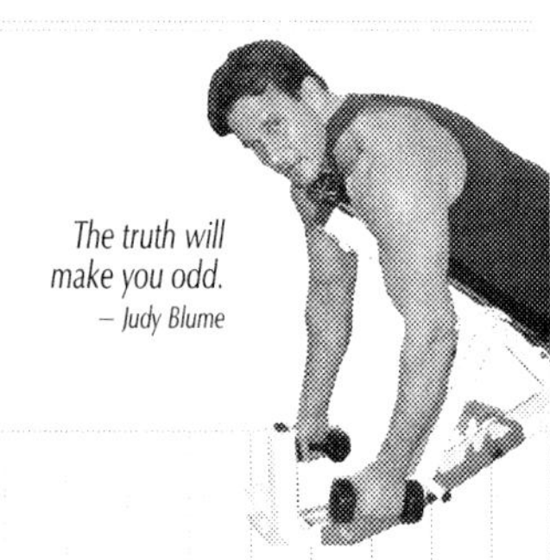

DATE

Steps Walked:

Cardio Workout:

Strength Training:

Calories Consumed:

Calories Burned:

Difference:

Weight / Body fat:

Write it down & get it done.

1

2

3

4

5

6

7

8

9

10

Read it, live it, love the results.

Exercise regularly.

Many studies have shown that exercise strengthens the heart and lungs, increases bone density, and wards off many unwanted medical issues, including diabetes, heart disease and stroke. Exercise also helps keep your weight under control, by burning calories. The more intensely you exercise, the more calories you burn — so keep your body moving and burn as many calories as possible.

Life's tough, get over it, she did!

Author, **Judy Blume**, a writer for the younger generation, began by writing stories for her own children. Her writings, which are based on real trials, made her a controversial writer and one of the most banned children's authors in the United States. Despite attempts at censorship Blume's young adult novels and books for children have sold 80 million copies world wide. She didn't let the opinions of others stop her.

What the mind of man can conceive and believe, it can achieve.
–Napolean Hill

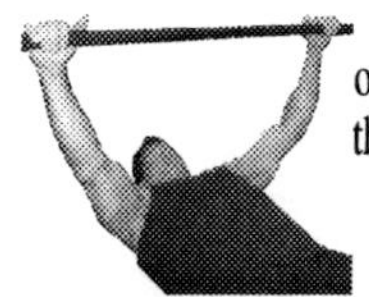

lying side to side pullup

Place a bar between two sturdy chairs, then lie on the floor face up, under the bar. Hold the bar with an overhand grip, with hands spread out wide. Slowly pull yourself up, keeping your body perfectly straight throughout the movement. Bring your chin up to touch the right side of bar. Hold here for 2-3 counts then slowly lower to starting position, then raise yourself to the left side of the bar. Repeat 10-15 times.

	DATE
Steps Walked:	
Cardio Workout:	
Strength Training:	
Calories Consumed:	
Calories Burned:	
Difference:	
Weight / Body fat:	

Eating healthy tastes great!

Raspberry Spinach Salad
3 tbs raspberry wine vinegar
3 tbs raspberry jam • 1/4 cup olive oil
8 cups baby spinach
1/4 cup macadamia nuts, chopped
1 cup fresh raspberries
3 kiwis, peeled and sliced
Whisk vinegar and jam in small bowl, add oil in thin stream, blending well; set aside. Toss remaining ingredients, then toss with dressing.

Read it, live it, love the results.

Believe in yourself.
Believe that you have the will power and knowledge to create a healthy lifestyle. See yourself as a happy, healthy person and you can become that person. Only you can change who you are. Know that you can do it, and make it happen. It's all in your attitude, no one can do it for you.

Write it down & get it done.

1
2
3
4
5
6
7
8
9
10

lying sternum pullup

Place a bar between two sturdy chairs, then lie on the floor face up, under the bar. Hold the bar with an underhand grip with hands shoulder-width apart. Slowly pull yourself up, leaning your head back and arching your back throughout the movement. Bring your lower chest or sternum up to touch the bar. Hold here for 2-3 counts then slowly lower to the starting position. Repeat 10-15 times. Keep your legs extended out straight, throughout the movement.

Do not let circumstances control you. You change your circumstances. –Jackie Chan

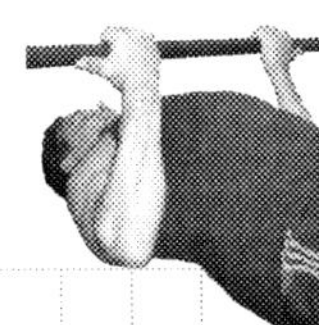

DATE

Steps Walked:
Cardio Workout:
Strength Training:
Calories Consumed:
Calories Burned:
Difference:
Weight / Body fat:

Write it down & get it done.

1
2
3
4
5
6
7
8
9
10

Read it, live it, love the results.

You can save a life with STR.
You could save the life of another by recognizing the signs of a stroke. Ask these three simple questions if you suspect someone is suffering a stroke.

S Ask the individual to **Smile.**
T Ask the person to **Talk** and repeat a simple sentence. (i.e.. It is sunny out today.)
R Ask them to **Raise** both arms straight up.

Be the change you want to see.

Actor, **Jackie Chan**, performs all of his own stunts. As a result he has broken dozens of bones in the process. However, this does not stop him from striving to be the greatest. He has become one of the best-known names worldwide in the areas of kung fu and action films. Whereas, he is known for his acrobatic fighting style, comic timing, use of improvised weapons and innovative stunts.

back

If you do not conquer self, you will be conquered by self. –Napolean Hill

one arm pullup

Place a bar between two sturdy chairs, then lie on the floor face up, under the bar. Hold the bar with the right hand using an overhand grip. The left hand may be used to help balance. Slowly pull yourself up, keeping your body perfectly straight throughout the movement, bring your chin up to touch the bar. Hold here for 2-3 counts then slowly lower and repeat 5-10 times. change hands and complete another 5-10 repetitions.

	DATE
Steps Walked:	
Cardio Workout:	
Strength Training:	
Calories Consumed:	
Calories Burned:	
Difference:	
Weight / Body fat:	

Eating healthy tastes great!

Barley and Edamame Salad
$^{2}/_{3}$ cups pearled barley
2 cups shelled edamame
1 cup carrots, shredded
3 cups cabbage, shredded
$^{1}/_{2}$ cup green onion, diced
low fat asian dressing
pepper to taste
Prepare barley and edamame according to package instructions. Toss all ingredients until dressing is evenly distributed.
Serve warm or cold.

Read it, live it, love the results.

Lower your cholesterol when you eat a diet high in fiber.
Studies show that people who ate a high-fiber diet of oats, barley, eggplant, okra, and other vegetables lowered their cholesterol by close to 30 percent after four weeks. In addition to improving digestive health and lowering cholesterol levels, a high-fiber diet can help you reduce the risk of heart disease and diabetes, and keep your weight in check. 25-35 grams of fiber are recommended daily.

Write it down & get it done.

1
2
3
4
5
6
7
8
9
10

mixed grip pullup

Place a bar between two sturdy chairs, then lie on the floor face up, under the bar. Hold the bar with an overhand grip with the right hand, an underhand grip with the left hand. Hands should be shoulder-width apart. Slowly pull yourself up, keeping your body perfectly straight throughout the movement, bring your chin up to touch the bar. Hold here for 2-3 counts then slowly lower and repeat 10 times. Change grip and complete another 10 repetitions.

A day will never be anymore than what you make of it. Practice being a "doer"!
–Josh S. Hinds

DATE

Steps Walked:
Cardio Workout:
Strength Training:
Calories Consumed:
Calories Burned:
Difference:
Weight / Body fat:

Write it down & get it done. Read it, live it, love the results. Your level of success is up to you.

1
2
3
4
5
6
7
8
9
10

Don't diet to lose weight.
There are countless diets and diet books, however most are unsuccessful in helping you lose weight in a heatlhy way, or keeping the weight off long term. *"Going on a diet"* implies that you will eventually *"go off"* the diet, regaining all of the weight you have lost. To lose weight in a healthy manner and keep it off, you must make lifestyle changes that include healthy eating and exercise.

Emmy Award-winning stand-up comedian and talk show host, **Jay Leno** a mild dyslexic, received mainly Cs and Ds in high school. When applying to Emerson College in Boston, he was denied. Determined, he sat outside the admission officers' office twelve hours a day, five days a week until he was accepted. He knew what he wanted and never gave up. With determination and drive, he moved on to become a huge success.

Cherish your visions and your dreams as they are the children of your soul; the blue prints of your ultimate accomplishments.
—Napoleon Hill

dry land breast stroke

Lie on the floor face down with hands extended out front, with legs flat on floor extended out back. Holding a dumbbell in each hand, simulate a breast stroke, as if you were in water. Bring the right hand back toward the shoulder, then lift and return to starting position. Repeat the movement with the left hand. Continue, alternating arms for 10-15 repetitions. Keep the glutes and abs tight throughout the exercise.

	DATE
Steps Walked:	
Cardio Workout:	
Strength Training:	
Calories Consumed:	
Calories Burned:	
Difference:	
Weight / Body fat:	

Eating healthy tastes great!

Cobb Salad
10 cups mixed greens
Dice or chop each ingredient for the salad; 2 chicken breasts, sautéd
2 hard-boiled eggs, 6 strips turkey bacon, 1/2 cup tomatoes, 1 large cucumber, 1 avocado, 1/4 cup onion,
3 tbsp white-wine vinegar
1 tbs dijon mustard • 1 tsp pepper
3 tbs olive oil • 1/2 cup light blue cheese
Combine vinegar, onion, mustard, pepper and oil. Mix well with greens, add remaining ingredients.

Read it, live it, love the results.

See yourself healthy and happy.
When you have visions and dreams you believe in, you will accomplish more than you ever thought possible. See yourself walking or jogging each day.
See yourself accomplishing those things which you desire most. You must have a vision of the finish line in order to reach it.

Write it down & get it done.

1
2
3
4
5
6
7
8
9
10

wall angels

Stand against a wall with feet slightly wider than shoulder-width apart, back straight, shoulders back and chest out, holding a dumbbell in each hand, bend your elbows to 90-degrees, level with your shoulders. While maintaining contact against the wall with your tailbone and shoulder blades, raise your arms above your head, keeping your elbows and wrists as close to the wall as possible. Hold for 2-3 counts at the top, then lower the dumbbells to starting position, repeat 10-15 times.

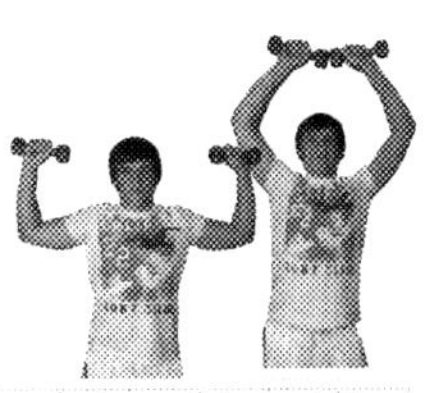

DATE

The foods that we eat today, and the foods that we feed our children, will determine the diseases that we develop tomorrow. – Delia M. Garcia M.D.

Steps Walked:
Cardio Workout:
Strength Training:
Calories Consumed:
Calories Burned:
Difference:
Weight / Body fat:

Write it down & get it done.

1
2
3
4
5
6
7
8
9
10

Read it, live it, love the results.

Think positive.
The subconscious mind makes no distinction between constructive and destructive thoughts. It only works with the information you feed it, through your thought impulses. Focus on feeding your mind only those thoughts which are positive and you will naturally aid in your growth mentally, emotionally and physically.

Doors open when least expected.

The printmaking firm, **Currier & Ives**, evolved by chance. Nathaniel Currier had begun the business, but wasn't successful until 20 years later when James Merritt Ives joined him as a bookkeeper. However, his art education led him to producing drawings. Today, original Currier and Ives prints are collectors items and modern reproductions of the prints are popular decorations.

If you want to succeed you should strike out on new paths rather than travel the worn paths of accepted success.
—John D. Rockefeller

bent over dumbbell row

Stand tall with dumbbells in each hand, palms facing forward, away from your body. Bend over at your waist, with the right foot in front of the left, knees bent, back straight, and abs tightened. From this position, lift the dumbbells up to chest height, near your hips, rotating the palms toward your body as you lift. Do not arch your back. Hold for 2-3 counts, then slowly return to starting position and repeat 10-15 times.

Steps Walked:
Cardio Workout:
Strength Training:
Calories Consumed:
Calories Burned:
Difference:
Weight / Body fat:

DATE

Eating healthy tastes great!

Chicken and Veggies
4 chicken breasts
2 tbs Mrs. Dash® original seasoning
1 tbs olive oil • 2 tbs minced garlic
1 onion and green pepper, diced
Preheat oven to 350°F. Place garlic, sliced onion and pepper in baking dish. Brush chicken with olive oil and Mrs. Dash, place on vegetables. Cover with foil, bake 15 minutes. Increase to 375°F, remove foil, turn chicken, and bake additional 15 minutes, or until chicken is done.

Read it, live it, love the results.

Be open, energetic and positive.
Successful people are not necessarily those who have the highest IQ, or who have come from wealthy families. Successful people are those who are energetic, open and positive. Change your thoughts and you can change your life. It's up to you to become the best person you can possibly be, no one can do it for you. Nor, can you blame others for your lack of success.

Write it down & get it done.

1
2
3
4
5
6
7
8
9
10

In order to succeed, your desire for success should be greater than your fear of failure.
– Bill Cosby

one-arm dumbbell row

Stand with the right foot slightly in front of the left, with the right hand resting on the right knee. Hold a dumbbell in the left hand with arm extended straight down. Keeping your back flat, pull the dumbbell up to chest height, near your hips. Hold here for 2-3 counts, then lower slowly to starting position. Focus on using the back muscles. Complete 10-15 repetitions, then perform a set on the opposite side.

DATE

Steps Walked:
Cardio Workout:
Strength Training:
Calories Consumed:
Calories Burned:
Difference:
Weight / Body fat:

Write it down & get it done.

1
2
3
4
5
6
7
8
9
10

Read it, live it, love the results.

Make education ongoing, attempt to learn something new each day.

"Many people make the mistake of assuming that, because Henry Ford had but little 'schooling,' he is not a man of 'education.' Those who make this mistake do not know Henry Ford, nor do they understand the real meaning of the word 'educate'."
–Napolean Hill

Life's tough, get over it, he did!

Comedian, actor, author, television producer and activist, **Bill Cosby**, left school after failing the tenth grade. He had been working before and after school to help out the family, it was all too much. After dropping out, he joined the Navy, and later received his GED. He then won an athletic scholarship to Temple University. While here, he worked as a bartendar and discovered his talent for comedy.

Just because you're a failure at a project, does not make you a failure at life.
– Phyllis Diller

one arm dumbbell row using a chair

Standing near a chair, place your right knee and hand on the chair, your left foot flat on the floor. Holding a dumbbell in your left hand, let the arm hang straight down, then, keeping your back flat, pull the dumbbell up to your chest. Hold here for 2-3 counts, then lower slowly to starting position and repeat. Focus on using the back muscles to move the dumbbell. Complete 10-15 repetitions, then perform a set on the opposite side.

	DATE
Steps Walked:	
Cardio Workout:	
Strength Training:	
Calories Consumed:	
Calories Burned:	
Difference:	
Weight / Body fat:	

Eating healthy tastes great!

Texas Chicken
4 chicken breasts
1 cup low sodium chicken broth
1 tbs Worcestershire sauce • 1 onion, diced
1 tsp horseradish • 1 packet Splenda®
cili powder, cayenne pepper and pepper
Preheat broiler. Place breasts in greased baking dish. Combine all remaining ingredients in saucepan and cook 10 minutes on low heat. Brush chicken with sauce, then place in broiler. Broil 10 minutes, remove, turn and brush again. Continue this until chicken is well done.

Read it, live it, love the results.

Focus on keeping your body healthy.
Though keeping your body healthy should be your top priority, many have let this priority fall from their list. Your body is a fine tuned machine which requires the best possible care, it's the only thing you are guaranteed to have for the rest of your life. Change the way you think about your body, and you'll change the way you eat.

Write it down & get it done.

1
2
3
4
5
6
7
8
9
10

close grip upright row

Stand with feet shoulder-width apart and knees slightly bent. Holding dumbbells with an overhand grip let arms hang straight down, resting on thighs. With your back straight raise the dumbbells to your chin, pressing the butts of the dumbbells together. Keep your elbows up high, lifting them above your ears. Hold for 2-3 counts, then return to starting position and repeat 10-15 times.

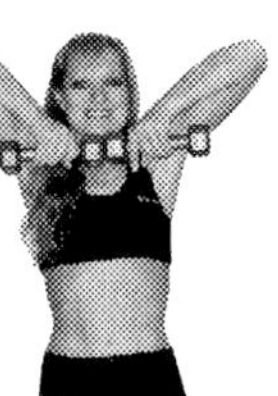

Not the senses I have but what I do with them is my kingdom.
–Helen Keller

DATE

Steps Walked:
Cardio Workout:
Strength Training:
Calories Consumed:
Calories Burned:
Difference:
Weight / Body fat:

Write it down & get it done.

1
2
3
4
5
6
7
8
9
10

Read it, live it, love the results.

Try Siberian Ginseng.
Research shows that Siberian Ginseng helps you in many ways. It boosts energy, works as an antiviral, strengthens the immune system, improves physical and mental performance, shortens recovery time after exercise or stressful situations, improves sexual function, supports the adrenal glands, increases stress resistance, extends endurance, and helps cancer patients tolerate chemotherapy treatment.

Doors open, when you work hard.

Golden Globe Award-nominated actor, **Patrick Dempsey**, famous for his role as Dr. Derek Shepherd on TV's Grey's Anatomy, actually spent several years in B-pictures and failed starts at television. However, he never gave up and today is regarded as a *"hunk"* and credible leading man. In 2007, he was ranked #2 in *People Magazine's* annual *"Sexiest Man Alive"* list.

back

Miracles sometimes occur, but one has to work terribly hard for them.
– Chaim Weizmann

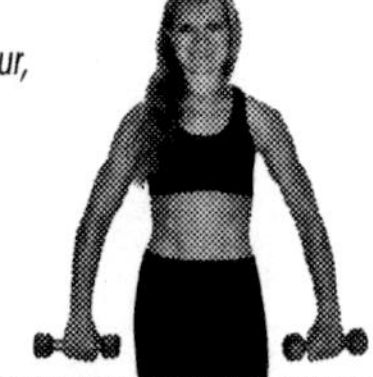

wide grip upright row

Stand with feet shoulder-width apart and knees slightly bent. Holding dumbbells with an overhand grip let arms hang straight down 4-5 inches away from thighs. With your back straight squeeze your shoulders and raise the dumbbells 3-4 inches. Hold for 2-3 counts, then return to starting position. Repeat 10-15 times.

	DATE
Steps Walked:	
Cardio Workout:	
Strength Training:	
Calories Consumed:	
Calories Burned:	
Difference:	
Weight / Body fat:	

Eating healthy tastes great!

Quesadillas
2-6" whole wheat tortilla • salsa
1/4 cup each diced; cooked chicken breast, green and red peppers, zucchini, tomatoes and onions
1/4 cup low fat monterey jack cheese
Sauté chicken and veggies, set aside. Place tortilla in skillet, top with sautéd mix and cheese, then top with another tortilla. Cook over medium heat until cheese begins to melt. Flip to brown other side.Cut into 6 triangles. Serve with salsa.

Read it, live it, love the results.

Work hard, be broad-minded, persistent and stick to a life-time of learning.
We all have the desire to be successful, though many fall short of reaching success, only because they give up too early. Successful people become successful because they have the philosphy of life-time learning, working hard to get what they want and never giving up.

Write it down & get it done.

1
2
3
4
5
6
7
8
9
10

lower back rotation
Lie on the floor, face up, arms at sides, knees bent, feet flat on the floor with shoulders pressed firmly into the floor. *(Place a dumbbell between your knees to increase the difficulty.)* Keeping your upper body still drop your knees to the right, hold here for 3 to 5 counts then rotate to the left and hold here. Repeat 10-15 times, alternating from the left to the right.

The hardships that I encountered in the past will help me succeed in the future.
— Philip Emeagwali

DATE

Steps Walked:
Cardio Workout:
Strength Training:
Calories Consumed:
Calories Burned:
Difference:
Weight / Body fat:

Write it down & get it done.

1
2
3
4
5
6
7
8
9
10

Read it, live it, love the results.

Discard negative thoughts.
When you fill your mind with positive thoughts and discard the negative, you are able to change the way you think and deal with any difficulties you may face. With a positive outlook, you will be amazed at how the problems you thought were huge will shrink down to practically nothing—allowing you to live a happier, less stressful life.

Doors open, when you work hard.

Super computing pioneer, **Philip Emeagwali**, the winner of several awards, including a Distinguished Scientist Award, came from a poor Nigerian family. He dropped out of high school because of the Nigerian-Biafran war and largely self-taught himself. After the war, he completed a high-school equivalency test through self-study and came to the United States to attend college on a scholarship. Determination and hard work brought him success.

When diet is wrong, medicine is no use; when diet is correct, medicine is of no need.
– Ancient Ayurvedic Proverb

flat leg lift

Lie on the floor, face down with your chin resting on your hands, palms down. With or without ankle weights, bend your right knee to 90-degrees, so your heel is facing the ceiling. Lift the right leg 6-8 inches off the floor, pressing your heel towards the ceiling as you press your hips into the floor. Hold here for 2-3 counts, lower, then lift your left leg and hold for 2-3 counts. Complete 10-15 repetitions of this alternating count.

DATE

Steps Walked:	
Cardio Workout:	
Strength Training:	
Calories Consumed:	
Calories Burned:	
Difference:	
Weight / Body fat:	

Eating healthy tastes great!

Cheesy Salsa Dip
8 oz package light cream cheese
15 oz can black beans, drained
4 oz can green chiles, diced
8 oz low fat monterey jack cheese
1 cup salsa
Baked tortilla chips
In microwave-safe bowl, combine all ingredients, except chips. Microwave on high 5-6 minutes, stirring every minute, until smooth and heated through. Serve with baked tortilla chips.

Read it, live it, love the results.

Build a relationship with your body.
Treat you body as if you really love it. We often treat our beloved pets better than we treat ourselves. You wouldn't dream of feeding your dog or cat a piece of chocolate cake, however you probably don't hesitate to devoure it yourself. Rule of thumb: if you wouldn't feed it to your pet, don't eat it yourself.

Write it down & get it done.

1
2
3
4
5
6
7
8
9
10

back

bent over row II

Place dumbbells on the floor in front of you, approximately 12-14 inches apart. Stand with feet shoulder-width apart with knees slightly bent. Bend down and grab the dumbbells with an overhand grip. Keeping your back parallel to the floor with a slight arch, head up, eyes looking straight ahead, slowly lift the dumbbells to the side of your chest. Hold 2-3 counts, then lower to the starting position without allowing dumbbells to touch the floor. Repeat 10-15 times.

There are two great days in a person's life…
The day we are born,
And the day we discover why.
—William Barclay

DATE

Steps Walked:
Cardio Workout:
Strength Training:
Calories Consumed:
Calories Burned:
Difference:
Weight / Body fat:

Write it down & get it done.

1
2
3
4
5
6
7
8
9
10

Read it, live it, love the results.

Eat plenty of fruit.
Studies show that fruits are fat free, low in calories, loaded with fiber, vitamins, and phytochemicals such as beta-carotene and flavonoids that may protect against heart disease and cancer. Additionally, diets rich in fruits have consistently been found to help protect against stroke, diabetes, cataracts and macular degeneration. You are in control of the foods you eat, are you making wise choices?

Life's tough, get over it, he did!

Musician and composer **Ray Charles** became blind at the age of seven. Despite this, he refused to give up his love of music. He attended a *School for the Deaf and the Blind* in St. Augustine where he developed his musical talent. During this time he performed on WFOY radio in St. Augustine. It was the first step in the making of a legend. He became one of the first African-American musicians to be given artistic control by a mainstream record company.

Whenever you do anything, act as if all the world were watching.
– Thomas Jefferson

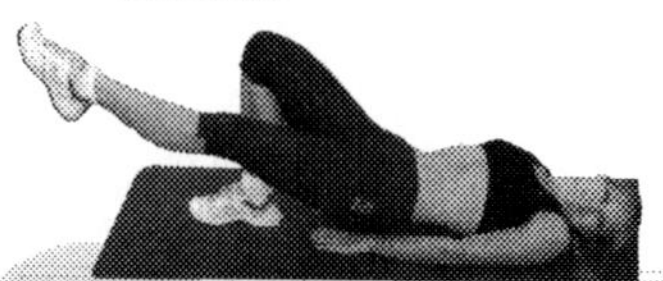

lower back leg raise

Lie on the floor, face up, arms folded across your chest or under your buttocks for support. With or without ankle weights, bend the left knee, placing the foot flat on the floor while extending the right leg out straight. As you tighten the abdominal muscles lift the right leg 5 to 12 inches off the floor. Hold here for 2-3 counts, lower and repeat 10-15 times, then complete a set with the left leg extended.

DATE

Steps Walked:
Cardio Workout:
Strength Training:
Calories Consumed:
Calories Burned:
Difference:
Weight / Body fat:

Eating healthy tastes great!

Mexican Breakfast Scramble
10 eggs • 1 green bell pepper, diced
1 onion, diced
$^1/_3$ cup skim milk
$^1/_2$ cup light cheddar cheese
$^1/_4$ cup chunky-style salsa
Saute bell pepper and onion in skillet. In bowl, mix egg, milk and pepper, then add to skillet. Once cooked, top with salsa and cheese. Cover and let set 4-5 minutes.

Read it, live it, love the results.

Enjoy a veggie scramble at least 2-3 days a week.
Fixing an omelet for breakfast takes a matter of minutes. Simply mix eggs with bell peppers, broccoli, spinach, mushrooms and/or tomatoes, place in glass bowl and microwave for two minutes. You are ready for a healthy breakfast. If you are in a big hurry, you may use frozen vegetables and/or *Egg Beaters* in an easy to pour carton.

Write it down & get it done.

1
2
3
4
5
6
7
8
9
10

reverse row

Lie on a bench, face down, with your chin over the edge. Straddle your legs on either side of the bench and place your feet on the floor. With a dumbbell in each hand, let your arms hang straight down with palms facing back. Pull the dumbbell up toward your chest, squeezing your shoulder blades together. Rotate your palms inward and keep your elbows in close to your body. Hold for 2-3 counts at the top and then slowly lower dumbbell to the starting position. Repeat 10-15 times.

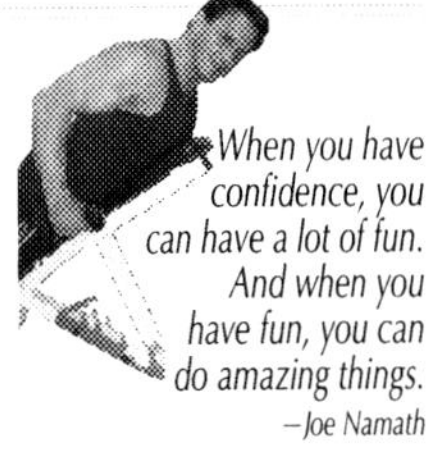

When you have confidence, you can have a lot of fun. And when you have fun, you can do amazing things.
—Joe Namath

DATE

Steps Walked:
Cardio Workout:
Strength Training:
Calories Consumed:
Calories Burned:
Difference:
Weight / Body fat:

Write it down & get it done.

1
2
3
4
5
6
7
8
9
10

Read it, live it, love the results.

Feeling stressed? Try snacking on cashews.
Studies show that cashews can improve baroreflex sensitivity. That is, when your blood pressure rises, cashews can tell your heart to calm down.
However, do keep in mind that they are high in fat and still contain calories, so don't consume the entire can at once!

Be the change you want to see.

Former St. Louis Cardinal **Mark McGwire** is best known for his home run records. During his career, he averaged a home run once every 10.61 at bats, the lowest ratio in baseball history—Babe Ruth is second with 11.80. However, perhaps even more important is the *"home run"* he has hit with many children with the *Mark McGwire Foundation for Children*, the organization which supports agencies that help children who have been sexually and physically abused.

The difficulties of life are intended to make us better, not bitter. –Mandie Ellingson

rear flye

Lie on the floor, face down with arms extended out perpendicular to your chest, holding dumbbells in each hand. Bend your elbows slightly, keeping your toes, hip bones and ribs on the floor at all times. Lift your arms 3-4 inches off the floor and hold 2-3 counts before lowering to starting position. Repeat 10-15 times.

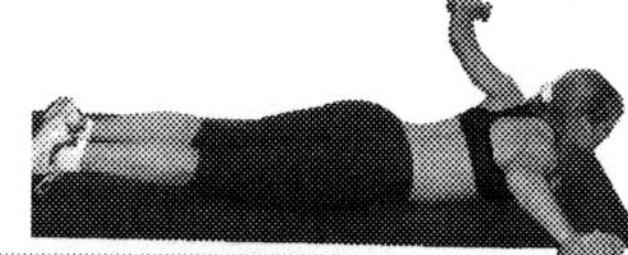

Steps Walked:

Cardio Workout:

Strength Training:

Calories Consumed:

Calories Burned:

Difference:

Weight / Body fat:

DATE

Eating healthy tastes great!

California Club Wrap

1 whole wheat low carb tortilla
$^1/_2$ turkey breast, sliced thin
2 strips turkey bacon
$^1/_2$ cup baby spinach
$^1/_4$ cup diced tomato
4 thin slices of cucumber
4 thin slices of avacado

Lay tortilla shell out flat, pile on the ingredients and roll, you have a great healthy sandwich.

Read it, live it, love the results.

Discard negative beliefs.

Negative beliefs may be keeping you from succeeding. If you believe you can't succeed, you won't succeed. When you fill your mind with negative thoughts, these thoughts will become self-fulfilled prophecy. Discard negative thoughts and fill your mind only with positive thoughts. You will be amazed how wonderful life can be when looking through "rose-colored glasses."

Write it down & get it done.

1
2
3
4
5
6
7
8
9
10

upper back press

Lie on the floor, face down with arms at sides holding dumbbells with palms facing up. Legs stretched out back with your forehead resting on the floor in alignment with the rest of your spine. Lift the dumbbells 5-10 inches, squeezing your shoulder blades together. Hold here for 2-3 counts, lower and repeat, completing 5-10 repetitions.

We come to love not by finding the perfect person, but by learning to see an imperfect person perfectly.
–Angelina Jolie

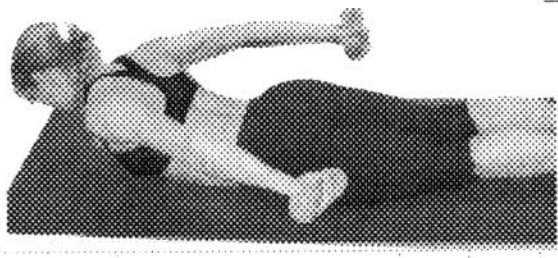

DATE

Steps Walked:

Cardio Workout:

Strength Training:

Calories Consumed:

Calories Burned:

Difference:

Weight / Body fat:

Write it down & get it done.

1

2

3

4

5

6

7

8

9

10

Read it, live it, love the results.

Replace butter and margarine with healthier choices.

Margarine often contains trans fats, which are as bad or worse than the saturated fats in butter. Olive, Canola and Soybean Oil would be much healthier choices. Studies show that these oils, which are high in omega-3 fatty acids, may help maintain normal heart function, prevent platelets from clotting, and promote healthy blood pressure.

Life's tough, get over it, she did!

Actress **Angeline Jolie**, was not always the *"beauty queen"*. While attending Beverly Hill High, Jolie was often teased by other students for wearing second-hand clothes, being extremely thin, and wearing glasses and braces. Today she is cited as one of the world's most beautiful women. She has also received three *Golden Globe Awards,* two *Screen Actors Guild Awards* and an *Academy Award.*

Building strong chest muscles not only gives you a great chiseled chest with cleavage, but also helps you perform everyday activities, such as mowing the grass and carrying laundry. As we age these "simple" tasks become more and more difficult, making it essential to maintain muscle. According to Michael J. Joyner, MD, a physiologist at Mayo Clinic in Rochester, Minnesota. "70% of 70-year-olds can't get up off the floor. They're not strong enough." Neglecting to keep yourself strong and fit is voluntarily imprisoning yourself. As you age, and muscle strength continues to decline, you will find yourself unable to sustain an independent life and having to rely upon the kindness of others to get even minor tasks completed.

DATE

Steps Walked:
Cardio Workout:
Strength Training:
Calories Consumed:
Calories Burned:
Difference:
Weight / Body fat:

Eating healthy tastes great!

Thai Tuna Salad
12 oz can tuna, drained
1/2 cup red onion, diced
1 tsp ginger
1 tsp red pepper flakes
2 tbs lime juice
1/4 cup cilantro
2 tbs olive oil
1/4 cup peanuts
white pepper to taste
Mix all ingredients. Serve chilled on bed of spinach, with rice crackers or on whole wheat toast.

Read it, live it, love the results.

Develop a desire to be healthy.
Anyone who truly understands the importance of being healthy, wants to be healthy. Though wanting and wishing will not make you healthy. You must have a true desire to be healthy, a desire so strong that it becomes an obsession. An obsession that leads you to create a healthy lifestyle plan and the persistence to stick with that plan, no matter what happens.

Write it down & get it done.

1
2
3
4
5
6
7
8
9
10

beginner pushups

If you are a beginner, perform push-ups on your hands and knees. Hands should be 6-24 inches apart. Keeping your head in line with your spine, lower your body, hovering inches above the floor. Hold for 2-3 counts, then push back to start. Repeat 10-15 times. Keep elbows out to the sides to stress the pectoral muscles. Keep at sides to work the triceps.

It is better to aim at perfection and miss, than to aim at imperfection and hit it.
— T. J. Watson, Sr.

DATE

Steps Walked:
Cardio Workout:
Strength Training:
Calories Consumed:
Calories Burned:
Difference:
Weight / Body fat:

Write it down & get it done.

1
2
3
4
5
6
7
8
9
10

Read it, live it, love the results.

Don't smoke, exercise regularly, eat plenty of fruits and vegetables, and drink alcohol in moderation.
After tracking more than 20,000 people aged 45 to 79 years in the United Kingdom from about 1993 to 2006, Kay-Tee Khaw of the University of Cambridge and colleagues found that people who adopted these four healthy habits lived an average of 14 years longer than those who didn't.

Life's tough, get over it, he did!

Welsh pop music singer **Tom Jones** had a rough start into stardom. At the age of sixteen, long before becoming a pop idol, he got married and had a son. He also dropped out of high school and took on a variety of jobs including, a builder's laborer and door-to-door vacuum salesman. Despite the rough times, he never gave up on his dreams. His desire and passion to become a singer eventually paid off.

Use incredible thoughts to manifest an incredible life. Your life will follow your thoughts. If you think it, and believe it, then you will see it.
—Hooman Hamzehloui

push-ups with elbows in

On the floor, support yourself on hands and knees just as you would a beginner pushup—with hands positioned just below your shoulders. Keeping your elbows close to your sides, drop your chest hover 1-2 inches from the floor. Hold your body in this position for 8-10 counts. Repeat 2-3 times.

	DATE
Steps Walked:	
Cardio Workout:	
Strength Training:	
Calories Consumed:	
Calories Burned:	
Difference:	
Weight / Body fat:	

Eating healthy tastes great!

Creole Chicken
4 chicken breasts, sautéed
6 slices turkey bacon, cooked
1/2 cup low fat ham, diced
2 cups okra sliced
1 cup onion, diced
2 cups tomatoes, diced
1 tsp parsley • 1/2 tsp thyme
1/2 tsp Tobasco® Sauce
2 cups water • 2 tbs minced garlic
Place all ingredients in large pot, cook on low for 30-45 minutes.

Read it, live it, love the results.

Listen to yourself.
One of the first steps to creating a healthy lifestyle is to listen to what you say and pay attention to your actions. What you say is a reflection of what you believe. When you say you cannot change your health because of your age or family history, you install this belief. Change your thoughts, and you'll change your health.

Write it down & get it done.

1
2
3
4
5
6
7
8
9
10

advanced push ups

If you are advanced, perform push-ups on your hands and toes. Hands should be 6-24 inches apart. Keeping your head in line with the spine, lower your body, hovering inches above the floor. Hold for 2-3 counts, then push back to start. Repeat 10-15 times. Keep elbows out to the sides to stress the pectoral muscles. Keep at sides to work the triceps.

Don't give up at half time.
Concentrate on winning the second half.
–Coach Paul "Bear" Bryant

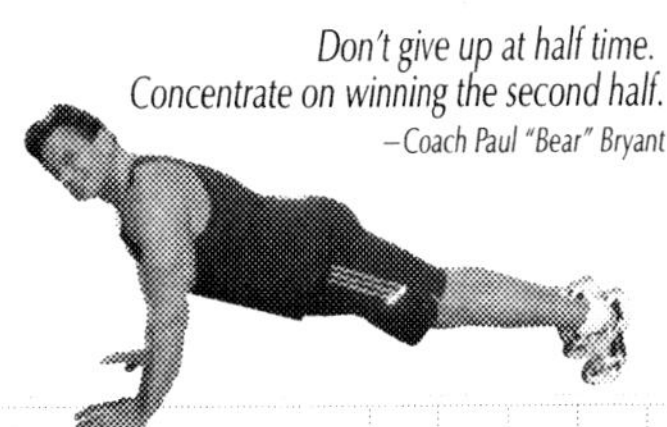

DATE

Steps Walked:
Cardio Workout:
Strength Training:
Calories Consumed:
Calories Burned:
Difference:
Weight / Body fat:

Write it down & get it done.

1
2
3
4
5
6
7
8
9
10

Read it, live it, love the results.

Try Vicks Vaporub for a cough. Studies show that you may be able to stop nighttime coughing by putting Vicks Vaporub on the bottom of the feet, then covering with socks.
Some feel this is even more effective than strong prescription cough medicines, which may cause more harm than good due to the chemical makeup of these drugs.

Doors open when least expected.

Actor **Michael Keaton** had originally sought to become a stand-up comedian, however he was unsuccessful. As a result he became a TV cameraman at a local public television station. While there he was given the opportunity to appear on the Mister Rogers Show and came to realize that he wanted to work in front of the cameras. He then headed to Los Angeles. Since then he's appeared in ten television roles and in over forty movies.

The quality of a person's life is in direct proportion to their commitment to excellence, regardless of their chosen field of endeavour.
– Vince Lombardi

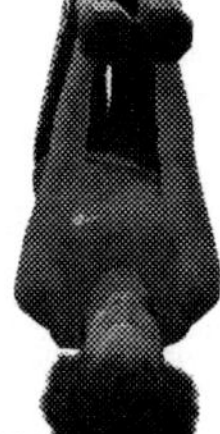

inside dumbbell press

Lie on a bench, face up, knees bent, with feet flat on bench or floor. With palms facing and a dumbbell in each hand, extend arms straight above your chest. Pressing the dumbbells together, lower them to your chest, then slowly return to starting position. Repeat 10-15 times.

DATE

Steps Walked:

Cardio Workout:

Strength Training:

Calories Consumed:

Calories Burned:

Difference:

Weight / Body fat:

Eating healthy tastes great!

Egg Foo Yung

½ cup each finely chopped; sautéd chicken breasts, cooked shrimp, mushrooms, green onions, celery and bean sprouts.
12 eggs • peanut oil

Mix all ingredients, except peanut oil. Heat peanut oil in skillet, then pour about ⅓ cup of mix into skillet. Brown 1-2 minutes on each side. Place in oven at 200°F to keep warm until each is cooked.

Read it, live it, love the results.

Take charge of your life.

Your background and circumstances may have influenced who you are, however, you are responsible for who you become. Don't live an unhealthy life simply because it's how you were brought up. You, and only you, have control over who you become. Take charge and love the control you have when you create a healthy lifestyle.

Write it down & get it done.

1
2
3
4
5
6
7
8
9
10

dumbbell bench press

Lie on a bench or the floor, face up with feet flat on the floor or bench. Holding a dumbbell in each hand, extend arms straight up with palms facing feet. Keeping your lower back pressed flat, lower dumbbells until they are at chest level, just above the shoulders, then return to starting position, pressing the ends of the dumbbells together once they reach the top. Complete 10-15 repetitions.

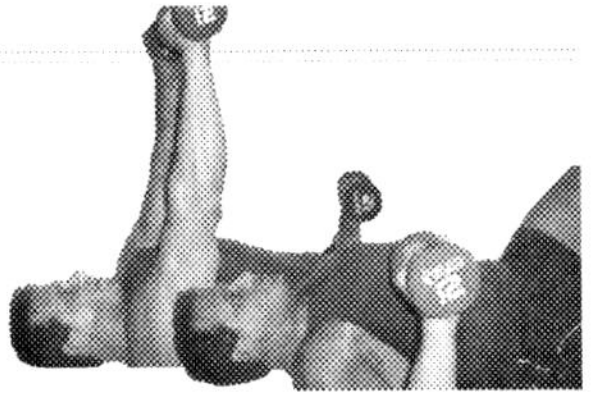

Remember this: your body is your slave; it works for you. —Jack LaLanne

DATE

Steps Walked:
Cardio Workout:
Strength Training:
Calories Consumed:
Calories Burned:
Difference:
Weight / Body fat:

Write it down & get it done.

1
2
3
4
5
6
7
8
9
10

Read it, live it, love the results.

Exercise regularly.
Studies indicate that the risk of high blood pressure increases with age. However this is not an inevitable medical condition. With regular exercise you can prevent high blood pressure, which in return reduces your risk of cardiovascular disease and stroke. If your blood pressure is already high, exercise can help you bring it back under control.

Be the change you want to see.

Founder of the Ford Motor Company and father of modern assembly lines, **Henry Ford**, was poor and uneducated when he dreamed of a horseless carriage. He went to work with the tools he possessed and now evidence of his dream encompasses the world. He has put more vehicles into operation than any man who ever lived, simply because he had a dream, and a desire to make that dream come true.

The man who can drive himself further once the effort gets painful, is the man who will win. —Roger Bannister

burpees

Stand with feet shoulder-width apart and toes pointed straight ahead. Drop to your hands in a squatting position, then push your feet back into a full push-up position. From here, pull your feet back in and stand up as quickly as you can, repeat 10-15 times. This high intensity exercise will take some practice.

	DATE
Steps Walked:	
Cardio Workout:	
Strength Training:	
Calories Consumed:	
Calories Burned:	
Difference:	
Weight / Body fat:	

Eating healthy tastes great!

Roasted-Spiced Almonds

2 cups whole almonds
1 tbs chili powder
1 tbs olive oil
½ tsp of each; ground cumin, ground coriander, cinnamon and black pepper

Preheat oven to 350ºF. Mix all ingredients, except almonds. Add almonds and toss to coat. Place in baking pan and bake about 10 minutes or until almonds are toasted, stirring twice.

Read it, live it, love the results.

Give your immune system a boost when you eat foods rich in vitamin E.

Vitamin E gives your immune system a powerful defense against free radicals which can challenge your immunity; it also reduces production of certain prostaglandins that interfere with the work of T cells. Good sources of Vitamin E include wheat germ, sunflower seeds, pine nuts, sun-dried tomatoes and almonds.

Write it down & get it done.

1
2
3
4
5
6
7
8
9
10

straight arm flye
Lie on the floor, face up, arms extended straight above the chest with a dumbbell in each hand, palms pressed together. Keeping your arms fairly straight, with a slight bend in the elbows, open your arms, bringing the dumbbells down to your sides 1-2 inches above the floor. Hold here for 2-3 counts, then return to the starting position, pressing the dumbells together above your chest. Complete10-15 repetitions.

A lot of people are afraid to say what they want. That's why they don't get what they want.
–Madonna

DATE

Steps Walked:
Cardio Workout:
Strength Training:
Calories Consumed:
Calories Burned:
Difference:
Weight / Body fat:

Write it down & get it done.

1
2
3
4
5
6
7
8
9
10

Read it, live it, love the results.

Keep your fitness program exciting.
Don't let yourself get bored with your workout or the healthy foods you eat. Check-out local and national resources for healthy activities and organizations, try new exercise equipment, eat new low-fat foods and continually set new goals. If you can keep it exciting, you are more likely maintain a healthy lifestyle.

Be the change you want to see.

Recording artist and entertainer **Madonna**, moved to New York City in 1977 to pursue a dance career. She said, *"When I came to New York, it was the first time I'd ever taken a plane, the first time I'd ever gotten a taxi-cab, the first time for everything. And I came here with $35 in my pocket. It was the bravest thing I'd ever done."* She didn't let fear stop her from achieving her dreams. Today she's noted as the world's most successful female recording artist of all time.

Every block of stone has a statue inside it and it is the task of the sculptor to discover it.
—Michelangelo

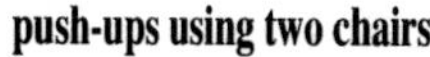

push-ups using two chairs

Using two sturdy chairs, place them facing each other, with enough space between so that you may drop your chest between them. With a hand on each chair, extend your legs straight out behind you, balancing on your toes. With head in line with the spine and elbows out to sides, lower your body, to the chair seat level, or slightly below. Hold for 2-3 counts, then push back to start. Repeat 10-15 times.

	DATE
Steps Walked:	
Cardio Workout:	
Resistance Workout:	
Calories Consumed:	
Calories Burned:	
Difference:	
Weight / Body fat:	

Eating healthy tastes great!

Mediterranean Tuna Spread

6 1/2 oz tuna, drained
1/2 cup low fat cottage cheese
1/2 cup fat free mayonnaise
2 tbs lemon juice
1 tsp Dijon mustard
1 tsp dried tarragon

In food processor, blend tuna, cottage cheese, mayonnaise, lemon juice, tarragon and mustard. Serve chilled.

Read it, live it, love the results.

Make each day a day to work on your masterpiece—your body. Michelangelo did not create his masterpieces in a day or even weeks, they took time. Imagine your body a huge piece of stone to be sculpted. Instead of using a chisel, you will use healthy eating and workout habits. Take photos along the way, and watch the progress as the weeks pass.

Write it down & get it done.

1
2
3
4
5
6
7
8
9
10

push-ups against wall
Standing 2-3 feet from a wall with feet shoulder-width apart, lean into the wall placing your hands on the wall 6-24 inches apart. Keeping your head in line with your spine and holding your elbows out to sides, lower your body, hovering inches from the wall. Hold for 2-3 counts, then push back to starting position. Repeat 10-15 times.

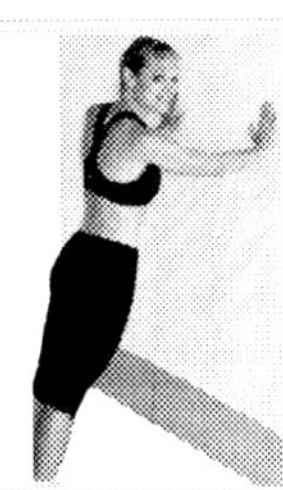

Here's proof that if you live long enough, anything is possible.
—Barry Manilow

DATE

Steps Walked:
Cardio Workout:
Strength Training:
Calories Consumed:
Calories Burned:
Difference:
Weight / Body fat:

Write it down & get it done.

1
2
3
4
5
6
7
8
9
10

Read it, live it, love the results.

Let your imagination go wild. The quality of any given item, depends upon the quality of imagination and judgement that goes into creating that item. Let your imagination go wild. Don't limit yourself to that which you think you can achieve, shoot for that which you never thought attainable. You will be amazed at what happens when you don't set limits on yourself.

Doors open when least expected.

Singer-songwriter, musician, **Barry Manilow**, was raised by his mother and grandparents after his parents divorced when he was two. It was they who encouraged him to take up his first musical instrument. Later, when his mother remarried, it was his stepfather who introduced him to jazz and swing and gave him a piano for his thirteenth birthday. Manilow went on to become very successful, with album sales of more than 76 million worldwide.

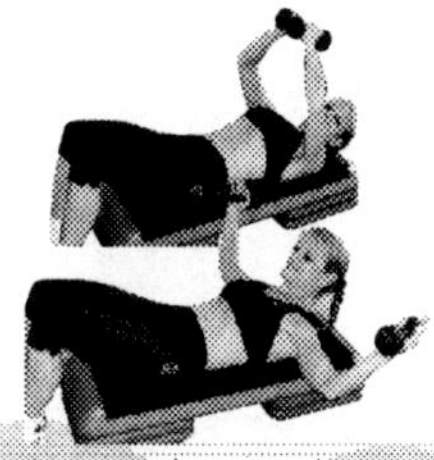

crunch and flye

Lie on a bench, face up, with knees bent, feet flat on the floor. Hold a dumbbell in each hand above your chest with palms facing in. Keeping elbows slightly bent, lower your arms outward until the elbows are just below the level of the bench. Contract your abs and crunch, lifting your shoulders, head and neck 3-4 inches off bench. At the same time, bring arms back to starting position. Imagine you are hugging a big barrel. Lower slowly and repeat 10-15 times.

	DATE
Steps Walked:	
Cardio Workout:	
Strength Training:	
Calories Consumed:	
Calories Burned:	
Difference:	
Weight / Body fat:	

All that mankind needs for good health and healing is provided by God in nature... the challenge to science is to find it.
—Paracelsus, the father of Pharacology

Eating healthy tastes great!

Refreshing Frozen Fruit Salad

1/2 cup each diced; peaches, strawberries, cherries and blackberries.
9 oz can crushed pineapple, drained
1 cup blueberries
1/4 cup Sweet & Low®
2 tbs lemon juice
1 pint fat free sour cream
Blend sour cream, Sweet & Low®, and lemon juice in blender.
Pour into 9" pan, stir in fruit and freeze until firm.

Read it, live it, love the results.

Eat even more fish, fruits and vegetables when injured.

Studies show that the phytochemicals and omegas found in fruits, vegetables and fish serve as powerful, anti-inflammatories which help your body heal. If you ignore inflammation you may be putting yourself at risk for artery, nerve cell and immune system damage. Inflammation also attributes to Alzheimer's, obesity, diabetes and heart disease.

Write it down & get it done.

1
2
3
4
5
6
7
8
9
10

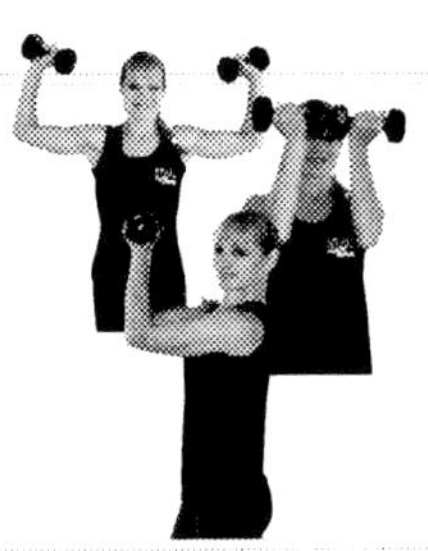

butterfly chest press
Stand with feet shoulder-width apart, one foot slightly in front of the other, shoulders back, chest out and abs in. With a dumbbell in each hand, hold arms straight out to sides, elbows bent 90-degrees with palms facing forward. Bring the arms together, rotating the dumbbells so palms face body and the ends butt together. Squeezing the elbows and dumbbell butts together, hold for 2-3 counts, then return to starting position. Repeat 10-15 times.

DATE

To be a leader, you have to make people want to follow you, and nobody wants to follow someone who doesn't know where he is going. –Joe Namath

Steps Walked:
Cardio Workout:
Strength Training:
Calories Consumed:
Calories Burned:
Difference:
Weight / Body fat:

Write it down & get it done.

1
2
3
4
5
6
7
8
9
10

Read it, live it, love the results.

Keep nutrition in your foods until they are eaten.
Here are a few tips in maintaining the nutritional value of foods.

- Keep fruit and vegetables cool.
- Do not slice or dice until needed– unless you freeze them.
- Use a minimum amount of water when cooking.
- Use low temperature methods of cooking. (ie: bake instead of frying)
- Cook as little as possible, eat as many foods raw as possible.

Be the change you want to see.

Hall of Fame quarterback **Joe Namath** was rejected by Maryland University because his college-board scores were 20 points below the school's requirements. Futunately, the University of Alabama offered him a full-ride scholarship. During his time at Alabama, he led the team to a 29–4 record over three seasons, and a *National Championship* in 1964. Despite a serious knee injury his senior year, Namath was drafted by both football leagues!

Great people talk about ideas. Average people talk about events. Small people talk about other people.
—Tobias S. Gibson

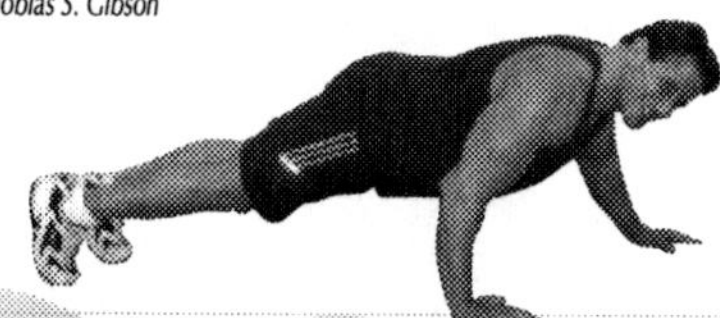

offset push-up

On the floor support yourself on hands and toes just as you would an advanced push-up, with hand positioned just below shoulders. Move the left hand back towards your abs 4-6 inches. Complete 10-15 push-ups with hands in this position, then change the position of the hands and perform an additional 10-15 repetitions.

DATE

Steps Walked:

Cardio Workout:

Strength Training:

Calories Consumed:

Calories Burned:

Difference:

Weight / Body fat:

Eating healthy tastes great!

Grilled Asparagus
1 bunch asparagus, *about 22 spears with ends trimmed*
2 tsp olive oil • pepper to taste
cooking spray and aluminum foil
Layer 2 large sheets of foil, folding sides up to form edges. Coat with cooking spray. Place asparagus on foil in single layer, don't overlap. Drizzle olive oil over each spear. Salt and pepper to taste. Place on grill, away from direct heat. Cook 10 minutes until tender.

Read it, live it, love the results.

Try asparagus for kidney, rheumatic and arthritic pains.
A remedy used by many of the "old-timers" may be just what you need to relieve the pain.
How does it work? Chemists have reported that the juice of the asparagus helps break up the oxalic acid crystals in the kidneys as well as elsewhere in the muscles of the body.

Write it down & get it done.

1
2
3
4
5
6
7
8
9
10

suicide pushup

Success is a journey, not a destination.
– Ben Sweetland

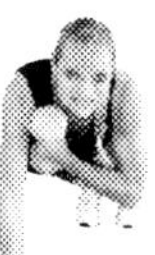

On the floor, support yourself on knees with hands holding 5-10 pound dumbbells positioned just below your shoulders, similar to a beginner push-up. Perform a push-up, keeping elbows close to your body, drop your chest to within 2-3 inches of the floor, then push back up. As you straighten your arms, lift the right dumbbell to the left side of your chest, then the left dumbbell to the right side of your chest, holding each up for 2-3 counts; then complete another push-up and repeat the movement. Complete 10-15 repetitions.

DATE

Steps Walked:
Cardio Workout:
Strength Training:
Calories Consumed:
Calories Burned:
Difference:
Weight / Body fat:

Write it down & get it done.

1
2
3
4
5
6
7
8
9
10

Read it, live it, love the results.

Diabetics MUST exercise regularly. Studies show that having diabetes increases your risk of high blood pressure, heart attack, stroke and other cardiovascular diseases. Exercise counteracts the risk by improving blood flow, increasing your heart's pumping power and improving your cholesterol levels.

Life's tough, get over it, he did!

Author, political activist, and lecturer **Helen Keller** became deaf and blind when she was just ninteen months old. Despite this, she became the first deafblind person to earn a Bachelor of Arts degree, she never let her handicap get in the way. In addition to being a well traveled, prolific author, she became a member of the Socialist Party USA and the Wobblies. She campaigned against the war, for women's suffrage, workers' rights, and socialism, as well as many other leftist causes.

There's only one corner of the universe you can be certain of improving, and that's your own self.
—Aldous Huxley

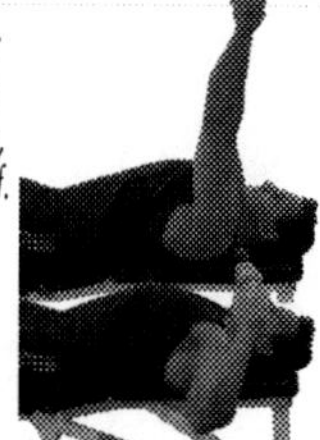

dumbbell neck press

Lie on a bench, face up with feet flat on the floor or on bench. Holding a dumbbell in each hand, with palms facing feet, extend arms straight up. Keeping your back pressed into the bench, lower dumbbells until they are even with your neck. Hold 2-3 counts, then return to the starting position, pressing the ends of the dumbbells together once you reach the top. Complete 10-15 repetitions.

	DATE
Steps Walked:	
Cardio Workout:	
Strength Training:	
Calories Consumed:	
Calories Burned:	
Difference:	
Weight / Body fat:	

Eating healthy tastes great!

Tuna Tarts

3 1/2 oz water-packed tuna, drained
2 eggs • 1/4 cup fat free sour cream
1/4 tsp Dijon mustard
1/4 tsp oregano
1 tbs whole wheat breadcrumbs
Preheat oven to 400ºF. Mix tuna, eggs, sour cream, mustard and oregano. Spray 2-cup casserole dish with nonstick cooking spray, then coat with bread crumbs. Add the tuna mixture. Bake 25 minutes until firm.

Read it, live it, love the results.

Read as much as you can on health and fitness.

The more you know about your body, the more prepared you are to take care of your body. When you know the negative results of eating certain foods, you may be less inclined to eat them, therefore, reducing your risk of disease. When you know the benefits of exercise, you may be more likely to stay active.

Write it down & get it done.

1
2
3
4
5
6
7
8
9
10

lying angel

Lie on a bench, face up with legs extended straight out. With a dumbbell in each hand, hold them at sides, hovering just above the floor with palms facing body. Keeping the dumbbells hovering, make a big circle, moving the dumbbells above your head. As you do this, lift your legs 1-2" and open them into a big inverted "V". Without letting the legs or arms return to the floor, hold here for 2-3 counts then return to starting position and repeat. If you can, don't allow the arms or legs to touch the floor throughout the entire exercise. Complete 10-15 repetitions.

DATE

I always want to learn but I am sure on my dying day I will feel like I left something in the bucket. – Tim McGraw

Steps Walked:

Cardio Workout:

Strength Training:

Calories Consumed:

Calories Burned:

Difference:

Weight / Body fat:

Write it down & get it done.

1
2
3
4
5
6
7
8
9
10

Read it, live it, love the results.

Watch your alcohol intake. Studies show that alcohol is the liver's worst enemy—however problems are not often detected until ninety percent of the liver is destroyed. Alcohol detroys liver cells, which the liver then regenerates, and in doing so, produces connective tissue. This over-abundance of connective tissue results in the blockage of circulation through the liver and eventually liver failure.

Be the change you want to see.

Country musician **Tim McGraw** went to college on a baseball scholarship to study sports medicine. While there he learned to play guitar, frequently performing for tips, though he claims his friends often hid the guitar because he was so bad. When his hero Keith Whitley died, McGraw dropped out of college and went to Nashville to follow his dream. It was one of the best decisions he ever made.

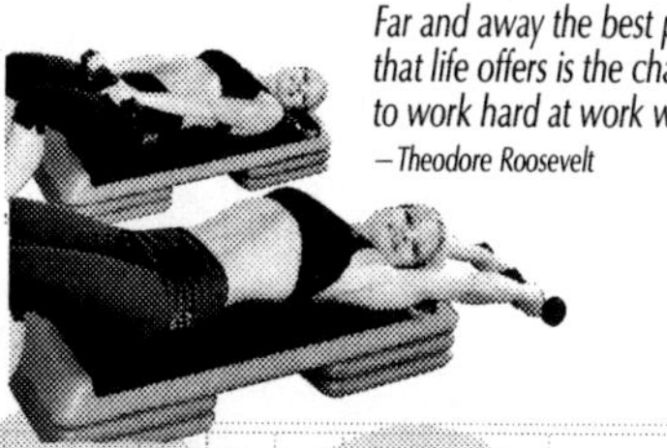

Far and away the best prize that life offers is the chance to work hard at work worth doing.
—Theodore Roosevelt

front raise with pullover

Lie on a bench, face up with feet flat on the floor. Holding dumbbells, let your hands rest on your upper thighs with palm down. Keeping your arms straight, raise the dumbbells over your head, then lower behind your head as far as possible. Hold here for 2-3 counts then return to the starting position. Repeat 10-15 times.

	DATE
Steps Walked:	
Cardio Workout:	
Strength Training:	
Calories Consumed:	
Calories Burned:	
Difference:	
Weight / Body fat:	

Eating healthy tastes great!

Honey Italian Grilled Chicken
4 chicken breasts
1/2 cup honey
1/2 cup Italian dressing

Combine honey and Italian dressing, pour over chicken. Marinate overnight. Grill 5-8 minutes on each side or until chicken is fully cooked.

Read it, live it, love the results.

Don't mistake activity for achievement.
When you take the time to workout, make it count. Don't spend a half-hour walking on the treadmill at a speed of 1.5 if it takes 3.5 to get your heart rate up. Your time is very valuable, use it wisely. Remember, you get out of your workout what you put into it. When you intensify your workouts you will burn many more calories, and isn't that what you want?

Write it down & get it done.

1
2
3
4
5
6
7
8
9
10

plyo-pushup

On the floor support yourself on hands and toes just as you would an advanced push-up, with hands positioned just below shoulders. Keeping your elbows close to your body, drop your chest to within 2-3 inches of the floor then push up explosively lifting both hands off the floor, clapping and returning to floor. Complete 10-15 push-ups in this manner.

You can grow without destroying the things that you love.
–Ed McMahon

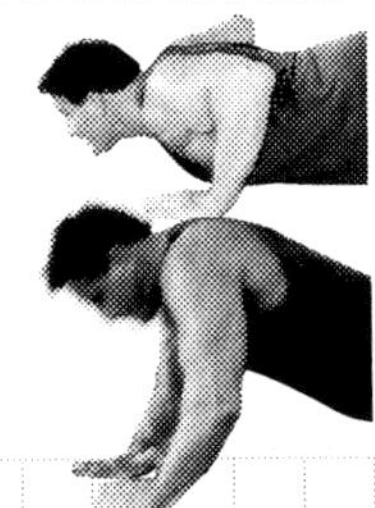

DATE

Steps Walked:
Cardio Workout:
Strength Training:
Calories Consumed:
Calories Burned:
Difference:
Weight / Body fat:

Write it down & get it done.

1
2
3
4
5
6
7
8
9
10

Read it, live it, love the results.

Try cloves to stop smoking. Some have found cloves to be beneficial in giving up smoking. Studies show that the nicotine taste left in the mouth after smoking is one of the causes for reaching for another. Cloves have a neutralizing effect on this taste. Keep a small clove branch in your mouth for a couple hours, discard and use another fresh branch. This inexpensive method is certainly worth trying to improve your health.

Doors open, when you work hard.

TV personality **Ed McMahon**, best known as Johnny Carson's sidekick, had begun his "*showbiz*" career as a bingo caller at the young age of fifteen. He also worked as a carnival barker for three years when he was teenager. Then, to pay his way through college, he worked as a pitchman for vegetable slicers on the Atlantic City boardwalk. He knew what he wanted and he worked hard to achieve everything he desired.

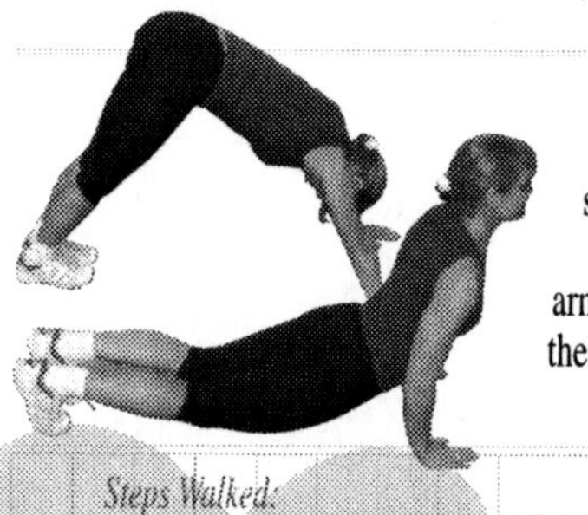

downward facing dog push-up

On the floor, start in downward-facing dog position with hands slightly wider than shoulder-width apart, hips up, balancing on toes with heels pressing down. Slowly push chest forward and through arms, bringing the chest between your hands, with hips 2-3 inches off the floor, arch your back . Hold this position for 2-3 counts, then push yourself back to starting position, completing 10-15 repetitions.

DATE

Steps Walked:
Cardio Workout:
Strength Training:
Calories Consumed:
Calories Burned:
Difference:
Weight / Body fat:

One important key to success is self-confidence. An important key to self-confidence is preparation. —Arthur Ashe

Eating healthy tastes great!

Baked Salmon with Herbs
2 lbs salmon fillets
1/2 cup onion, finely diced
2 tbs minced garlic
1 tbs parsley
1/2 tps each; basil, thyme, oregeno and pepper
1/4 cup light butter, softened
3 tbs lemon juice
Place salmon in baking pan. Combine remaining ingredients and spread over salmon. Bake 25-30 minutes, until fish flakes.

Read it, live it, love the results.

Salmon may help reduce your LDL cholesterol.
Salmon is a great source of protein and omega-3 fatty acids, which has been shown to decrease LDL cholesterol and raise HDL cholesterol.
The American Heart Association recommends eating at least two servings of fish a week, particularly fatty fish such as salmon.

Write it down & get it done.

1
2
3
4
5
6
7
8
9
10

reverse dumbbell flye

Lie on a bench, face up with feet flat on the floor. With a dumbell in each hand, extend arms up with elbows bent, as if wrapped around a big barrel, palms facing feet. Keeping your lower back pressed into the bench, lower dumbbells until they are slightly below chest level. Hold for 2-3 counts, then return to the starting position, pressing the ends of the dumbbells together once you reach the top. You should be able to feel your chest rise. Complete 10-15 repetitons.

Put your trust in the Lord and go ahead. Worry gets you no place. *– Roy Acuff*

DATE

Steps Walked:
Cardio Workout:
Strength Training:
Calories Consumed:
Calories Burned:
Difference:
Weight / Body fat:

Write it down & get it done.

1
2
3
4
5
6
7
8
9
10

Read it, live it, love the results.

Exercise to lower blood pressure. Studies show that a stronger heart can pump more blood with less effort, reducing the force and pressure that's exerted on your arteries. Becoming more active can lower your blood pressure by an average of 10 millimeters of mercury (mm Hg). That's the same effect as some blood pressure medications, making it possible for many to stop taking medications once they start working out.

Doors open when least expected.

Country musician **Roy Acuff** was known around the world as the "King of Country Music." Ironically, baseball was his first love. He played semi-professional, however, a sunstroke in 1929 and a nervous breakdown in 1930 ended his aspirations to play for the New York Yankees. This turned out to be a great new beginning. Roy, turning his attention to his father's fiddle, played in a traveling medicine show, and became one of the greatest musicians of his time.

If constructive thoughts are planted positive outcomes will be the result. Plant the seeds of failure and failure will follow.
–Sidney Madwed

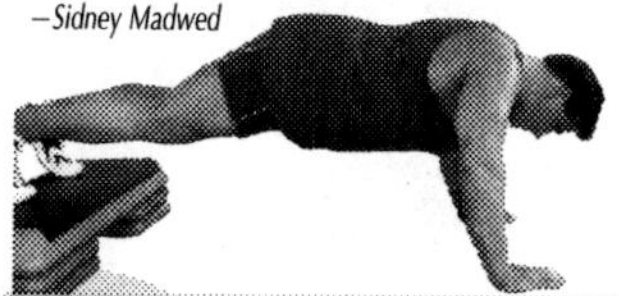

push-ups with feet elevated

On the floor, support yourself on your hands, with toes resting on step, just as you would an advanced push-up. Hands are positioned 6-24 inches apart. Lower your body, touching your chin to the floor, hold for 2-3 counts, then press yourself upwards, fully extending your elbows, as you return to the start position. Complete10-15 repetitions.

Steps Walked:
Cardio Workout:
Strength Training:
Calories Consumed:
Calories Burned:
Difference:
Weight / Body fat:

DATE

Eating healthy tastes great!

Garlic Mashed Potatoes
4 cups potatoes, cubed
2 tbs minced garlic
1/3 cup skim milk
1 tbs light butter
2 tbs Parmesan cheese
black pepper to taste

Boil garlic and potatoes, then simmer 20 minutes and drain. Add remaining ingredients and blend with mixer.

Read it, live it, love the results.

Try garlic to reduce High Blood Pressure.
If you suffer from hypertensive high blood pressure, garlic may be a helpful addition to your diet. Though not all people respond as well as others, many have found this old-time remedy to be very beneficial. You may take garlic capsules or use liberally on the foods you would normally eat.

Write it down & get it done.

1
2
3
4
5
6
7
8
9
10

squat thrusts with pushup

Stand with your feet 3-5 inches apart, shoulders back, chest out and abs in. Drop down, placing your palms on the floor, simultaneously kicking your feet out behind you into a pushup position. Perform a full body pushup, then bring your body back to the squatting position and stand. Repeat 10-15 times.

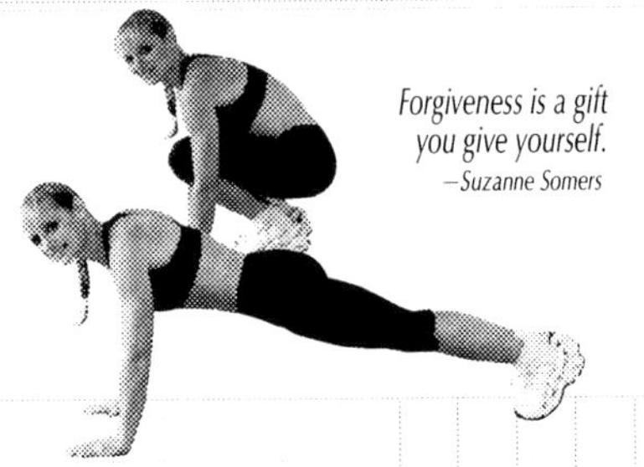

Forgiveness is a gift you give yourself.
—Suzanne Somers

DATE

Steps Walked:
Cardio Workout:
Strength Training:
Calories Consumed:
Calories Burned:
Difference:
Weight / Body fat:

Write it down & get it done.

1
2
3
4
5
6
7
8
9
10

Read it, live it, love the results.

Eat healthy, it's not as difficult as you might think.
Simply eat a variety of foods, including vegetables, fruits and whole-grain products, lean meats, poultry, fish, beans, low fat dairy products and, drink plenty of water. Avoid too much salt, sugar, alcohol, saturated fat and trans fats. The rewards you reap from eating healthy far outweigh the instant gratification you receive from eating foods which destroy your body.

Life's tough, get over it, she did!

Actress and author **Suzanne Somers**, best known for her role on *Three's Company*, grew up with an alcoholic father—who she would often hide from, when he would become violent. It was these life events that she based her first autobiography, *Keeping Secrets*. This autobiography eventually became a made-for-TV-movie starring Somers herself. Remember, it's not what happens to you that matters, it's how you respond.

The way to gain a good reputation, is to endeavor to be what you desire to appear.
– Socrates

stepped push-up

On the floor near a step or bench, support yourself on hands and toes just as you would an advanced pushup, or on your knees as you would a beginner pushup. With one hand on the step, place the other hand on the floor. Slowly lower your body to within inches of the floor, then press back to starting position. Complete 10-15, then change the position of the hands and perform an additional 10-15 repetitions.

	DATE
Steps Walked:	
Cardio Workout:	
Strength Training:	
Calories Consumed:	
Calories Burned:	
Difference:	
Weight / Body fat:	

Eating healthy tastes great!

Exotic Chicken Salad
4 chicken breasts, sautéd and diced
1/2 cup each, diced;
celery, green pepper and onion
2 cups concord grapes, halved
2 cups pineapple chunks, drained
1 cup almonds, slivered
2/3 cup fat free mayonnaise
1/4 cup fat free sour cream
2 tbs vinegar • pepper to taste
Combine all ingredients, chill, serve over a bed of lettuce with celery sticks on the side.

Read it, live it, love the results.

Celery may relieve your arthritis pain and stiffness.
Celery, which contains sodium, potassium, calcium, chlorine, phosphorus, sulfur, magnesium and iron – in addition to vitamins A, B, C and E, can do wonders for your body. Studies show that drinking six ounces of celery juice a day may help severe arthritis stiffness. You may also get these benefits by eating the leaves and stalks.

Write it down & get it done.

1
2
3
4
5
6
7
8
9
10

dumbbell flyes

The beautiful thing about learning is nobody can take it away from you.
—B. B. King

Lie on a bench, or the floor face up with feet flat on the floor or bench. With a dumbbell in each hand and palms facing, extend arms up with elbows bent, as if wrapped around a big barrel. Keeping your lower back pressed into the bench and elbows bent, lower dumbbells until they are slightly below chest level. Hold for 2-3 counts, then return to starting position, pressing the dumbbells together once you reach the top. You should be able to feel your chest rise. Complete 10-15 repetitions.

DATE

Steps Walked:
Cardio Workout:
Strength Training:
Calories Consumed:
Calories Burned:
Difference:
Weight / Body fat:

Write it down & get it done.

1
2
3
4
5
6
7
8
9
10

Read it, live it, love the results.

Get rid of clutter in your life.
What you own soon owns you. Having too much clutter in your life consumes much of your energy for cleaning and maintenance, in addition to making you disorganized and increasing your stress level.Cut back and let go. A good rule of thumb is *"anything you haven't used in six months can be given away to a charity."*
It will do your body good, as well as benefit others.

Doors open, when you work hard.

American blues guitarist **B. B. King**, didn't do so well on his first trip to Memphis. He tried to work as a musician but was rejected, and after a few months of hardship, went back to Mississippi. However, he didn't give up on his dream, instead, he worked to improve himself, then returned to Memphis two years later. As a result, he became one of the greatest guitarists of all time. Rolling Stone magazine named him the third out of the "Top 100 greatest."

Life's like a boom-a-rang. The more good you throw out, the more you receive in return.
—Josh S. Hinds

push-ups on chair

Place a sturdy chair against a wall. Place your hands on the chair, extending your legs straight out behind you, balancing on your toes. Hands should be at least six inches apart, though you may also spread them as far apart as the chair permits. With head in line with the spine and elbows out to sides, lower your body, hovering inches above the chair seat. Hold for 2-3 counts, then push back to the starting position. Repeat 10-15 times.

DATE

Steps Walked:
Cardio Workout:
Strength Training:
Calories Consumed:
Calories Burned:
Difference:
Weight / Body fat:

Eating healthy tastes great!

Fresh Mushroom Salad
1 lb fresh mushrooms, sliced
6 green onions, minced
1/2 cup low fat sour cream
1/4 tsp Sweet and Low®
salt and white pepper
Combine 2 cups water and 2 tsp lemon juice in pan, bring to boil. Add mushrooms, cover, simmer three minutes, drain, then cool. Once mushrooms have cooled combine all ingredients and chill. Serve over a bed of lettuce.

Read it, live it, love the results.

Focus on the positive.
When you focus on good thoughts and actions, you will of course produce good results. However, focus on bad thoughts and actions, and you will ultimately produce bad results. It's a basic principle, unfortunately there are many who choose the bad over the good. Which do you choose?

Write it down & get it done.

1
2
3
4
5
6
7
8
9
10

dumbbell flye crossover Lie on a bench, face up with feet flat on the floor or on the bench. With a dumbbell in each hand and palms facing, extend arms up with elbows bent, as if wrapped around a big barrel. Drop arms, crossing the right in front of left, with elbows lined up. Drop dumbbells slightly below chest level. Hold for 2-3 counts, then return to the starting position. Be careful not to hit fingers with dumbells as you cross them. Complete 10-15 repetitons.

Winners, I am convinced, imagine their dreams first. They want it with all their heart and expect it to come true. There is, I believe, no other way to live.
—Joe Montana

DATE

Steps Walked:
Cardio Workout:
Strength Training:
Calories Consumed:
Calories Burned:
Difference:
Weight / Body fat:

Write it down & get it done.

1
2
3
4
5
6
7
8
9
10

Read it, live it, love the results.

Take responsibility.
When you blame your circumstances on outside conditions, you will never be able to take control and make changes in your life. Knowing you are in control of what happens to you gives you the power to change and grow in a positive manner. When you blame your misfortunes on others, you give them the power to control your life. This is not the way you want to live.

Doors open, when you work hard.

Pro Football Hall of Famer **Joe Montana** wasn't always in the spotlight. He spent much time on the bench his first two years of high school. Then in his junior and senior years he was starting quarterback. His hard work, talent and dedication earned him a scholarship to play for Notre Dame University—after which he went pro. In 1999, he was ranked third in The Sporting News *"Football's 100 Greatest Players."*

A gem cannot be polished without friction, nor man perfected without trials.
– Chinese Proverb

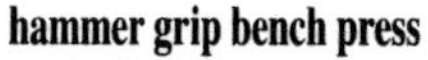

hammer grip bench press

Lie on a bench or the floor, face up with feet flat on the floor or bench. Holding a dumbbell in each hand, extend arms straight up with palms facing each other. Keeping your lower back pressed into the bench, lower the dumbbells until they are at chest level, just above the shoulders, then return to starting position. Complete 10-15 repetitions.

	DATE
Steps Walked:	
Cardio Workout:	
Strength Training:	
Calories Consumed:	
Calories Burned:	
Difference:	
Weight / Body fat:	

Eating healthy tastes great!

Broccoli-Cauliflower Salad

1 cup broccoli florets
1 cup cauliflower florets
2 hard boiled eggs, diced
1 cup shredded low fat mozzarella
1/4 cup raisins
1/4 cup sunflower seeds
1 cup fat free mayonnaise
1/4 cup Splenda®
2 tbs white wine vinegar

Whisk mayonnaise, Splenda® and vinegar. Mix well with other ingredients, then chill.

Read it, live it, love the results.

Embrace positive thoughts, your attitude and health will follow.

Many people find themselves eating unhealthy when they are feeling down and depressed. This is not unusual. Studies show that when an individual is happy, they are more likely to treat their body well and eat healthy. *"Each of us literally chooses, by his way of attending to things, what sort of universe he shall appear to himself to inhabit." – William James*

Write it down & get it done.

1
2
3
4
5
6
7
8
9
10

flat chest press

Lie on a bench or the floor, face up with feet flat on the floor or bench. Hold a dumbbell in each hand with elbows bent at 90-degrees, parallel to the floor with palms facing up.Bring the arms together so dumbbells and elbows touch just above chest. Squeezing them together, hold for 2-3 counts, then return to starting position. Repeat 10-15 times.

No matter what people tell you, words and ideas can change the world.
– Robin Williams

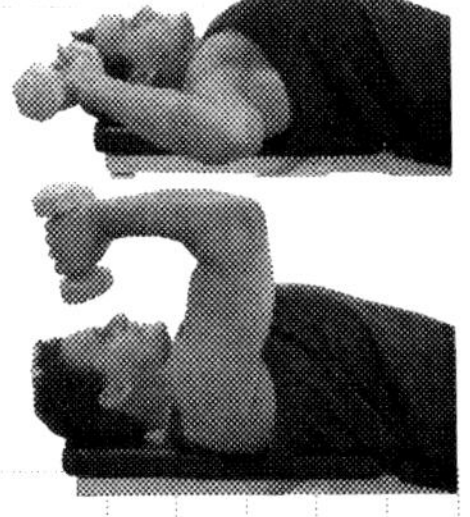

DATE

Steps Walked:
Cardio Workout:
Strength Training:
Calories Consumed:
Calories Burned:
Difference:
Weight / Body fat:

Write it down & get it done.

1
2
3
4
5
6
7
8
9
10

Read it, live it, love the results.

Regular exercise may ease chronic pain.
When suffering from chronic pain, exercise may be the last thing you want to do. However, studies show exercise is a great way to ease chronic pain and improve your condition. When inactive, your muscles, including your heart, lose strength and work less efficiently, you also become more fatigued and stressed.

Life's tough, get over it, he did!

Actor and comedian, **Robin Williams**, describes himself as a quiet child, whose first imitation was of his grandmother to his mom. He didn't overcome his shyness until he became involved with the high school drama department. Unfortunately, the only high school award he won was for "Most Likely To Not Succeed." My guess is that he's now the "Most Successful", with many Awards to show for it.

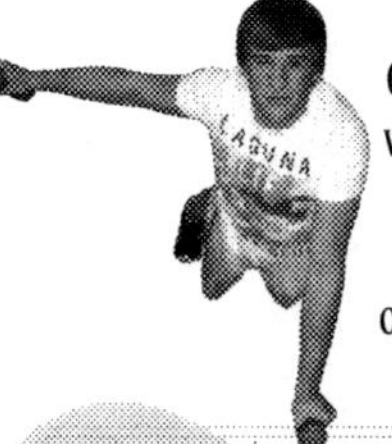

push-up with lateral raise

On the floor support yourself on hands and knees, just as you would a beginner push-up, with hands positioned just below your shoulders, holding dumbbells. Perform a push-up, keeping elbows close to your body, droping your chest to within 2-3 inches of the floor. As you straighten your arms to return to the starting position, lift the right hand straight out to the side, turning the thumb towards the floor, hold for 2-3 counts. Perform another push-up, lifting the left hand straight out to side. Complete 10-15 repetitions.

	DATE
Steps Walked:	
Cardio Workout:	
Strength Training:	
Calories Consumed:	
Calories Burned:	
Difference:	
Weight / Body fat:	

Trust in yourself. Your perceptions are often far more accurate than you are willing to believe.
—Claudia Black

Eating healthy tastes great!

Ocean Cod Supreme

2 lbs cod • 1 cup dry white wine
1/4 cup wheat bread crumbs
1 cup low fat plain yogurt
1 cup green onion, minced

Preheat oven 400°F. Place fish in baking dish with wine. Marinate in refrigerator 15 -30 minutes. Discard wine. Pat fish dry, then coat with bread crumbs. Combine yogurt and green onion. Spread over fish. Sprinkle with paprika. Bake 15-20 minutes until fish

Read it, live it, love the results.

Don't live in fear.

Studies show that if you live in fear of disease, you are likely to end up suffering from disease. The anxiety you feel towards the imprisonment of a disease can actually disable your body's ability to fight it off. When thoughts are positive and pure, your body is strengthened.

Write it down & get it done.

1
2
3
4
5
6
7
8
9
10

flye with a twist

Lie on a bench, or the floor face up with feet flat on the floor or on the bench. With a dumbbell in each hand and palms facing feet, extend arms up with elbows bent, as if wrapped around a big barrel. Keeping your lower back pressed into the bench, turn palms to face your body as you lower them just slightly below chest level. Hold for 2-3 counts, then return to the starting position, pressing the dumbbells together once you reach the top. You should be able to feel your chest rise. Complete 10-15 repetitions.

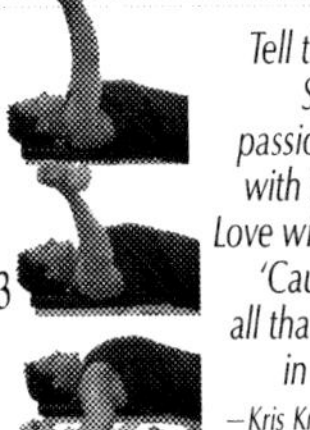

Tell the truth. Sing with passion. Work with laughter. Love with heart. 'Cause that's all that matters in the end.
– Kris Kristofferson

DATE

Steps Walked:
Cardio Workout:
Strength Training:
Calories Consumed:
Calories Burned:
Difference:
Weight / Body fat:

Write it down & get it done.

1
2
3
4
5
6
7
8
9
10

Read it, live it, love the results.

Keep protein bars, yogurt and other healthy snacks on hand. When you are hungry reach for a high nutrition snack, instead of chips or cookies. The healthier snacks will fill you up with nutritional calories and help energize your body and mind. Snacks high in fat and empty calories will only make you feel tired and run down.
How you feel is up to you!

Doors open, when you work hard.

Writer, actor, and musician, **Kris Kristofferson**, went through some hard times, but never gave up on his dream. While sweeping floors at Columbia Studios in Nashville, he met Johnny Cash and gave him some of his songs; Cash ignored them. To get Cash's attention he unexpectedly landed a helicopter in Cash's yard and gave him some tapes, it worked. He eventually became very successful, winning many awards, in addition to being inducted into the Country Music Hall of Fame in 2004.

wide stance push-up

This is an advanced pushup, performed on your hands and toes. Hands should be placed 8-12 inches wider than your shoulders. Keeping your head in line with your spine, lower your body, hovering 2-3 inches above the floor. Hold for 2-3 counts, then return to the "up position". Repeat 10-15 times.

Great achievement is usually born of great sacrifice, and is never the result of selfishness.
—Napoleon Hill

Steps Walked:
Cardio Workout:
Strength Training:
Calories Consumed:
Calories Burned:
Difference:
Weight / Body fat:

DATE

Eating healthy tastes great!

Fruit and Yogurt Parfait

1/4 cup of each sliced fruit; strawberries, blueberries, peaches and bananas
4 oz fat free vanilla yogurt
1 tbs wheat germ

In glass goblet, layer fruit, yogurt and wheat germ. Chill before serving.

Read it, live it, love the results.

Look great in your skin.

When you enjoy a diet of high antioxidant foods, you will look and feel better than ever, as they fight against the free radicals leaving you with healthy, younger looking skin. Antioxidant foods include: beans, artichokes, prunes, strawberries, raspberries, wild blueberries, black plums, plums, gala apples, granny smith apples, blueberries, cranberries, blackberries and russet potatoes.

Write it down & get it done.

1
2
3
4
5
6
7
8
9
10

biceps

Biceps are the large muscles located to the front of the upper arms. This two 'headed' muscle flexes the forearm and draws it up, making it possible to do everything from lifting a gallon of milk to making your bed. Of course bicep exercises also make your arms look great. In addition, as with all other exercises, bicep exercises offer many great benefits, from lowering your blood pressure to relieving depression and improving self-esteem. Most importantly, the longer you remain strong and healthy the longer you remain independent of having to rely upon others to get things done. Bicep exercises can easily be performed while watching TV or working at your desk. Keep your arms in shape and you will love the way you look and the things you can do.

DATE

Real success is not on the stage, but off the stage as a human being, and how you get along with your fellow man.
–Sammy Davis, Jr.

Steps Walked:
Cardio Workout:
Strength Training:
Calories Consumed:
Calories Burned:
Difference:
Weight / Body fat:

Write it down & get it done.

1
2
3
4
5
6
7
8
9
10

Read it, live it, love the results.

Make sacrifices to achieve your desires.
To achieve that which you desire, you must put forth an honest effort. Without sufficient effort and directed thought, you will have little chance of succeeding. When you sacrifice much, you will achieve much; sacrifice little, and you will achieve little. So, get off your buns and do something constructive; make an effort to acheive your goals!

Be the change you want to see.

Entertainers, **Dean Martin** and **Frank Sinatra** were largely responsible for the integration of Las Vegas, simply by refusing to appear anywhere that barred their friend, **Sammy Davis Jr.** With their protest, they forced the casinos to open their doors to African-American entertainers and patrons, and to drop restrictive covenants against Jews. It's amazing what a difference people can make when they fight for what they believe in.

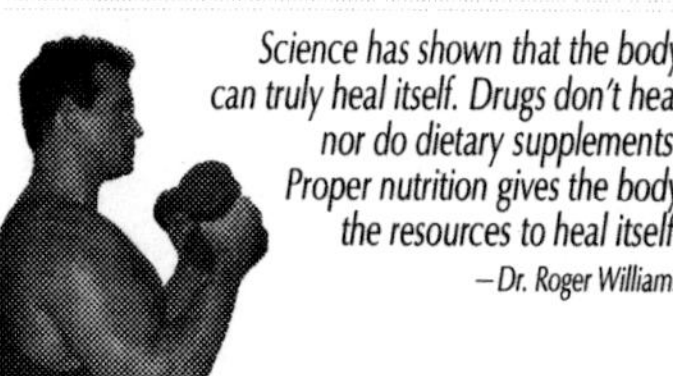

dumbbell curl

Stand with one foot slightly in front of the other, back straight, shoulders back and chest out. With a dumbbell in each hand, let arms hang at sides with palms facing forward. Contract your biceps as you bend your elbows, curling the dumbbells up toward your shoulders, hold 2-3 counts, squeezing the bicep, then lower slowly to starting position. Repeat 10-15 times.

	DATE
Steps Walked:	
Cardio Workout:	
Resistance Workout:	
Calories Consumed:	
Calories Burned:	
Difference:	
Weight / Body fat:	

Eating healthy tastes great!

Sauerkraut Relish Salad

2 stalks celery, cut diagonal
1 canned pimiento, diced
1 green pepper, diced
1 onion, sliced thin
14 oz can sauerkraut, drained
1/3 cup vinegar
3 tbs olive oil
1/4 cup Sweet and Low®
1/4 cup water

Combine all ingredients, cover and refrigerate at least 8 hours.

Your never too old to change.

Don't diet.

If you want to create a healthy lifestyle, don't go on a diet. Changing your health by going on a diet is like stopping a dripping faucet by putting a cup under the drip. It's a temporary fix. You must change your thoughts and attitude in order to change your life. Direct your thoughts towards a healthy lifestyle, and your body will crave healthy foods.

Write it down & get it done.

1
2
3
4
5
6
7
8
9
10

concentration curl

Sit to the front edge of a chair with legs open and feet flat on the floor. Lean forward placing the right elbow against the inside hollow of your right knee. With a dumbbell in the right hand, allow the forearm to drop down, aligning with the side of the leg. Contract your bicep, as you slowly lift the dumbbell to the front of the shoulder. Hold here for 2-3 counts then slowly lower to starting position. Repeat 10-15 times, then complete a set on the opposite side.

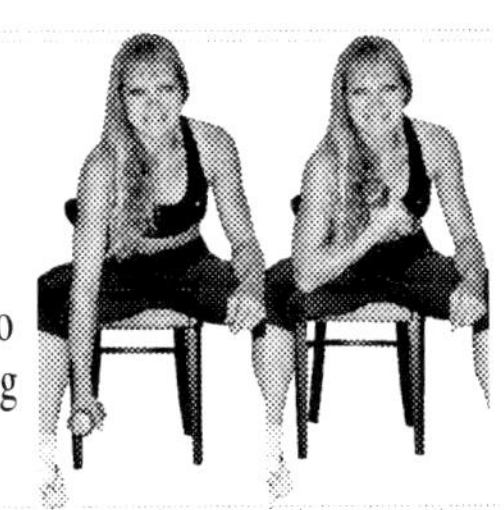

DATE

A man may conquer a million men in battle but one who conquers himself is, indeed, the greatest of conquerors. –Buddha

Steps Walked:
Cardio Workout:
Strength Training:
Calories Consumed:
Calories Burned:
Difference:
Weight / Body fat:

Write it down & get it done.

1
2
3
4
5
6
7
8
9
10

Read it, live it, love the results.

Practice meditation for health and wellness purposes.
The daily stress you face is responsible for destroying your health–and aging you more quickly than most would like. A daily meditation program is a great way to decompress and release tension at the end of a busy day, slowing the negative effects of this stress. Enjoy what others have used for thousands of years in religious and cultural settings throughout the world.

Your level of success is up to you.

Regarded as one of the best quarterbacks of his era, **Tom Brady** once struggled to get play time. During his first two years at the University of Michigan, he was backup, fortunately, he never gave up, and did became a starter. After college he was drafted by the Patriots. In 2004 and 2007, he was named *"Sportsman of the Year"* by The *Sporting News*, then in 2007 *NFL MVP*, as well as 2007 *Male Athlete of the Year* by *The Associated Press*.

A happy person is not a person in a certain set of circumstances but rather a person with a certain set of attitudes.
- Hugh Downs

outside curl

Stand with one foot slightly in front of the other, back straight, shoulders back and chest out. With a dumbbell in each hand, let arms hang at sides with palms facing away from your body. Contract your biceps as you bend your elbows, curling the dumbbells up toward your shoulders. Hold here for 2-3 counts, then lower the dumbbell slowly to the starting position. Repeat 10-15 times.

DATE

Steps Walked:
Cardio Workout:
Strength Training:
Calories Consumed:
Calories Burned:
Difference:
Weight / Body fat:

Eating healthy tastes great!

Fruit Kebabs
8 pineapple cubes *(1 inch)*
12 seedless concord grapes
8 papaya cubes *(1 inch)*
1 cup low fat vanilla yogurt
4 bamboo skewers

Slide fruit onto skewers, then chill. Serve with low-fat vanilla yogurt.

Read it, live it, love the results.

Enjoy papaya and pineapple as a dessert to aid digestion.
Studies show that pineapple and papaya eaten or drank (in juice form) after a meal can aid in digestion of the meal. The enzyme papain, found in the papaya and the enzyme, bromelain, found in pineapple are the digestive boosters. By eating these fruits, we inhibit the excessive acids and correct for over-acidity.

Write it down & get it done.

1
2
3
4
5
6
7
8
9
10

arm wrestling curl with dumbbell

Sit to the front edge of a chair near a table with feet flat on the floor. Holding a dumbbell in your right hand, rest your elbow on the table. Just as you would when arm wrestling, drop the dumbbell to within an inch of the table, hold here for 2-3 counts then slowly return to the starting position.
Repeat 10-15 times, then complete a set with the left arm.

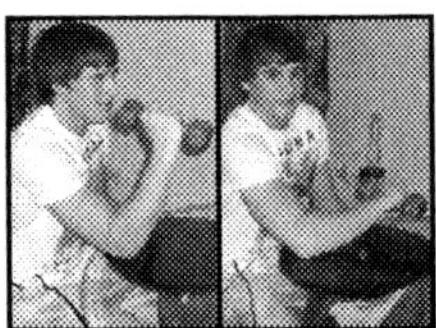

When I commit, I commit with my whole heart, my whole being. I know the Bible like the back of my hand.
—Barry White

DATE

Steps Walked:
Cardio Workout:
Strength Training:
Calories Consumed:
Calories Burned:
Difference:
Weight / Body fat:

Write it down & get it done.

1
2
3
4
5
6
7
8
9
10

Read it, live it, love the results.

Weight train on a regular basis. Studies show that weight training will help you maintain joint flexibility, increase bone density and help better manage your weight. Weight training also improves your mental health and reduces your risk of depression. Another huge advantage of weight training is, you don't need to join a gym or spend a ton of money to do it!

Be the change you want to see.

When record producer, songwriter and singer, **Barry White** was 16 he was sent to jail for 4 months. While there he listened to Elvis Presley on the radio, as he sang "It's Now or Never". This was an experience he later credited with changing the course of his life. After his release, he left gang life and began his own musical career, which proved to be quite successful, winning multiple Grammies.

Not everything that is faced can be changed; but nothing can be changed until it is faced.
—*James Baldwin*

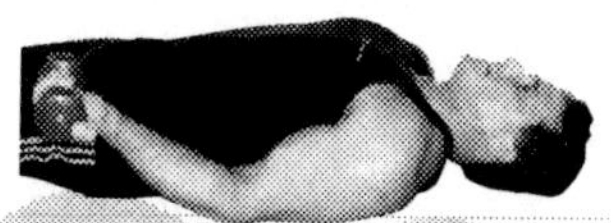

lying flat dumbbell curls

Lie on the floor, face up with a dumbbell in each hand, knees bent with feet flat on the floor. Position arms at sides with palms facing up. Press your elbows into the floor, while keeping the dumbbells suspended just above the floor. Holding the elbows steady, lift the dumbbells 7-10 inches from the floor, hold 2-3 counts then slowly return to starting position. Complete10-15 repetitions.

	DATE
Steps Walked:	
Cardio Workout:	
Strength Training:	
Calories Consumed:	
Calories Burned:	
Difference:	
Weight / Body fat:	

Eating healthy tastes great!

Pineapple Pound Cake

9 oz package sugar free vanilla instant pudding mix
1½ cups skim milk
½ tsp almond extract
20 oz can crushed pineapple, drained
¼ cup toasted almonds, chopped
12 oz fat free pound cake

Whisk first three ingredients. Let stand five minutes. Fold pineapple and almonds into mixture. Cut cake. Spread mixture on top. You may top with orange slices or strawberries.

Read it, live it, love the results.

Make small changes for big results.

When you begin to make life changes, the changes you make may seem small and trivial. However, they are very significant and extremely important in creating a base for the new you—these small changes are essential to creating the big changes you desire.

Write it down & get it done.

1
2
3
4
5
6
7
8
9
10

hammer curl

Stand with one foot slightly in front of the other, back straight, shoulders back and chest out. With a dumbbell in each hand let arms hang at sides with palms facing body. Contract your biceps as you curl the dumbbells toward your shoulders in a hammer motion. Once you reach the top, lower the dumbbell slowly to starting position. Repeat 10-15 times.

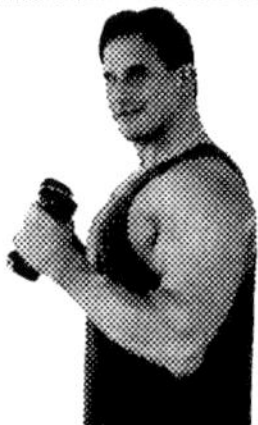

Our way is not soft grass, it's a mountain path with lots of rocks. But it goes upward, forward, toward the sun.
– Dr. Ruth

DATE

Steps Walked:
Cardio Workout:
Strength Training:
Calories Consumed:
Calories Burned:
Difference:
Weight / Body fat:

Write it down & get it done.

1
2
3
4
5
6
7
8
9
10

Read it, live it, love the results.

Drink plenty water and eat foods high in fiber.
Getting a sufficient amount of fiber and water in your diet is essential to keeping your body healthy. This combination keeps food bulky and soft, allowing it to move easily through your system without excessive pressure on your intestines. It also makes you feel fuller, keeping you from overeating, in turn aiding in overall health.

Life's tough, get over it, she did!

Sex therapist **Dr. Ruth Westheimer**, was just ten-years old when she was sent, without her parents, to Switzerland. She later learned that they had perished in the Holocaust. She joined the Haganah in Jerusalem and trained as a scout and sharpshooter. Unfortunately she was wounded and unable to walk for months. Eventually, she immigrated to the US where she became a talk show host and wrote several books on human sexuality.

We build too many walls and not enough bridges.
—Isaac Newton

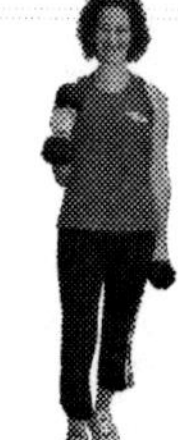

alternating hammer curl
Stand with one foot slightly in front of the other, back straight, shoulders back and chest out. With a dumbbell in each hand let arms hang straight down with palms facing your body. Contract your bicep and curl the right dumbbell toward your right shoulder, then lower slowly to the starting position and curl the left arm. Repeat this alternating count 10-15 times.

	DATE
Steps Walked:	
Cardio Workout:	
Strength Training:	
Calories Consumed:	
Calories Burned:	
Difference:	
Weight / Body fat:	

Eating healthy tastes great!

Austrian Cucumber Salad
1 cucumber, sliced thin
1 medium onion, sliced thin
2 tbs olive oil
2 tbs white vinegar
1/3 cup fat free sour cream
paparika, parsley and pepper to taste
Combine all ingredients and mix well. *(Add cucumbers and onions after mixing other ingredients first)* Cover and refrigerate 2 hours. Drain well and serve chilled.

Read it, live it, love the results.

Get started today.
Sir Isaac Newton stated that; "A body at rest tends to remain at rest and a body in motion tends to remain in motion." Taking the first steps towards creating a healthy lifestyle are certainly the hardest. However, once you have taken these steps, the hardest part is over. Get your body moving or you will never experience the changes you desire.

Write it down & get it done.

1
2
3
4
5
6
7
8
9
10

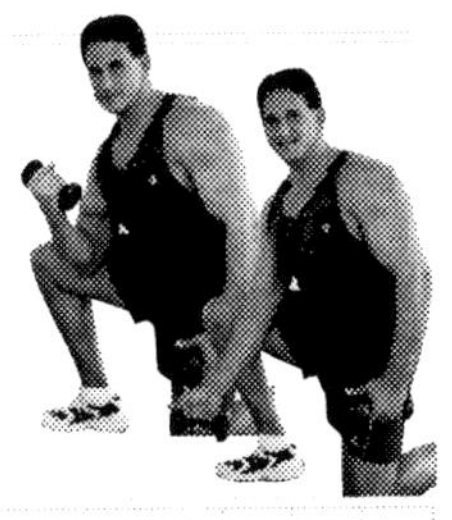

concentration curl kneeling

Kneel, placing the right knee on floor with the left knee at a 90-degree angle, foot flat on floor. Holding a dumbbell in the left hand with palm up, lean forward placing the left elbow against the inside hollow of left knee. Allow the forearm to drop down, aligning with the side of the leg. Contract the bicep, as you slowly raise the dumbbell to the front of your shoulder, hold here for 2-3 counts then slowly return to starting position. Complete 10-15 repetitions on each arm.

DATE

The world is round and the place which may seem like the end may also be only the beginning. – Ivy Baker Priest

Steps Walked:

Cardio Workout:

Strength Training:

Calories Consumed:

Calories Burned:

Difference:

Weight / Body fat:

Write it down & get it done.

1
2
3
4
5
6
7
8
9
10

Read it, live it, love the results.

Work on your attitude.
Creating a healthy lifestyle involves more than changing your eating habits and working out. It requires developing a healthy emotional attitude. When you have good emotional health, you are more in tune with your body, thoughts, feelings and behaviors. This is a huge step towards a long healthy life.

Doors open, when you work hard.

Comedy actor **Dana Carvey** failed with his first television efforts. In 1982 he starred in the sitcom *"One of the Boys,"* it was canceled after only eight months. Luckily this did not stop him from pursuing his career. He knew he wanted to be an actor and never gave up. In 1986, Carvey became a household name when he joined the cast of NBC's *"Saturday Night Live."* He later stared in the spin-off movie *"Wayne's World."*

One can choose to go back toward safety or forward toward growth. Growth must be chosen again and again; fear must be overcome again and again.
–Abraham Maslow

seated reverse curl

Sit on the front edge of a chair, feet flat on the floor with legs open. Holding a dumbbell in the right hand, rest the right elbow on the right knee, with the palm facing down. Place the left hand on the left thigh. Slowly lift the dumbbell, bringing it upright, then slowly lower through the same arc, resisting the weight all the way down, until your forearm is parallel to the floor. Complete 10-15 repetitions on each arm.

DATE

Steps Walked:

Cardio Workout:

Strength Training:

Calories Consumed:

Calories Burned:

Difference:

Weight / Body fat:

Eating healthy tastes great!

Hungarian Beef Strips
2 lbs of beef, cut into strips
1 onion, sliced thin
1/2 cup mushrooms, sliced
1 green pepper, sliced thin
1 red pepper, sliced thin
3 tbs olive oil
1 1/4 tsp paprika
black pepper to taste
Sauté beef strips and onions in 2 tbs olive oil. When done, add remaining ingredients and simmer 25-30 minutes. Serve hot.

Read it, live it, love the results.

Eat healthy to avoid wrinkles.
In a recent study researchers revealed that individuals who consumed a diet rich in vegetables, beans, olive oil, nuts, and multigrain breads were less likely to wrinkle, compared to those who ate red meat, butter, and sugary foods. Eating healthier and taking care of your body is much more economical and safer than getting plastic surgery.

Write it down & get it done.

1
2
3
4
5
6
7
8
9
10

zottman curls

Stand with one foot slightly in front of the other, back straight, shoulders back and chest out. With a dumbbell in each hand, let arms hang down with palms facing away from your body. Keeping the upper arms pressed against your body, curl the dumbbells up toward your shoulders. Once the dumbells reach your shoulders, rotate your wrists so the palms face the floor, then slowly return to starting position.

If you're never scared or embarrassed or hurt, it means you never take any chances.
—Julia Soorel

DATE

Steps Walked:
Cardio Workout:
Strength Training:
Calories Consumed:
Calories Burned:
Difference:
Weight / Body fat:

Write it down & get it done.

1
2
3
4
5
6
7
8
9
10

Read it, live it, love the results.

Fill your mind with positive thoughts.
Think positive thoughts and you will lead a healthier, happier life. Listen to motivational books on cd or an iPod while doing housework or in the car. Try christian radio for a positive change. These sources of strength and positive thinking will help you develop a positive outlook and maintain a healthy lifestyle.

Life's tough, get over it, he did!

Comedian **Chris Rock** spent much of his childhood in Brooklyn's notoriously tough Bedford-Stuyvesant neighborhood. Attending a nearly all-white public school, he was subjected to discrimination at an early age. It was these early bouts with racism that influenced his comedic material which has made him famous. Rock was voted by Comedy Central as the fifth greatest stand-up comedian of all time.

Each of us today has a real chance to live, and live very well to age 100 and beyond.
—Ronald Klatz, M.D

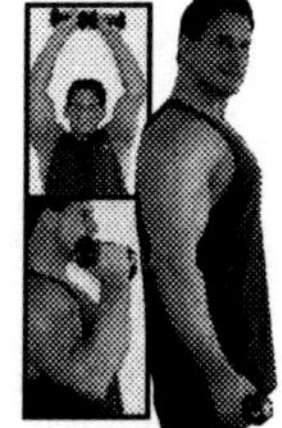

curl, twist & press

Stand with one foot slightly in front of the other, back straight, shoulders back and chest out. With a dumbbell in each hand let arms hang at sides with palms forward. Keeping the upper arms straight, curl the dumbbells up. When at the top of the curl, lift the dumbbells straight up and over your head, twisting so that palms face out. Hold briefly, then return to starting position. Repeat 10-15 times.

Steps Walked:
Cardio Workout:
Strength Training:
Calories Consumed:
Calories Burned:
Difference:
Weight / Body fat:

DATE

Eating healthy tastes great!

Lazy Cabbage Rolls

2 cups cabbage • 1 lb ground turkey
1 onion, diced • 3 tbs minced garlic
1 tbp worcestershire sauce
14 oz can crushed tomatoes
2 cups tomato juice
1 cup short grain brown rice, uncooked

Preheat oven to 325ºF. Place shredded cabbage in casserole dish. Saute meat with remaining ingredients, then pour over cabbage. Cover and bake 2 hours or until rice is tender.

Read it, live it, love the results.

See your entire body and you'll change the way you eat.

It's perhaps to your disadvantage that you're covered with an opaque layer of skin. You can't see the damage you do to your internal organs as the numbers increase on the scale. You don't see the fat layering your heart, increasing the risk of heart disease or the narrowing of your arteries. Envision what's happening inside, not just how you look on the outside.

Write it down & get it done.

1
2
3
4
5
6
7
8
9
10

reverse dumbbell curl
Stand with one foot in front of the other, back straight, knees slightly bent. With a dumbbell in each hand let arms hang in front of body, with palms facing thighs. Bending your elbows, contract the biceps as you curl the dumbbells toward your shoulders. Hold 2-3 counts, then lower the weight slowly to starting position. Repeat 10-15 times.

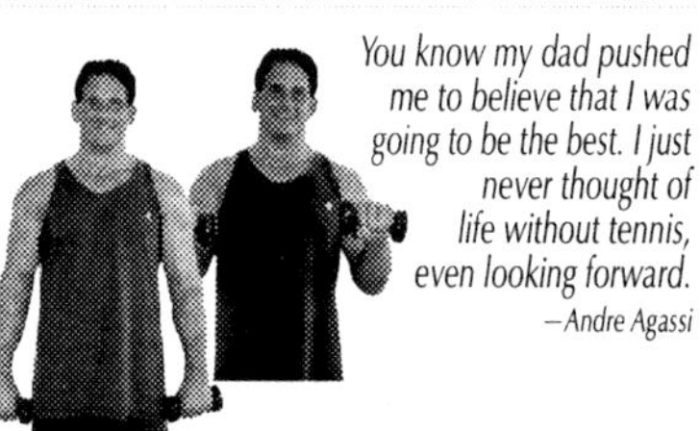

You know my dad pushed me to believe that I was going to be the best. I just never thought of life without tennis, even looking forward.
—Andre Agassi

DATE

Steps Walked:
Cardio Workout:
Strength Training:
Calories Consumed:
Calories Burned:
Difference:
Weight / Body fat:

Write it down & get it done.

1
2
3
4
5
6
7
8
9
10

Read it, live it, love the results.

Eat a balanced, healthy diet to maintain a healthy lifestyle.
This includes:
Proteins // fish, meat, beans, nuts, poultry, dairy products and eggs.
Fats //animal and dairy products, nuts and oils
Carbohydrates // vegetables, fruits, grains, beans and other legumes.
Vitamins // A, B, C, D, E, and K
Minerals //calcium, potassium and iron

Life's tough, get over it, he did!

Writer, poet, philologist, and university professor, **J. R. R. Tolkien**, best known as the author of The Hobbit and The Lord of the Rings, lost his father when he was just three. This left the family without an income, so his mother took him to live with her parents in Birmingham. Soon after, they moved to Sarehole, then a Worcestershire village. His exposure to these places served as inspiration for his books.

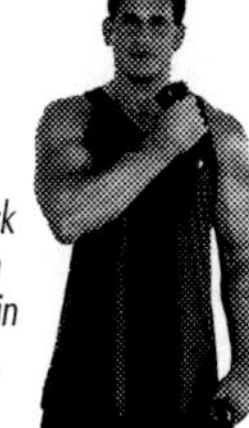

A rock pile ceases to be a rock pile the moment a single man contemplates it, bearing within him the image of a cathedral.
— Antoine de Saint-Exupéry

cross body hammer curl

Stand with one foot in front of the other, back straight and knees slightly bent. With a dumbbell in each hand let arms hang at sides with palms facing body. Contract your biceps as you curl the right dumbbell toward your left shoulder. Lower the dumbbell slowly to the starting position and repeat with the left dumbbell to the right shoulder. Repeat this alternating count 10-15 times.

	DATE
Steps Walked:	
Cardio Workout:	
Strength Training:	
Calories Consumed:	
Calories Burned:	
Difference:	
Weight / Body fat:	

Eating healthy tastes great!

Cucumber and Onion Salad
$2\frac{1}{2}$ cups cucumbers, thinly sliced
$\frac{1}{2}$ cup onions, thinly sliced
$\frac{1}{3}$ cup Splenda®
$\frac{1}{3}$ cup white vinegar
black pepper to taste
Place cucumbers and onions in a bowl. Combine remaining ingredients and pour over the cucumbers and onions.
Cover and refrigerate for at least two hours.
Stir occasionally, serve chilled.

Read it, live it, love the results.

Slow down when you eat!
With so much going on in our lives, many of us treat lunch and dinner as an olympic event, chowing down as quickly as possible. Not surprising, eating too quickly can cause issues with your digestion.
Remember the next time you grab that *quick meal*, poor eating habits are habits that should never be practiced...or taught to your children.

Write it down & get it done.

1
2
3
4
5
6
7
8
9
10

3-part curls "21's"

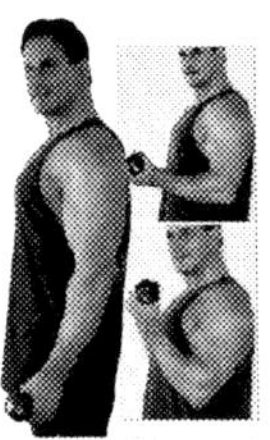

Stand with one foot slightly in front of the other, back straight, shoulders back and chest out. With a dumbbell in each hand let arms hang down with palms facing forward. Contract your biceps as you curl the dumbbells halfway up, pump twice, then drop back down. Repeat 7 times, then without pausing, curl the dumbbells all the way up, then halfway down with a 2 count pump at the halfway point. Complete 7 repetitions of this movement. Then finish off the exercise by performing 7 full-range dumbbell curls.

DATE

Steps Walked:
Cardio Workout:
Strength Training:
Calories Consumed:
Calories Burned:
Difference:
Weight / Body fat:

Write it down & get it done.

1
2
3
4
5
6
7
8
9
10

Read it, live it, love the results.

Act upon your dreams!
If you want to run a marathon, don't expect to do so by watching television and counting down the days. Instead, set up a training schedule and stick to it.
Do everything in your power to make your dream come true, don't sit around and wait for a miracle. Miracles are created with a lot of hard work.

Doors open, when you work hard.

Scientist, botanist, educator, and inventor who revolutionized agriculture in the Southern US, **George Washington Carver**, was born to slave parents then rescued from Confederate kidnappers. His education began while working as a farm hand and studying in a one-room schoolhouse. After graduating high school he was denied admission to Highland University because of his race, however, gained acceptance to Simpson College in Indianola, Iowa.

bent over curl

Let your food be your medicine, let your medicine be your food.
– Hippocrates

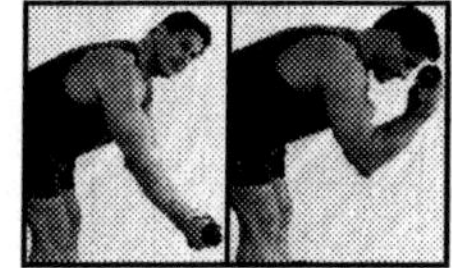

Stand with one foot slightly in front of the other, back straight, shoulders back and chest out. With a dumbbell in each hand, bend over almost 90-degrees at the waist with arms out front and palms facing away from your body. Contract your biceps as you curl the dumbbells toward your shoulders. Repeat 10-15 times.

Steps Walked:
Cardio Workout:
Strength Training:
Calories Consumed:
Calories Burned:
Difference:
Weight / Body fat:

DATE

Eating healthy tastes great!

Pumpkin Granola Bars
¾ cup pumpkin puree • 1 egg
¼ cup light butter • ¼ cup honey
2 tsp molasses • 2 cups rolled oats, uncooked • ¼ cup wheat germ
½ cups peanuts or walnuts, chopped
2 tbs unsweetened coconut, shredded
½ tsp ground cinnamon
1 tbs grated orange rind
Preheat oven at 350°F. Combine ingredients, spread mixture into a lightly greased pan. Bake 40 minutes or until golden brown.

Read it, live it, love the results.

Don't poison your body.
If gasoline tasted great would you drink it? Surprisingly, many people would. Too many people think because something tastes good, they deserve it, who cares what the results are. Think about all of the unhealthy foods you eat on a daily basis. Essentially you are poisoning yourself just as you would if you drank gasoline. Does this really make any sense at all?

Write it down & get it done.

1
2
3
4
5
6
7
8
9
10

triceps

Triceps are the smaller muscles located to the back of the upper arms. This three 'headed' muscle extends the forearm so it may be held straight. Triceps are used in conjunction with the biceps when lifting and lowering items. They also come in handy when pushing yourself up out of a deep sofa. And, as with the bicep exercises, tricep exercises make your arms look great.

If you can find a path with no obstacles, it probably doesn't lead anywhere. —author unknown

DATE

Steps Walked:
Cardio Workout:
Strength Training:
Calories Consumed:
Calories Burned:
Difference:
Weight / Body fat:

Write it down & get it done.

1
2
3
4
5
6
7
8
9
10

Read it, live it, love the results.

Reach deep within and discover the talents you need to succeed. Do you feel you lack that "special something" that would make you successful in leading a healthy lifestyle? A lack of willpower, knowledge or the right genes? In truth you possess everything you need, you must simply learn to use everything you have—and use it to your advantage.

Doors open when least expected.

"Queen of Country Music" **Kitty Wells**, was ready to abandon her career as a singer and focus on raising her family, when, despite her resistance, her husband sent a demo tape to Decca Records. Decca signed her, she recorded *"It Wasn't God Who Made Honky Tonk Angels"* and it immediately went to #1 on the country charts, catapolting her career to the top. She was the first female country singer to top the US Country Charts.

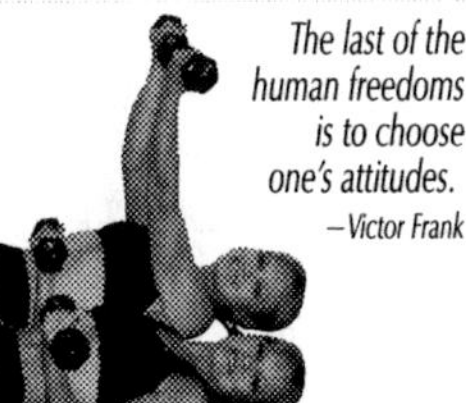

The last of the human freedoms is to choose one's attitudes.
– Victor Frank

reverse bench presses

Lie on a bench or the floor, face up with feet flat on the floor or on the bench. Holding dumbbells in each hand, extend arms straight up with the butts of the dumbells pressed together, palms facing towards your head. Bending your elbows, slowly lower the dumbbells to within an inch of your chest while keeping elbows in at your sides. Hold for 2-3 counts, then extend back up to the starting position, again keeping your elbows in.Repeat 10-15 times.

	DATE
Steps Walked:	
Cardio Workout:	
Strength Training:	
Calories Consumed:	
Calories Burned:	
Difference:	
Weight / Body fat:	

Eating healthy tastes great!

Simple Applesauce

3 lbs apples, peeled and chopped
3 cups water
1/4 cup Splenda®
1 tbs lemon juice
1 tsp ground cinnamon

Place apples in a large pan, barely covering with water. Simmer over medium-low heat 15 to 20 minutes until apples are tender. Place apples, Splenda®, lemon juice and cinnamon in blender and blend smooth. Serve chilled or frozen.

Read it, live it, love the results.

Enjoy apples for a healthier life!

Michigan State University did a study of five hundred students who ate two or three apples a day and compared them to a group who ate no apples.

Those who ate apples had;

- Fewer colds
- Fewer upper respiratory infections
- Fewer headaches
- Less nervousness
- Better ability to concentrate
- Fewer stomach and intestinal issues

Write it down & get it done.

1
2
3
4
5
6
7
8
9
10

overhead extension

Stand with one foot slightly in front of the other, back straight, shoulders back and chest out. Hold a single heavy dumbbell using both hands as pictured. Press the dumbbell overhead so the arms are fully extended and your palms are facing up. Bending your elbows, lower the dumbbell, while keeping your upper arms vertical, back straight, head up and elbows pointing toward the ceiling. Continue down until your biceps and forearms touch. Lift the dumbbell back to the starting position and repeat 10-15 times.

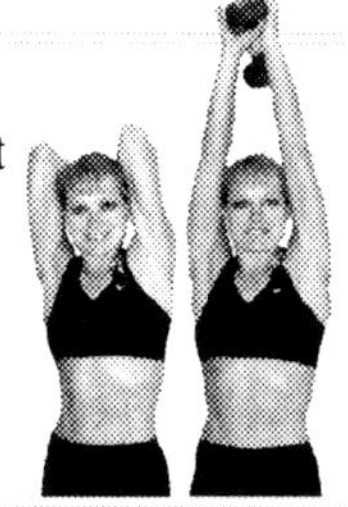

DATE

Back then, we didn't know we were poor, and people were more proud then.
– Loretta Lynn

Steps Walked:
Cardio Workout:
Strength Training:
Calories Consumed:
Calories Burned:
Difference:
Weight / Body fat:

Write it down & get it done.

1
2
3
4
5
6
7
8
9
10

Read it, live it, love the results.

Stay active and social.
Harvard studies have found that individuals with more social connections have a lower death rate than those who live an isolated life. If you don't have the opportunity to spend time with others—get a pet or plants. They too can eliminate loneliness, and boredom from your life—it's as essential to your life as regular exercise.

Life's tough, get over it, she did!

Revered country singing icon **Loretta Lynn**, faced several tragedies through the years, yet she never gave up. She grew up poor, then married at age 14 in an effort to "escape." It was a devoted but rocky marriage. These life experiences often provided the bases for her hit songs and her best-selling 1976 autobiography, *"Coal Miner's Daughter."* Lynn ruled the charts during the '60s and '70s, accumulating over 70 hits as a solo artist and a duet partner.

The greater part of our happiness or misery depends on our dispositions, and not on our circumstances.
–Martha Washington

seated one arm tricep extension
Sit on the front edge of a chair with a dumbbell in your right hand, extended straight above your head with your palm facing forward. Support the right elbow with the left hand to prevent the upper arm or elbow from moving. Slowly, drop the dumbbell until the forearm touches the bicep, then return to the starting position, flexing your tricep muscle at the top. Complete 10-15 repetitions on each arm.

DATE

Steps Walked:
Cardio Workout:
Strength Workout:
Calories Consumed:
Calories Burned:
Difference:
Weight / Body fat:

Eating healthy tastes great!

Cabbage Tomato Soup
1 cabbage, diced into bitesize pieces
4 cups low sodium chicken broth
1 onion, diced
2 carrots, sliced thin
28 oz can tomatoes, diced
1 cup green peppers, diced
3 tbs minced garlic • olive oil
Braise cabbage in olive oil for about 5 minutes. Then place all ingredients into big soup pot and simmer for 1.5 hours. Serve as is or add cooked beans.

Read it, live it, love the results.

Eat healthy throughout the day, especially when there's a party in the evening.
Many people starve themselves the day of a big party, just so they can splurge at the party. Bad idea. Eat breakfast and lunch, and have a piece of fruit or cheese before you leave home. You're, of course, more likely to overeat when you attend a party hungry. Endulge responsibly.

Write it down & get it done.

1
2
3
4
5
6
7
8
9
10

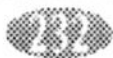

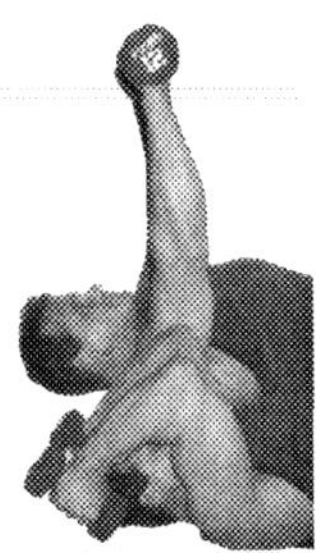

lying tricep extension
Lie on a bench or the floor, face up with feet flat on the floor or on the bench. Extend arms straight up, with a dumbbell in each hand, palms facing feet. While keeping your upper arms and elbows as still as possible, lower both dumbbells, twisting them as you do so that palms are facing as dumbbells drop to the side of your head. Make sure your elbows don't flair out during this movement. Return to the starting position, flexing your triceps as you reach the top. Complete 10-15 repetitions.

DATE

The man who does not read good books has no advantage over the man who can't read them. – Mark Twain

Steps Walked:
Cardio Workout:
Strength Training:
Calories Consumed:
Calories Burned:
Difference:
Weight / Body fat:

Write it down & get it done.

1
2
3
4
5
6
7
8
9
10

Read it, live it, love the results.

Keep your brain active.
Read fitness magazines, check out websites, attend seminars and classes. Do whatever you can do to learn everything you can about health and fitness. The more you know about health and fitness, the better you can take care of yourself. Continuing to learn is also a great way to reduce your risk of Alzheimer's.

Doors open when least expected.

Academy and *Golden Globe Award* winning actress, **Cate Blanchett**, first experienced acting when she was an extra for a crowd scene, making $10 a day. She ended up getting upset when the director yelled at her and walked off the set, yet it was the experience that developed her love for acting. Since then she has won various acting awards, including two *SAGs*, two *Golden Globe Awards* and two *BAFTAs*.

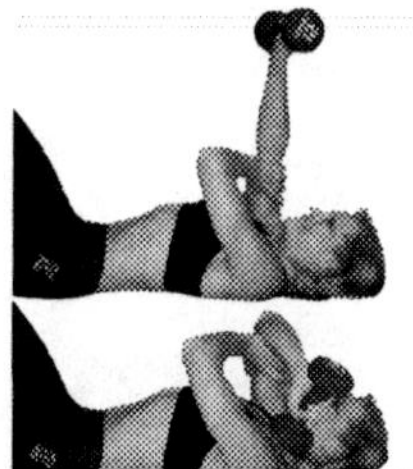

You are what you do when it counts.
—John Steakley

lying dumbbell tricep extension across face

Lie on a bench or the floor, face up with your feet flat on the floor or on the bench. Extend the right hand straight up, holding a dumbbell with palm facing feet. While keeping the upper arm and elbow completely still, lower the dumbbell across your chest. Hold for 2-3 counts, then return to the starting position, flexing the tricep as you reach the top. Complete 10-15 repetitions, then complete a set with the left arm.

	DATE
Steps Walked:	
Cardio Workout:	
Strength Workout:	
Calories Consumed:	
Calories Burned:	
Difference:	
Weight / Body fat:	

Eating healthy tastes great!

Chicken Sukiyaki
4 chicken breasts, diced
1/2 cup each; sliced mushrooms, diced green onions, bean sprouts, 5oz can bamboo shoots
2 cups fresh baby spinach

combine before adding:
1/3 cup soy sauce • 2 tbs sherry wine
1 packet Splenda® • 2 tbs peanut oil
1/2 cup low sodium chicken broth

Sauté chicken, then add remaining ingredients *(except spinach)*. Bring to boil, then add spinach. Simmer 3-5 minutes.

Read it, live it, love the results.

Never give yourself a reason to treat your body badly.
There may be times when you feel the world is against you, that nothing seems to work out the way it should. It's at those times that you become weak and treat your body badly. Instead of resorting to binging, go for a walk or run to clear your head and regain control, you'll love yourself when you do. There's nothing so horrible in your life, that you should treat yourself badly.

Write it down & get it done.

1
2
3
4
5
6
7
8
9
10

dip with two chairs

Place two sturdy chairs about 2½-3 feet apart. Place your feet on one chair and your hands on the other. Keep your legs together and your hands just a bit narrower than shoulder-width apart. With arms straight, position your body so it's at an "L" shape between the two chairs. Bending your elbows, slowly lower your body between the chairs as far as comfortable. Hold this position for 2-3 counts, then straighten the arms and push yourself back up to starting position. Complete 10-15 repetitions.

The world is full of magical things patiently waiting for our wits to grow sharper.
–Bertrand Russel

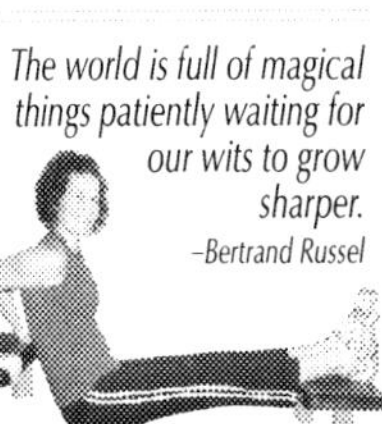

DATE

Steps Walked:
Cardio Workout:
Strength Training:
Calories Consumed:
Calories Burned:
Difference:
Weight / Body fat:

Write it down & get it done.

1
2
3
4
5
6
7
8
9
10

Read it, live it, love the results.

You are responsible for your future.
No matter what you've been through, the past is the past, get over it and move forward. Very few have traveled through life without enduring hard times. Don't let the past determine your future, everyday is a new opportunity for you to become an even bigger success. If you spend too much time worrying about the past, you'll miss opportunities of the present and future.

Doors open when least expected.

One of Hollywood's highest paid actors, **Renée Zellweger**, had originally gone to college to major in English. It wasn't until she took a drama class, to fulfill the fine arts credit she needed to graduate, that she realized how much she loved acting. As an actor she's won several awards including *Academy, BAFTA, SAG,* and *Golden Globe Awards*.
You never know where life will take you.

It is not what they take away from you that counts. It's what you do with what you have left.
–Hubert Humphrey

dips off chair

Position yourself in front of a sturdy, stationary chair. With hands on the chair, extend your legs straight out, placing your weight on the heels. Keep legs together and your hands just a bit narrower than shoulder-width apart. Bending your elbows, slowly lower your body as far as comfortable without touching the floor. Hold this position for 2-3 counts, then straighten your arms, pushing yourself back to the starting position. Repeat 10-15 times.

DATE

Steps Walked:
Cardio Workout:
Strength Workout:
Calories Consumed:
Calories Burned:
Difference:
Weight / Body fat:

Eating healthy tastes great!

Mixed Greens with Fruit
$^{1}/_{2}$ cup orange juice
$^{1}/_{2}$ cup honey
1 tsp ground cinnamon
6 oranges, peeled and sliced
6 kiwifruit, peeled and sliced
8 cups torn mixed salad greens
$^{1}/_{2}$ cup dried cranberries
Blend orange juice, honey and cinnamon for dressing. Combine greens with fruit, then toss with the dressing.

Read it, live it, love the results.

Treat your body as you would a best friend.
You wouldn't poison the food or drink of a friend, yet when your diet is filled with unhealthy foods and drinks, you poison your own body. You are the only one who can determine what you eat and drink. It's up to you to make these choices healthy. Fill your body with unhealthy choices now, and you will pay the penalty later.

Write it down & get it done.

1
2
3
4
5
6
7
8
9
10

standing kickback

Keeping your back straight, bend over with your left leg slightly bent and the right leg shifted back 15-18 inches. Holding a dumbbell in each hand, bend your elbows to 90-degrees, holding the elbows in at your sides. Without moving the upper arms, press the lower arms back until the dumbbell is pointing away from your body, as if you are handing off a relay baton. Flex here 2-3 counts then return to the starting position, repeat 10-15 times.

I'm tough, ambitious, and I know exactly what I want.
– Madonna

DATE

Steps Walked:

Cardio Workout:

Strength Training:

Calories Consumed:

Calories Burned:

Difference:

Weight / Body fat:

Write it down & get it done.

1
2
3
4
5
6
7
8
9
10

Read it, live it, love the results.

Know that all endings, become beginnings.
Whether it be the end of a relationship, job or friendship, these endings make room for new beginnings. Don't retreat in despair, instead step boldly into the world and discover that which awaits you. When one door closes there is always another awaiting to be opened.It's up to you to continue opening these doors.

Life's tough, get over it, she did!

Widely considered one of the greatest baseball players of all time **Hank Aaron** grew up in a poor family with seven siblings. He spent his childhood working on a farm picking cotton, many say that it was this work that strengthened his hands so he could hit more home runs. His family couldn't afford baseball equipment, so he made his own bats and balls from materials he found on the streets–he practiced by hitting bottle caps with sticks.

single arm kickback

Keeping your back straight, bend over with your left leg slightly bent and the right leg shifted back 15-18 inches. Holding a dumbbell in your right hand, bend your elbow 90-degrees and place the elbow at your side, while resting your left hand on your left thigh. Without moving your upper arm, move the dumbbell back until it is pointing away from your body, as if you are handing off a relay baton. Hold this position 2-3 counts, then return to the starting position. Complete10-15 repetitions on each side.

Steps Walked:
Cardio Workout:
Strength Workout:
Calories Consumed:
Calories Burned:
Difference:
Weight / Body fat:

DATE

Our lives improve only when we take chances—and the first and most difficult risk we can take is to be honest with ourselves. —Walter Anderson

Eating healthy tastes great!

Triple-Berry Granola Crisp
8 oz bag frozen blueberries
10 oz bag frozen strawberries
10 oz bag frozen raspberries
1/4 cup sugar • 2 tbs wheat flour
1 1/2 cups oats & honey granola
Preheat oven to 375ºF. In ungreased 8-inch square glass baking dish, mix frozen berries, sugar and flour until fruit is coated. Bake 20 minutes, then sprinkle with granola. Bake another 15 to 20 minutes or until light golden brown. Cool before serving.

Read it, live it, love the results.

Keep frozen blueberries on hand.
Blueberries contain more cell-damage-fighting antioxidants than almost any other fruit or vegetable. Just one cup provides 9% of your daily vitamin A and 5% of your daily vitamin C. They also pack 17% of your daily fiber into a mere 79 calories. Try topping your breakfast cereal, oatmeal, or low fat yogurt with a handful of the blueberries, you'll love the way they taste and the way they make you feel.

Write it down & get it done.

1
2
3
4
5
6
7
8
9
10

lying one arm side push-up

Lie on the floor on your right side. With bottom leg slightly bent, prop yourself up with your left arm. Wrap the right arm around your waist. Bending the left elbow, slowly lower your body to the floor, then push up to return to the starting position. Complete 10-15 repetitions on each side.

If you always do what interests you at least one person is pleased.
– Katharine Hepburn

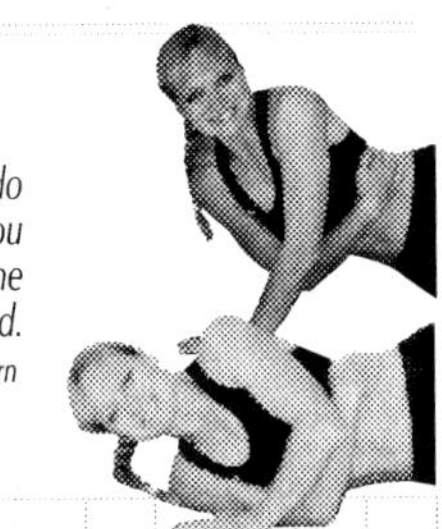

DATE

Steps Walked:
Cardio Workout:
Strength Training:
Calories Consumed:
Calories Burned:
Difference:
Weight / Body fat:

Write it down & get it done.

1
2
3
4
5
6
7
8
9
10

Read it, live it, love the results.

Don't set limits on yourself.
The only limitations you have are those you set on yourself. When you learn to live life without limits, you will accomplish things you never thought possible.
No one else can be blamed for your failures or your successes. See yourself as successful, and you can become successful; see yourself a failure, and you are guaranteed a failure.

Your level of success is up to you.

Actress **Katherine Hepburn** began her career badly. Her first leading role was a huge disaster. Terror stricken when she was thrown into the leading role Hepburn arrived late, flubbed her lines, tripped over her feet and spoke so rapidly it was hard to understand her. She was fired, but never gave up. Today, Hepburn holds the record for the most Best Actress Oscar wins with four, from twelve nominations.

It's not what you are that holds you back, it's what you think you're not.
– Denis Waitley

kickouts from chest

Lie on a bench or the floor, face up with feet flat on the floor or on the bench. Holding a dumbbell in each hand, place the dumbbells on your chest, next to each other. Elbows should be pointing straight out from your body, with the palms facing your feet. Without moving your upper arms or elbows, extend the dumbbells straight up and out, flexing here for 2-3 counts. Then slowly return dumbbells to starting position and repeat 10-15 times.

DATE

Steps Walked:
Cardio Workout:
Strength Workout:
Calories Consumed:
Calories Burned:
Difference:
Weight / Body fat:

Eating healthy tastes great!

Sloppy Joe—Turkey Style
2 lbs lean ground turkey
1/2 cup of each diced;
onion, green pepper, tomatoes and mushrooms.
2-15 oz can tomato juice
paprika, chili powder and white pepper to taste
Sauté turkey, onion and green pepper until lightly browning. Add remaining ingredients. Simmer 15 to 20 minutes. Serve over toasted whole wheat buns.

Read it, live it, love the results.

Know you are worthy.
If you don't see yourself worthy of having a great healthy body, you will never achieve a healthy body. Sadly, there are many who feel this way; they don't feel worthy and deserving of anything good. And, if they do happen to achieve success, they will often unconsciously find a way to sabotage this success. Know that you are worthy and deserving of all that is good, including a healthy life.

Write it down & get it done.

1
2
3
4
5
6
7
8
9
10

reach out

Standing, with one foot in front of the other to support your lower back, hold a dumbbell in each hand, placing them behind your head with the palms facing your head. Raise the dumbbells up and out, then slowly return to starting position. Repeat 10-15 times.

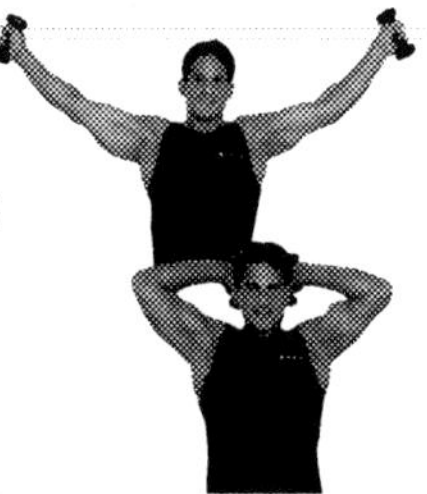

I think beauty comes from within. If you're happy and look at life in the best way you can, even when there are problems, it can make you beautiful on the outside.
—Faith Hill

DATE

Steps Walked:
Cardio Workout:
Strength Training:
Calories Consumed:
Calories Burned:
Difference:
Weight / Body fat:

Write it down & get it done.

1
2
3
4
5
6
7
8
9
10

Read it, live it, love the results.

Focus on yourself and set an example which others may follow. You must realize that others know what is best for themselves. If your significant other does not feel the need to eat healthy and workout, don't make it your job to change him or her. Your positive example will do more than endless nagging. The next best thing to leading a healthy lifestyle is getting others to do the same—simply by example.

Doors open when least expected.

Country singer **Faith Hill** quit college to become *"famous."* However, when she auditioned to be a backup singer and failed, she began selling t-shirts and became a secretary at a music publishing firm. Fortunately, a co-worker heard Hill singing to herself. Soon the head of the publishing company encouraged her to become a demo singer for the firm. From there, her fame grew, selling more than 35 million records with 11 number-one country singles.

True morality consists, not in following the beaten track, but in finding out the true path for ourselves and in fearlessly following it.
—Mohandas Gandhi

behind back tricep press

Stand with one foot slightly in front of the other, back straight, shoulders back and chest out. Hold a large dumbbell with both hands, palms facing in. With the dumbbell behind you, let it rest on your buns. Keeping your arms straight, raise the dumbbell as far back and high as possible, squeezing your shoulder blades together while opening your chest. Hold for 2-3 counts, repeat 10-15 times.

Steps Walked:
Cardio Workout:
Strength Training:
Calories Consumed:
Calories Burned:
Difference:
Weight / Body fat:

DATE

Eating healthy tastes great!

Carrots in Sauce
1 lb frozen carrots
4 whole cloves • 1 bay leaf
2 tbs light butter
2 tbs wheat flour
1 cup skim milk
cayenne pepper and parsley to taste
Melt butter in sauce pan, then blend in flour. Add milk and one cup water, cook until thickened. Add carrots and seasonings and cook additional 5-10 minutes, until carrots are hot.

Read it, live it, love the results.

Carrots really can help your eyesight!
Carrots are an old-time remedy for poor eyesight. Studies show that drinking a five ounce cup of carrot juice twice a day for two weeks, brings definate improvement. Scientists feel it's the special vitamin A ingredient carotene that helps with vision. So, if you can't eat enough carrots, give the juice a try—it tastes great and works!

Write it down & get it done.

1
2
3
4
5
6
7
8
9
10

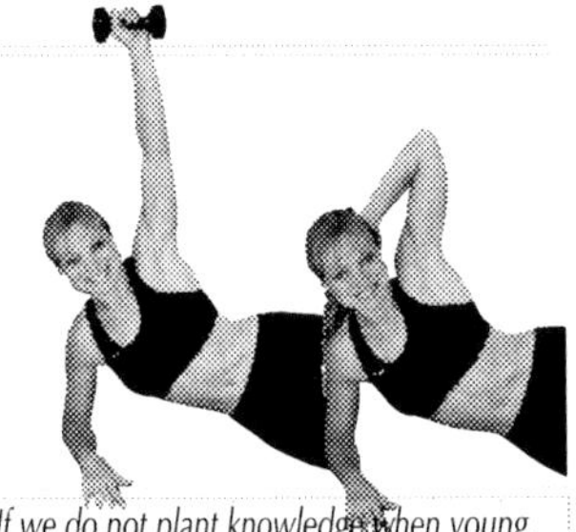

one arm overhead extension on side

Lie on the floor on your right side. With the bottom leg slightly bent, support yourself on your right elbow. Extended the left arm straight up, with a dumbbell in hand. Bending your elbow, moving only the forearm, lower the dumbbell behind your head. Hold for 2-3 counts then push up to starting position, flexing the tricep. Complete 10-15 repetitions with each arm.

If we do not plant knowledge when young, it will give us no shade when we are old.
— Lord Chesterfield

DATE

Steps Walked:
Cardio Workout:
Strength Training:
Calories Consumed:
Calories Burned:
Difference:
Weight / Body fat:

Write it down & get it done.

1
2
3
4
5
6
7
8
9
10

Read it, live it, love the results.

Be flexible. Resist the temptation to break.
There will be times when circumstances arise that you can't control. Circumstances which my cause you to stray from your goals. However, this does not give you permission to give up. You must be flexible, bend, then snap back and start again. It's not what happens to you that matters, it's how you respond to that which happens. Don't ever let yourself be broken.

Doors open when least expected.

Entertainer **Dean Martin** worked for various bands throughout the early 1940's, surviving mostly on looks and personality rather than vocal ability, as he didn't develop his smooth singing style until later. His big break came in 1943 when he opened for Frank Sinatra and flopped—it was the setting for the two men's introduction. Together they formed *"The Rat Pack"* and soon he was a *"household name"*.

Blessed are the flexible, for they shall not be bent out of shape.
—Anon

Shoulder exercises are important to maintaining upper body strength, giving you the ability to lift things above your head and safely remove items from upper cabinets and shelves. Physically, shoulder exercises make your body look better proportionately, as wide shoulders will make your waist look thinner. Most of the exercises in this section may be performed anywhere, making it inexcusable not to have strong healthy shoulders.

Steps Walked:
Cardio Workout:
Strength Workout:
Calories Consumed:
Calories Burned:
Difference:
Weight / Body fat:

DATE

Eating healthy tastes great!

Sunshine Morning Granola
2 cups Quaker® Oats, uncooked
1/3 cup honey • 1/4 cup pecans. diced
2 tbs olive oil • 1 tsp vanilla
2 tsp orange peel, grated
1/4 tsp ground cinnamon
2/3 cup dried mixed fruit
Preheat oven to 350°F. Combine all ingredients except dried fruit in large bowl. Mix well, then spread evenly in baking pan. Bake 20 to 25 minutes or until brown, stirring once after 10 minutes. Cool, then stir in dried fruit.

Read it, live it, love the results.

Don't forget about water—it's a great weight loss tool.
Not only is it an excellent appetite suppressant, it also has the advantage of having zero calories. Enjoy a free glass of ice cold, no fat, no calorie, no carbs, no sugar, water, and your body will thank you. Remember, *"a penny saved is a penny earned,"* and *"a calorie you don't consume is one you don't have to burn."*

Write it down & get it done.

1
2
3
4
5
6
7
8
9
10

lying front raise
Lie on the floor, on your right side. With bottom leg slightly bent, prop yourself up on the right elbow. Holding a dumbbell in your left hand, support it straight out front about an inch above the floor. Keeping your arm straight, raise the dumbbell directly out until it is parallel to the floor. Hold for 2-3 counts, then slowly lower to the starting position. Complete 10-15 repetitions on each side.

Losing doesn't eat at me the way it used to. I just get ready for the next play, the next game, the next season.
– Troy Aikman

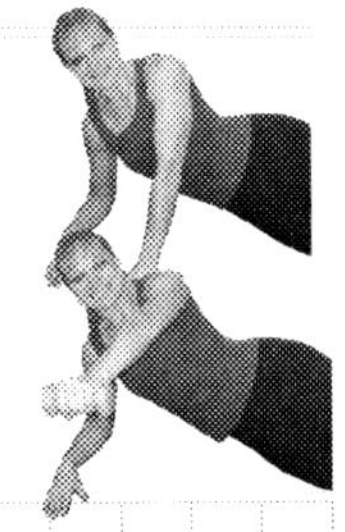

DATE

Steps Walked:
Cardio Workout:
Strength Training:
Calories Consumed:
Calories Burned:
Difference:
Weight / Body fat:

Write it down & get it done.

1
2
3
4
5
6
7
8
9
10

Read it, live it, love the results.

Exercise to avoid depression medications.
Studies reveal that an exercise program can produce a drastic decline in depression, similar to that seen in antidepressant medications. Unfortunately, research also indicates that despite the effectivness of exercise and the fact that it doesnt have bad side effects, it's often underused as a treatment. Individuals instead choose to medicate.

Doors open when least expected.

Quarterback **Troy Aikman**, thought his athletic career was over, when at the age of twelve his family moved from California to a farm in Oklahoma. However, while in Oklahoma, he made high school All-State in both football and baseball. Today, he is considered among the best NFL quarterbacks of all time, and was elected to the Pro Football Hall of Fame in 2006.

You will never find time for anything. If you want time you must make it.
—Charles Buxton

big circles

Sit tall with feet flat on the floor, shoulders back, chest out and abs in. Holding 3 or 5 pound dumbbells, extend arms straight out to sides and slowly make circles about one foot in diameter. Complete 10-15 circles clockwise, then 10-15 circles counter-clockwise. You may also perform this exercise standing.

	DATE
Steps Walked:	
Cardio Workout:	
Strength Training:	
Calories Consumed:	
Calories Burned:	
Difference:	
Weight / Body fat:	

Eating healthy tastes great!

Great Greek Stew

6 chicken breasts, diced
$2^1/_2$ lbs onions, diced
$^1/_3$ cup light butter
6 oz can tomato paste • $^1/_3$ cup red wine
2 tbs wine vinegar
$^1/_2$ tbs Splenda® brown sugar
2 bay leaves • $^1/_2$ tsp whole cloves
1 cinnamon stick

Preheat oven to 250ºF. Place chicken and onions in roaster, top with remaining ingredients. *DO NOT STIR.* Cover and bake for 5 hours.

Read it, live it, love the results.

Invest in your health.

Do you spend much of your time and energy building financial investments which will take you safely into the future? Investing in your future is great, however if you neglect to put the same time and energy into your health, you may find yourself spending your *nest-egg* on a nursing home, instead of vacations and good times.

Write it down & get it done.

1
2
3
4
5
6
7
8
9
10

around the world

Sit in a chair with feet flat on the floor, hands resting on your upper thighs with palms up, holding dumbbells. With the elbows slightly bent, lift the dumbbells up and around as if you were drawing an angel in the snow– bringing the dumbbells behind your head so they touch. Return to the starting position and repeat, 10-15 times.

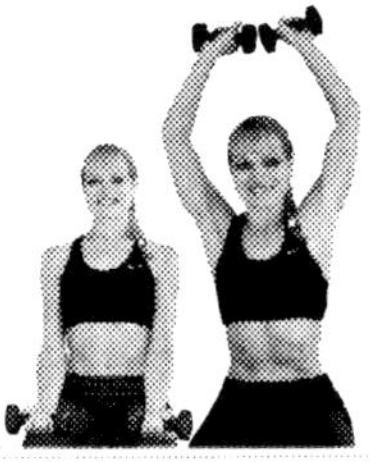

Failures do what is tension relieving, while winners do what is goal achieving.
–Dennis Waitley

DATE

Steps Walked:
Cardio Workout:
Strength Training:
Calories Consumed:
Calories Burned:
Difference:
Weight / Body fat:

Write it down & get it done.

1
2
3
4
5
6
7
8
9
10

Read it, live it, love the results.

Don't deprive yourself of sleep. In a study of nearly 10,000 adults between the ages of 32 and 49, those who slept less than seven hours a night were significantly more likely to be obese. Some researchers suggest that sleeping less may affect the body's metabolic rate or that it made people move around less during the day, burning fewer calories, while others feel the lack of sleep disrupts hormones which regulate the appetite.

Life's tough, get over it, he did!

NFL Hall of Famer **Terry Bradshaw**, had a rough first year in the NFL. He threw many interceptions and was widely ridiculed by the media for his rural roots and a perceived lack of intelligence. It took Bradshaw a few seasons to adjust to the pro game but once he did, he became a superstar. In four career *Super Bowl* appearances he passed for 932 yards and nine touchdowns, both were *Super Bowl* records at the time of his retirement.

Determine what you want, then resolve to pay the price to get it.
—Bunker Hunt

shoulder press

Stand with feet shoulder-width apart, one foot slightly in front of the other, shoulders back, chest out and abs in. Holding a dumbbell in each hand, bend elbows to 90-degrees, and place at your sides with palms facing your body. Keeping your elbows at the 90-degrees, slowly raise straight out to sides, until arms are parallel to floor. Hold for 2-3 counts, then lower slowly. Repeat 10-15 times.

Steps Walked:
Cardio Workout:
Strength Workout:
Calories Consumed:
Calories Burned:
Difference:
Weight / Body fat:

DATE

Eating healthy tastes great!

Spanish Green Peas
16 oz can peas, drained
2 canned pimientoes, chopped
1/4 cup ripe black olives
2 tbs olive oil
pepper and oregano to taste

Sauté onion with spices in olive oil. Add peas, pimientos and olives. Toss lightly, simmer 8-10 minutes until peas are hot.

Read it, live it, love the results.

Aloe Vera can be used for stomach irritations and ulcers.
Many have grown to know the benfits of using Aloe Vera to aide in the healing of burns. However, what you may not know is that Aloe may also be used for stomach irritations and ulcers. Simply remove a mature leaf from the plant, squeeze some of the "gel" into a glass of water, and drink.

Write it down & get it done.

1
2
3
4
5
6
7
8
9
10

military press

Stand with feet shoulder-width apart, shoulders back, chest out and abs in. Holding dumbells with an overhand grip, lift them to eye level, with the upper arms parallel to floor, elbows pointing straight out. Slowly press the weight overhead, keeping your shoulders down by pressing your shoulder blades together. Once you reach the top, lower slowly to the starting position and repeat 10-15 times.

May the best from your past be the worst of your future.
–from The Long Kiss Goodnight

DATE

Steps Walked:
Cardio Workout:
Strength Training:
Calories Consumed:
Calories Burned:
Difference:
Weight / Body fat:

Write it down & get it done.

1
2
3
4
5
6
7
8
9
10

Read it, live it, love the results.

Use your time wisely in becoming that which you desire. Don't waste time thinking about what you could have, or should have, done and become. Use your time wisely in becoming the person you desire to be today. Focus your energy on the here and now. You will get much more accomplished when you do so.

Doors open when least expected.

Actor, director, producer and composer, **Clint Eastwood** was encouraged to enroll in school plays, but he loved music. He wanted to attend college and major in music theory, however, was drafted by the U.S. Army. After serving, he managed apartments in Beverly Hills by day and worked at a gas station by night. It was by chance that he was discovered by Universal Studios. They felt he was *"the sort of good looking young man that has traditionally done well in the movies"*.

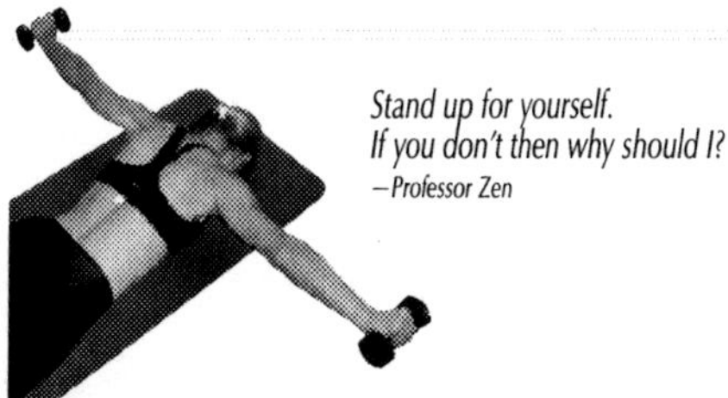

Stand up for yourself.
If you don't then why should I?
—Professor Zen

face down lateral lift

Lie on the floor, face down, with your forehead resting on a rolled-up towel. With a dumbbell in each hand, extend your arms straight out to sides. Keep your arms straight as you raise the dumbbells off the floor, hold for 2-3 counts, then slowly return to starting position. Perform 10-15 repetitions.

DATE

Steps Walked:
Cardio Workout:
Strength Workout:
Calories Consumed:
Calories Burned:
Difference:
Weight / Body fat:

Eating healthy tastes great!

Honey Nut Peach Shake
$1\frac{1}{3}$ cups fat free vanilla yogurt
$1\frac{1}{2}$ cups Honey Nut Cheerios®
15 oz can sliced peaches, drained
1 cup skim milk
1 banana
$\frac{1}{8}$ tsp ground cinnamon
2 scoops vanilla protein

Place all ingredients in blender and blend until smooth.
I recommend that women use soy protein and men use whey protein.

Read it, live it, love the results.

Eat nutrient rich, low calorie foods.
Studies, performed by the scientists at Washington University School of Medicine, show that blood pressure is significantly lower in people who follow a balanced calorie restricting diet. As long as you consume at least 1200 calories a day, you should be able to keep your metabolism up while building a healthier body.

Write it down & get it done.

1
2
3
4
5
6
7
8
9
10

front raises

Stand with one foot in front of the other with knees slightly bent. Holding a dumbbell in each hand with palms facing your body, let the dumbbells rest on your thighs. Keeping your arms straight, raise the dumbbells directly in front of you, parallel to the floor. Hold for 2-3 counts then lower slowly to the starting position, avoiding the tendency to arch your lower back. Repeat 10-15 times. right.

I can accept failure, everyone fails at something. But I can't accept not trying.
– Michael Jordan

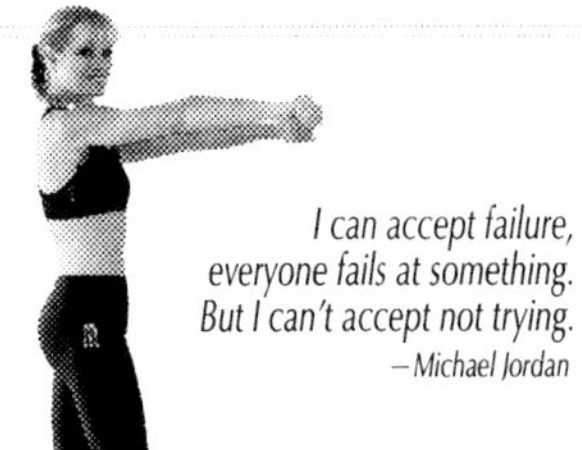

DATE

Steps Walked:
Cardio Workout:
Strength Training:
Calories Consumed:
Calories Burned:
Difference:
Weight / Body fat:

Write it down & get it done.

1
2
3
4
5
6
7
8
9
10

Read it, live it, love the results.

Help others achieve their health and fitness goals, and you will get better results yourself. When you help others, you help yourself. Enjoy the company of a workout partner and the satisfaction of helping another improve their life. In the long run, you may even be responsible for saving a life or two.

Your level of success is up to you.

Basketball superstar **Michael Jordan** had tried out for the varsity basketball team during his sophomore year of high school, but at 5'11", he was too short and cut from the team. The following summer he grew four inches and practiced religiously. Due to his persistance he earned a spot on the varsity team and grew into the greatest basketball player of all time.

Progress involves risks. You can't steal second with your foot on first.
– Fred Wilcox

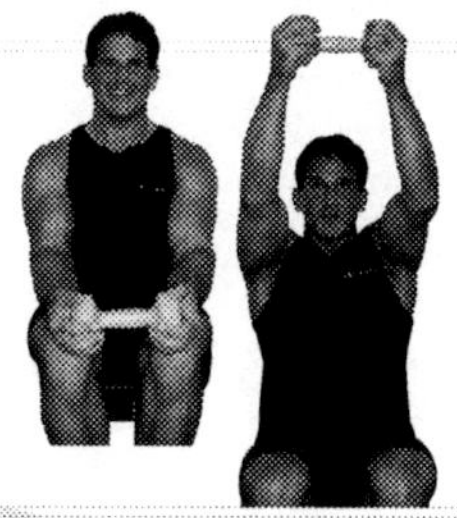

overhead hammer

Sit tall, abs in, shoulders back, chest out, feet flat on floor. Rest a large dumbbell on your knees. Cupping the ends with both hands and keeping the arms straight, slowly lift the dumbbell above your head, hold for 2-3 counts then slowly return to the starting position. Repeat 10-15 times.

DATE

Steps Walked:
Cardio Workout:
Resistance Workout:
Calories Consumed:
Calories Burned:
Difference:
Weight / Body fat:

Eating healthy tastes great!

Fruit and Spice Oatmeal

3/4 cup oatmeal
2 1/4 cups water
1 tart apple, diced
1/4 cup raisins • 3 tbs honey
1 tsp pumpkin pie spice
1/2 tsp ground ginger

Bring water to a boil, stir in oats, reduce heat and simmer, stirring occasionally. Stir in apple, raisins, honey, pie spice and ginger. Cover and simmer for 15 minutes or until oats are tender.

Read it, live it, love the results.

Eat an apple a day.

A new study shows that an apple a day may do much more than keep the doctor away. Researchers speculate that the high levels of brain-protecting antioxidants packed into apples may reduce the effects of age-related brain disorders such as Alzheimer's disease. Apples are also fat free and a great source of fiber, pectin, potassium, and vitamins A and C.

Write it down & get it done.

1
2
3
4
5
6
7
8
9
10

bent over shoulder raise
Stand with one foot in front of the other with knees slightly bent. Bend from the waist until your back is nearly parallel to the floor. With a dumbbell in each hand, let arms hang down in front with palms facing. Raise dumbbells laterally until your arms are parallel to the floor. Hold for 2-3 counts, then slowly lower to starting position. Repeat 10-15 times.

I believe that good things come to those who work.
– Wilt Chamberlain

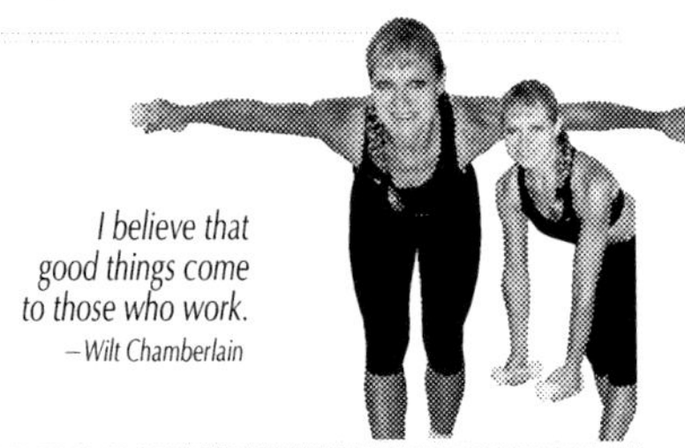

DATE

Steps Walked:
Cardio Workout:
Strength Training:
Calories Consumed:
Calories Burned:
Difference:
Weight / Body fat:

Write it down & get it done.

1
2
3
4
5
6
7
8
9
10

Read it, live it, love the results.

Walk every day for at least thirty minutes.
Studies show that daily moderate aerobic exercise, such as walking, has cardio-protective effects and may ward off degenerative brain diseases such as Alzheimer's and cognitive decline. Researchers also discovered that people with early Alzheimer's disease may be able to preserve their brain function for a longer period of time by exercising regularly.

Life's tough, get over it, he did!

Les Brown, one of my favorite motivational speakers, was born in an abandoned building and later adopted by a 38 year old single woman, who had very little education or financial means; however, she had a very big heart. In school Les was mistakenly declared *"educably mentally retarded"* and referred to as *"D .T."* for *"Dumb Twin"*. The label and stigma severely damaged his self-esteem for many years.

My riches consist not in the extent of my possessions, but in the fewness of my wants.
–J. Brotherton

bent-over single-arm lateral raise

Another version of the bent over lateral raise is to perform the exercise with a single arm. Stand with feet shoulder-width apart, knees bent with the right hand on your lower right thigh. Hold a dumbbell in your left hand, resting it against the right calf. Keeping the left arm straight, raise the dumbbell out to the side until parallel to the floor, hold for 2-3 counts, then slowly lower to starting position. Perform 10-15 repetitions on each arm.

Steps Walked:
Cardio Workout:
Resistance Workout:
Calories Consumed:
Calories Burned:
Difference:
Weight / Body fat:

DATE

Eating healthy tastes great!

Deviled Eggs
6 hard boiled eggs
3 tbs fat free mayonnaise
1 tbs red pepper, finely diced
1 tbs green onion, finely diced
1 tsp yellow mustard
white pepper to taste
Cut eggs lengthwise in half. Remove yolks and mix with remaining ingredients in zip lock bag. Mash and mix well, then cut corner of bag and squeeze mixture into egg half. Cover and refrigerate.

Read it, live it, love the results.

Eggs are great for your body!
Studies show an egg a day may prevent macular degeneraton and cataracts due to the carotenoid content, specifically lutein and zeaxanthin. Both nutrients are more readily available to our bodies from eggs than from other sources. Eggs are also a great source of protein and amino acides—one egg contains 6 grams of high-quality protein and all 9 essential amino acids.

Write it down & get it done.

1
2
3
4
5
6
7
8
9
10

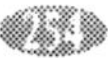

external rotation

Stand with feet shoulder-width apart, one foot slightly in front of the other, shoulders back, chest out and abs in. With a dumbbell in each hand, palms down, bend your elbows so the dumbbells touch in front of your ribcage. Roll your shoulders back so the shoulder blades squeeze together. Keeping your forearms level with the floor, wrists straight and abs in, press dumbbells behind you. Hold here for 2-3 counts, then slowly return to starting position. Complete 10-15 repetitions.

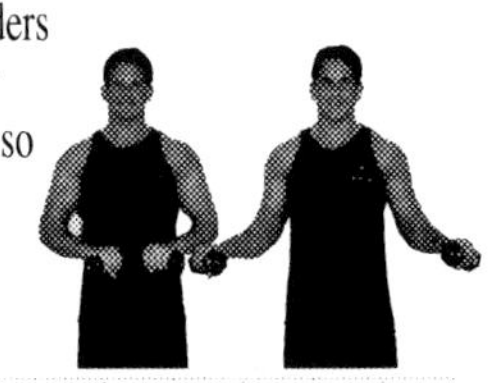

DATE

Self-praise is for losers. Be a winner. Stand for something. Always have class, and be humble.
–John Madden

Steps Walked:
Cardio Workout:
Strength Training:
Calories Consumed:
Calories Burned:
Difference:
Weight / Body fat:

Write it down & get it done.

1
2
3
4
5
6
7
8
9
10

Read it, live it, love the results.

Know the steps to take in order to achieve your goals.
When you know what you want and the exact steps it will take to get what you want, you are more likely to succeed.
A vague idea with hazy direction will get you nowhere but frustrated. By now you should know the importance of writing down your goals. If not, than let me tell you again.... "*Write it down if you want to make it happen!*"

Doors open when least expected.

A former NFL coach and one of the top NFL broadcasters, **John Madden**, was an incredible player who had his playing career cut short by a knee injury, just one year after he was drafted by the Philadelphia Eagles. However, in a way it was the start of his footcall career. First, as the head coach of the Oakland Raiders then, as a TV football commentator for *NBC Sunday Night Football*, author, and commercial pitchman.

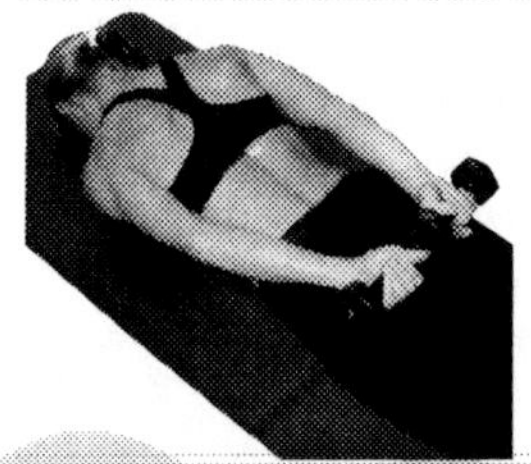

Goals are the fuel in the furnace of achievement.
—Brian Tracy

face down rear lift
Lie on the floor, face down, with your forehead resting on a mat or rolled-up towel. Holding dumbbells, reach back, resting the dumbbells on your buns with palms up. Raise the dumbbells 2-3 inches and hold for 2-3 counts, then slowly return to starting position. Perform 10-15 repetitions.

	DATE
Steps Walked:	
Cardio Workout:	
Resistance Workout:	
Calories Consumed:	
Calories Burned:	
Difference:	
Weight / Body fat:	

Eating healthy tastes great!

Vegetable Medley
1 cup of each diced or sliced; potatoes, carrots, onions, green peppers, eggplant, zucchini, summer squash
1/4 cup olive oil
8 oz can tomato sauce
3 tbs minced garlic • 1 cup water
tobasco and pepper to taste
Sauté garlic and onion in olive oil. Add remaining ingredients, bring to boil, reduce heat, cover and simmer 15-20 minutes.

Read it, live it, love the results.

Choose a healthy lifestyle.
Just as you can't accurately predict the weather, you can't accurately predict how your life will evolve. However, unlike mother nature, of which you have no control, you do have control of the lifestyle you choose. Making healthy choices greatly increase your odds of many "sunny" days ahead.

Write it down & get it done.

1
2
3
4
5
6
7
8
9
10

advanced t-pushup

On floor support yourself on hands and toes as you would a regular pushup, with hands positioned just below shoulders, supporting yourself on 5-10 pound dumbbells. With your abdominals engaged, rotate your entire body to the right, reaching towards the ceiling with the right hand, while holding the dumbbell. With the legs and feet stacked, hold for 2-3 counts, then lift the right leg 12-15 inches and hold for another 2-3 counts. Lower leg and hand and perform a push-up, bending elbows to 90-degrees. Return tostarting position and repeat the same movement on the left side. Complete 10-15 reps.

DATE

Steps Walked:
Cardio Workout:
Strength Training:
Calories Consumed:
Calories Burned:
Difference:
Weight / Body fat:

It's a funny thing about life; if you refuse to accept anything but the best, you very often get it.
—W. Somerset Maugham

Write it down & get it done.

1
2
3
4
5
6
7
8
9
10

Read it, live it, love the results.

Focus on the positive.
You were brought into this world with the ability to live a happy, healthy life. You will encounter circumstances which bring sorrow and unhappiness, however, you control the way these issues affect your life. Focus on the negative and you slowly destroy yourself, focus on the positive and you enhance your life.

Your level of success is up to you.

Actor, comedian, writer, playwright, producer, musician and composer, **Steve Martin**, actually developed his talents for magic, juggling, playing the banjo and creating balloon animals when he was a teenager, working at Disneyland in the Magic Shop. The hard work he put in as a teenager paid off well in later years. In a 2005 poll of The Comedian's Comedian, Martin was voted one of the top 15 Greatest Comedy Acts Ever.

Shoot for the moon. Even if you miss it you will land among the stars.
—Les Brown

dumbbell boxing

Stand with feet shoulder-width apart, one foot slightly in front of the other, shoulders back, chest out and abs in. With a dumbbell in each hand, position hands near your chin. Starting with the right, punch out to the left, extending the arm until nearly straight, without fully hyperextending your elbow or shoulder. Your body should twist with the movement, working the obliques. Complete 25-50 punches with the right, then complete a set with your left.

	DATE
Steps Walked:	
Cardio Workout:	
Resistance Workout:	
Calories Consumed:	
Calories Burned:	
Difference:	
Weight / Body fat:	

Eating healthy tastes great!

Spinach-Cheddar Frittata

2 eggs
1 oz low fat shredded cheddar cheese
1 cup baby spinach
black pepper to taste
nonstick cooking spray

Preheat the oven to 350ºF. Whisk egg with other ingredients and pour into small casserole dish that has been sprayed with nonstick cooking spray. Bake for 15 minutes or until firm.

Read it, live it, love the results.

Take control of your life.

There are millions of people who suffer from high blood pressure, heart disease, diabetes and many other health issues. These are often a result of poor lifestyle choices. When you choose to eat healthy and maintain a healthy lifestyle you are in control of your life. When you make poor choices you lose control. The choice is yours.

Write it down & get it done.

1
2
3
4
5
6
7
8
9
10

forward raise

Stand with one foot in front of the other, knees slightly bent, to support your lower back. Holding dumbbells, let arms hang straight down with palms facing upper thighs. Keeping wrists straight, raise the dumbbells straight out in front of you, then over your head. Once dumbbells are extended straight overhead, lower to starting position. Repeat 10 to15 times.

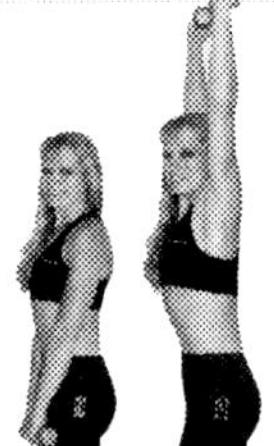

If you really want something you can figure out how to make it happen. –Cher

DATE

Steps Walked:
Cardio Workout:
Strength Training:
Calories Consumed:
Calories Burned:
Difference:
Weight / Body fat:

Write it down & get it done.

1
2
3
4
5
6
7
8
9
10

Read it, live it, love the results.

Fidget.
Overweight people tend to sit still all day, while thin people tend to pace and fidget, spending two hours more on their feet each day. The difference translates into about 350 calories a day.

Life's tough, get over it, she did!

Academy, Grammy, Golden Globe and Emmy Awards holder, **Cher**, had a pretty tough childhood. Her parents divorced when she was young and she was raised primarily by her mother, who was forced to place her in foster care for a time. Cher also suffered from severe dyslexia and dropped out of high school at the age of 16. However, she never gave up on herself—she simply took a different road to her success.

We must not allow other people's limited perceptions to define.
— *Virginia Satir*

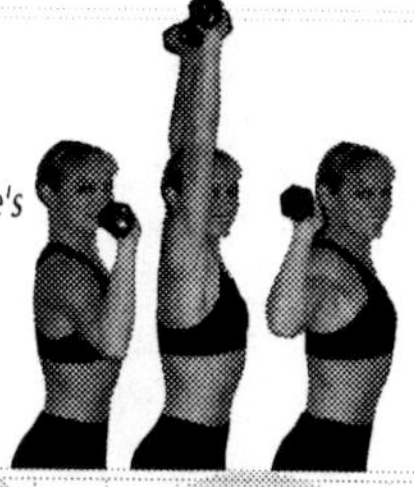

front to back press

Stand with feet shoulder-width apart, shoulders back, chest out and abs in. Holding dumbells with an overhand grip, lift them to eye level, with the upper arms parallel to floor, elbows pointing straight out. Press the dumbbell to arm's length overhead, then lower dumbbells behind your head to your ears. Press the dumbbells back to arm's length overhead and then lower to starting position. Complete 10-15 repetitions.

	DATE
Steps Walked:	
Cardio Workout:	
Resistance Workout:	
Calories Consumed:	
Calories Burned:	
Difference:	
Weight / Body fat:	

Eating healthy tastes great!

Souffléed Cauliflower

20 oz frozen cauliflower
10 oz can low fat mushroom soup
2 tbs sherry wine • 2 eggs
1 tbs light cream cheese
½ cup low fat cheese
pepper and paprika to taste
Preheat oven to 425°F.
Cook cauliflower as directed on package, drain and place in casserole dish. Beat eggs and add remaining ingredients. Pour mixture over cauliflower. Bake 20 minutes.

Read it, live it, love the results.

Cauliflower and other foods rich in vitamin K can slow bone loss.
Vitamin K is necessary for normal blood clotting and the synthesis of proteins found in plasma, bone, and kidneys. This aids in slowing bone loss and speeding the healing of fractures. Great sources of vitamin K include; spinach, lettuce, kale, cabbage, cauliflower, wheat bran, organ meats, cereals, some fruits, meats, dairy products and eggs.

Write it down & get it done.

1
2
3
4
5
6
7
8
9
10

lateral raise

Stand with one foot slightly in front of the other, back straight, shoulders back and chest out. With a dumbbell in each hand let arms hang at sides with palms facing thighs. Raise the dumbbells slightly higher than the shoulders, turning wrists so the back of the dumbbells are somewhat higher than the front. Hold for 2-3 counts, then lower slowly to starting position, repeat 10-15 times.

If life isn't about human beings and living in harmony, then I don't know what it's about.
–Orlando Bloom

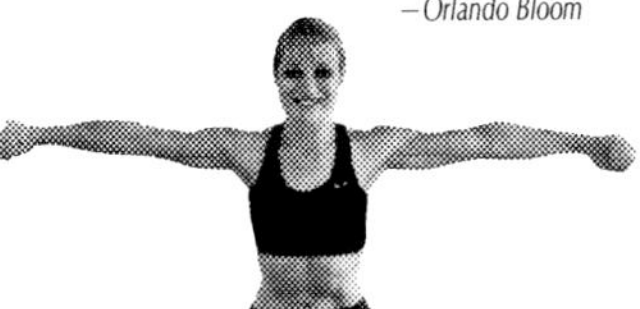

DATE

Steps Walked:
Cardio Workout:
Strength Training:
Calories Consumed:
Calories Burned:
Difference:
Weight / Body fat:

Write it down & get it done.

1
2
3
4
5
6
7
8
9
10

Read it, live it, love the results.

Focus on how your actions can take you closer to your goals. It's the little things that make a big difference. Skip putting the extra pat of butter on your baked potato, pass on dessert, drink water instead of soda, take the stairs instead of the elevator. All of these little changes add up to make big changes in your life. You, and only you, are responsible for your health.

Be the change you want to see.

An American patriot during the American Revolution, and participant in the *"Boston Tea Party"*, **Paul Revere** is best known for his ride through the night to warn people that the British were coming. Unfortunately his role was not particularly noted during his life. It wasn't until about forty years after his death–when the ride became the subject of the poem *"Paul Revere's Ride"*–that Revere became famous for his contribution as an American patriot.

lateral raise

Stand with one foot slightly in front of the other, back straight, shoulders back and chest out. With a dumbbell in each hand, extend the arms straight out to sides with palms up. Keeping your elbows still, curl the dumbbells toward your shoulders. Hold and squeeze for 2-3 counts then return to the starting position. Repeat 10-15 times.

Tomorrow isn't promised to any of us.
– Kirby Puckett

Steps Walked:
Cardio Workout:
Resistance Workout:
Calories Consumed:
Calories Burned:
Difference:
Weight / Body fat:

DATE

Eating healthy tastes great!

Stuffed Zucchini Boats

2 zucchini, sliced in half • 1 celery stalk
2 chicken breasts, cooked & shredded
2 hard boiled eggs • 3/4 cup cracker crumbs
1 tbs wheat flour • 2 green onions
1tbs light butter • 1/2 cup skim milk
parsley, chives, white pepper and nutmeg to taste // Preheat oven to 375ºF.
Scoop out Zucchini pulp, boil in water then simmer 5 minutes. In skillet, combine butter, milk and flour. Cook until thick. Add remaining ingredients, including pulp. Mix well & place in Zucchini. Bake 30 minutes.

Read it, live it, love the results.

Eat Zucchini and other foods which are rich in antioxidants.

When you choose to eat unhealthy foods, you build an army of free radicals which destroy your body. It's similar to placing termites in the walls of your home. When you eat healthy foods rich in antioxidants, you build a lifesaving army—which enhances your body and makes you feel great. *Zucchini* contains antioxidants Beta-Carotene Vitamin C, Folic Acid and Calcium.

Write it down & get it done.

1
2
3
4
5
6
7
8
9
10

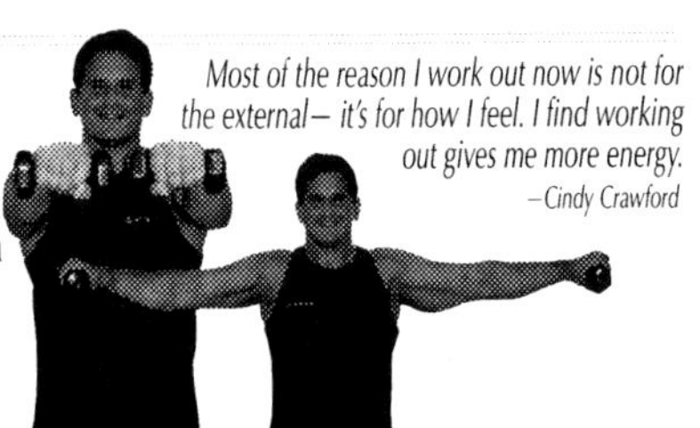

Most of the reason I work out now is not for the external– it's for how I feel. I find working out gives me more energy.
–Cindy Crawford

chest pull
Stand with feet shoulder-width apart, one foot slightly in front of the other, shoulders back, chest out and abs in. Holding dumbbells, extend your arms straight out front with palms down. Keeping your arms parallel with the floor, move the dumbbells to your sides, hold for 2-3 counts, then return slowly to the starting position. Repeat 10-15 times.

DATE

Steps Walked:
Cardio Workout:
Strength Training:
Calories Consumed:
Calories Burned:
Difference:
Weight / Body fat:

Write it down & get it done.

1
2
3
4
5
6
7
8
9
10

Read it, live it, love the results.

Dream BIG!
This is your life, make it the best it can be. You're limited only by your thoughts and dreams so dream really, really big and get excited about the changes you can make in your life. When you become excited about your future, you will do everything in your power to make that future a reality.

Doors open when least expected.

Model **Cindy Crawford** was discovered at the age of 16 when a newspaper photographer took a photo of her pollinating corn; it was her summer job. The positive feedback she received from the photo was enough to convince her to take up modeling. Who would have thought pollinating corn would lead to a successful modeling career? During the 1980s and 1990s, Crawford was among the most popular supermodels.

In the middle of difficulty lies opportunity.
—Albert Einstein

shoulder abduction

Stand with feet shoulder-width apart, one foot slightly in front of the other, shoulders back, chest out and abs in. Holding dumbbells, let arms hang straight down, palms facing thighs. Keeping the butts of the dumbbells pressed together and arms straight, lift dumbbells up to the right as far as possible. Hold here for 2-3 counts then return to starting position. Repeat 10-15 times on each side.

Steps Walked:

Cardio Workout:

Strength Training:

Calories Consumed:

Calories Burned:

Difference:

Weight / Body fat:

DATE

Eating healthy tastes great!

Crockpot Turkey

5 pound frozen turkey breast, NOT thawed, bone-in
16 oz can cranberry sauce
1 envelope dry onion soup mix
Put all ingredients in 5-6 quart crockpot, cover, and cook for 2 hours on high. Reduce heat to low and cook 4-5 hours additional hours, until turkey is 170ºF on instant meat thermometer.

Read it, live it, love the results.

Turkey may improve your mood!

Studies show that turkey is a great source of the amino acid tryptothan, an amino acid which has shown, in some studies, to be effective as a sleep aid– especially in normal patients. It has also been shown to have considerable promise as an antidepressant alone and as an "augmenter" of antidepressant drugs.

Write it down & get it done.

1
2
3
4
5
6
7
8
9
10

arnold press

Stand with feet shoulder-width apart, one foot slightly in front of the other, shoulders back, chest out and abs in. Hold dumbbells at chest level with palms facing chest. Press the dumbbells up, rotating them as you fully extend your arms, palms will be facing out. Lower slowly, with reverse rotation to original starting position. Complete 10-15 repetitions.

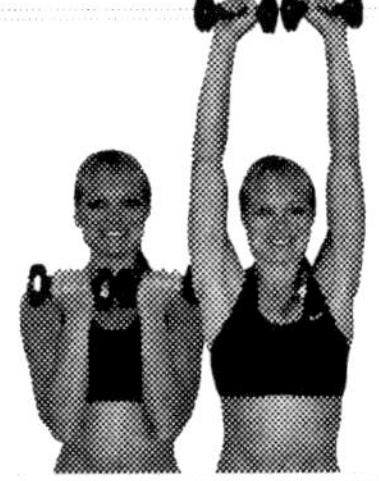

The purpose of education is to replace an empty mind with an open one.
– Malcom Forbes

DATE

Steps Walked:
Cardio Workout:
Strength Training:
Calories Consumed:
Calories Burned:
Difference:
Weight / Body fat:

Write it down & get it done.

1
2
3
4
5
6
7
8
9
10

Read it, live it, love the results.

Strive for order in your life. When things are unorganized you cannot feel your best or do your best. When your home is tidy, your checkbook balanced, your desk cleared and your closets cleaned you are mentally ready to "take on more", giving you a better state of mind to focus on your body. Don't be afraid to tell people "no", if you don't have the time. You must focus on you, before you can focus on others.

Doors open, when you work hard.

Grammy Award winning rock star, **Eric Clapton**, had received an acoustic Spanish Hoya guitar and a marimba for his thirteenth birthday. He found learning the instruments very difficult and nearly gave up. However, he continued practicing long hours, and eventually became a "natural". Today, Clapton is viewed by critics and fans alike as one of the greatest guitarists of all time.

Make a habit of doing things other people aren't willing to do. And that's our game here.
—Bob Bowman, Michael Phelps coach

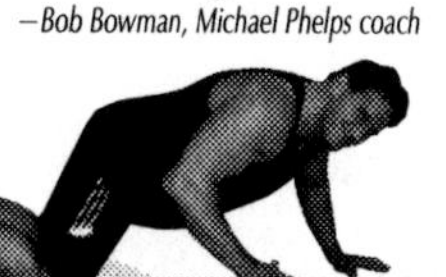

beginner single arm push-up

On floor support yourself on hands and knees, just as you would a beginner pushup, with hands positioned just below shoulders. Perform a pushup, keeping elbows close to your body, dropping your chest to within 2-3 inches of the floor before pushing back up. As you straighten your arms, lift the right hand 3-4 inches off the floor, then the left hand, holding each up for 2-3 counts. Perform another pushup and repeat hand movement, complete 10-15 repetitions.

Steps Walked:
Cardio Workout:
Resistance Workout:
Calories Consumed:
Calories Burned:
Difference:
Weight / Body fat:

DATE

Eating healthy tastes great!

Mexican Style Fish
2 lbs fish fillets
1 onion, minced • 1/4 cup olive oil
1/2 green pepper, minced
1 canned pimiento, minced
3 tbs wheat bread crumbs
chili powder, thyme and pepper
Preheat oven 425°F. Place fish fillets in baking dish. Combine remaining ingredients well and spread over fillets. Bake 25-30 minutes until fish flakes.

Read it, live it, love the results.

To get the body you've never had, you have to do things you've never done.
Good health is not a gift, it's something you must work towards. Eat healthier than you've ever eaten and stay active doing things you've never done. You will be amazed at what happens to your body—and your life!

Write it down & get it done.

1
2
3
4
5
6
7
8
9
10

axe chop

Stand with one foot in front of the other, knees slightly bent. Cupping the ends of a dumbbell, position it close to your right shoulder. Straightening your arms move the dumbbell down to the left thigh, then bring to your left shoulder and down to your right thigh. Return to the right shoulder and repeat 10-15 times.

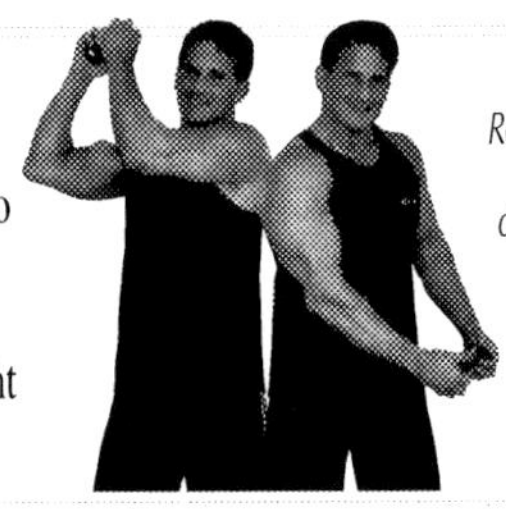

Really try to follow what it is that you want to do and what your heart is telling you to do.
—Jennifer Aniston

DATE

Steps Walked:

Cardio Workout:

Strength Training:

Calories Consumed:

Calories Burned:

Difference:

Weight / Body fat:

Write it down & get it done.

1
2
3
4
5
6
7
8
9
10

Read it, live it, love the results.

Take time for solitude.
When you take time to enjoy solitude you are able to reflect and contemplate all of the incredible possibilities that await you. Getting to know your inner self through solitude is the key to enriching your life and your relationships. It's also a great way to destress. "*...our society is so geared toward attachment and engagement and 'busyness,' that alonetime has been lost.*"
—Esther Buchholz, Ph.D.

Success is the reward of hard work.

Actress **Jennifer Anniston** had nearly given up on her acting career after struggling through four failed television series and an appearance in a critically derided horror film. Fortunately, she stuck it out, auditioned for *"Friends,"* and turned her career around. From the mid 1990's to the early 2000's Anniston played the role of Rachel in the popular sitcom *"Friends."* She won an *Emmy* and *Golden Globe Award* role for this part.

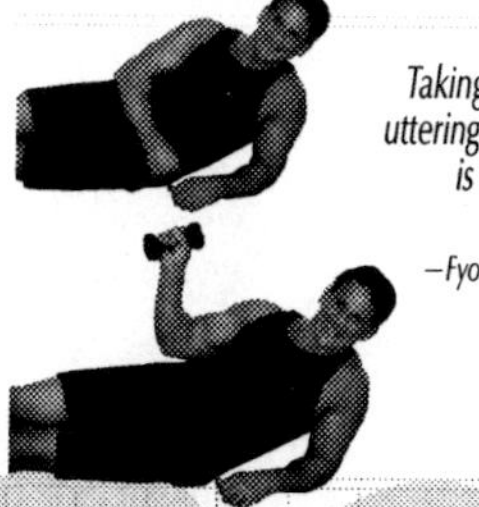

Taking a new step, uttering a new word is what people fear most.
–Fyodor Dostoyevski

lying front rotation

Lie on the floor, on your right side. With your bottom leg slightly bent, prop yourself up on the right elbow. Keeping your left elbow at your side, hold a dumbbell 2-3 inches above the floor. Twisting the arm, without removing the elbow from your side, raise the dumbbell towards the ceiling, hold for 2-3 counts then lower to starting position. Complete 10-15 repetitions on each side.

	DATE					
Steps Walked:						
Cardio Workout:						
Strength Training:						
Calories Consumed:						
Calories Burned:						
Difference:						
Weight / Body fat:						

Eating healthy tastes great!

Banana Chips

2 large, firm bananas
2 tbs fresh lemon juice

Preheat oven to 200ºF. Cut bananas diagonally into $^{1}/_{8}$-inch slices. Dip slices in lemon juice. Place slices on baking sheet coated with vegetable cooking spray. Bake for 2 hours; turn over and bake $1^{1}/_{2}$ to 2 hours or until slices are crisp. Place on wire rack to cool. Store in an airtight container.

Read it, live it, love the results.

Good health starts in your mind.
Americans spend more than $33 billion per year on weight loss products and services, and most have attempted at least one diet. However, what most people don't realize is that there's not enough money in the world to make you healthy, until you change your thoughts and attitude. When you change your thoughts, you will change your life.

Write it down & get it done.

1
2
3
4
5
6
7
8
9
10

lying lateral raise
Lie on the floor, on your right side. With your bottom leg slightly bent, prop yourself up on the right elbow. Holding a dumbbell in your left hand, let it hover about an inch above your leg. Keeping your arm straight, raise the dumbbell above your head, hold for 2-3 counts, then slowly lower to the starting position. Repeat 10-15 times on each side.

A wise man will make more opportunities than he finds.
– Francis Bacon

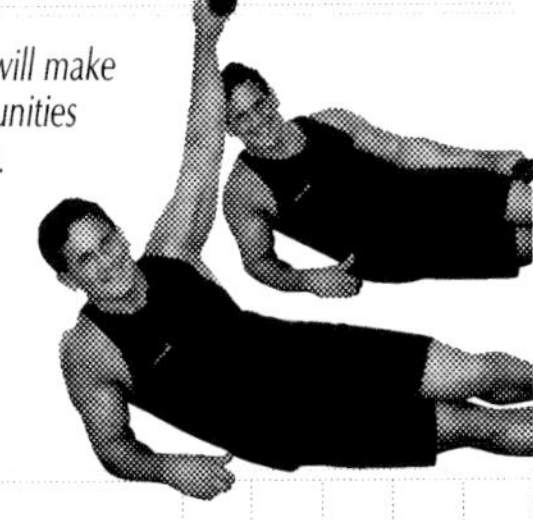

DATE

Steps Walked:
Cardio Workout:
Strength Training:
Calories Consumed:
Calories Burned:
Difference:
Weight / Body fat:

Write it down & get it done.

1
2
3
4
5
6
7
8
9
10

Read it, live it, love the results.

Take control of your life.
When in a canoe you must paddle to stay the course, this is similar to your journey through life. Don't allow the currents to control your journey. Pick up your paddle and move in the direction which makes you happy. If you allow yourself to be swept up in the currents, you may end up at the bottom of a waterfall.

Be the change you want to see.

President of the U.S., **Barack Obama**, lived with his maternal grandparents in Hawaii when he attended a private college preparatory school, from the fifth grade until his graduation from high school.
It was during these high school years that he used alcohol, marijuana and cocaine to *"push questions of who I was out of my mind."* At the 2008 Civil Forum on the Presidency, Obama identified his high-school drug use as his *"greatest moral failure."*

Take your life in your own hands and what happens? A terrible thing: no one to blame.
—Erica Jong

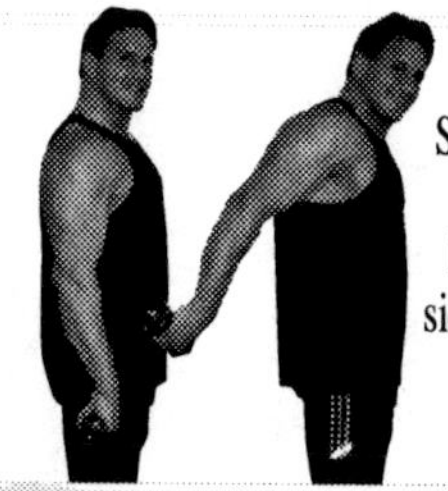

rear raises

Stand with feet shoulder-width apart, one foot slightly in front of the other, shoulders back, chest out and abs in. Holding a dumbbell in each hand, let your arms hang at sides with palms facing back. Lift your arms up and back as high as possible. Hold for 2-3 counts, then slowly return to the starting position. Repeat 10-15 times.

	DATE
Steps Walked:	
Cardio Workout:	
Strength Training:	
Calories Consumed:	
Calories Burned:	
Difference:	
Weight / Body fat:	

Eating healthy tastes great!

Chinese Green Beans

1 pound fresh green beans
3 tbs peanut oil
4 oz can sliced mushrooms
1 packet Sweet and Low®
1/3 cup low sodium chicken broth
1 tsp cornstarch with 1 tbs broth

Mix cornstarch with 1 tbs broth, set to side. Destem and cut beans in 2" pieces. Sauté beans in peanut oil 3-4 minutes. Add remaining ingredients, cook another 5 minutes. Add cornstarch to mix, stirring constantly.

Read it, live it, love the results.

Worried about cholesterol? Add green beans to your diet.

Studies show that eating beans, which are high in fiber,will help lower cholesterol.

Due to their rich source of fiber, beans also prevent blood sugar levels form rising too rapidly after a meal. This also makes them an excellent choice for individuals with diabetes, insulin resistance, or hypoglycemia.

Write it down & get it done.

1
2
3
4
5
6
7
8
9
10

rear rotation

Stand with feet shoulder-width apart, one foot slightly in front of the other, shoulders back, chest out and abs in. Holding a dumbbell in each hand, let your arms hang at your sides with palms facing back. Bending your elbow, bring the right dumbbell up behind your back to the left, hold for 2-3 counts, then slowly return to starting position. Repeat this with the left arm. Complete 10-15 alternating repetitions.

You don't paddle against the current, you paddle with it. And if you get good at it, you throw away the oars.
—Kris Kristofferson

DATE

Steps Walked:

Cardio Workout:

Strength Training:

Calories Consumed:

Calories Burned:

Difference:

Weight / Body fat:

Write it down & get it done.

1
2
3
4
5
6
7
8
9
10

Read it, live it, love the results.

Weight train on a regular basis. As you age your lean muscle mass naturally decreases. Fortunately, you can reverse this muscle loss by working out with weights. Studies show that weight training and other types of strength training can improve muscle tone, quality of life and the ability to complete daily tasks—even for those in their 80's and 90's. If you want to remain independent into your later years keep your body strong.

Be the change you want to see.

Prominent *American civil rights leader,* **Susan B. Anthony** was very self-conscious of her looks and speaking abilities when younger. As a result she long resisted public speaking for fear she would not be sufficiently eloquent. Thankfully for many this was something she overcame, and as an adult traveled the United States and Europe for forty-five years, giving 75 to 100 speeches each year on women's rights!

*Come forth into the light of things,
let nature be your teacher.*
–*William Wordsworth*

reverse dumbbell laterals

Stand with feet shoulder-width apart, one foot slightly in front of the other, shoulders back, chest out and abs in. Holding a dumbbell in each hand, let your arms hang at your sides with palms facing out. Slowly lift the dumbbells up, bringing them together over your head. Hold here for 2-3 counts, then slowly lower to starting position and repeat, completing 10-15 repetitions.

DATE

Steps Walked:
Cardio Workout:
Strength Training:
Calories Consumed:
Calories Burned:
Difference:
Weight / Body fat:

Eating healthy tastes great!

Cottage Potatoes

2 potatoes, cut into 3/8 inch strips
3 sprigs parsley, sniped
1 tbs light butter
1/4 cup low fat sour cream
1/4 cup Parmesan cheese
Preheat oven to 425ºF.
Place potato stips in casserole dish. Mix remaining ingredients spread over strips.
Cover and bake 40-45 minutes until potatoes are tender.

Read it, live it, love the results.

Alfalfa, it's not just for horses!

According to herbalists, alfalfa is one of the richest land-grown plants—containing more subnutritional trace minerals than any other plant. Due to the bad taste alfalfa tablets are available. The benefits of taking alfalfa tablets include; reduction of fatigue, tension and stiffness. Kidney and bladder problems are alleviated. It also adds strength to the heart muscle, in addition to relieving arthritis and lowering blood pressure.

Write it down & get it done.

1
2
3
4
5
6
7
8
9
10

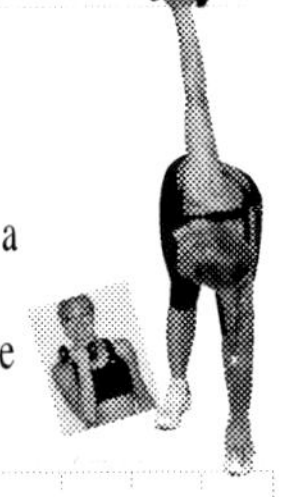

corkscrew press
Stand with feet shoulder-width apart, with the right foot turned slightly in and the left foot turned approximately 90-degrees to the side. With a dumbbell in your right hand hold it just below your chin, with your palm facing your body. As you begin lifting the dumbbell up with a corkscrew movement, reach down to your left foot with your left hand, hold this position for 2-3 counts, then return to the starting position, in a reverse corkscrew movement. Maintain eye contact with the dumbbell throughout the lift. Complete 10-15 repetitions on each side.

DATE

Growing up is not being so dead-set on making everybody happy. –Reba McEntire

Steps Walked:
Cardio Workout:
Strength Training:
Calories Consumed:
Calories Burned:
Difference:
Weight / Body fat:

Write it down & get it done.

1
2
3
4
5
6
7
8
9
10

Read it, live it, love the results.

Burn more calories than you eat. If you want to maintain your weight, you must balance calories consumed with calories burned. If you spend more time eating than moving – you will gain weight. However, if you eat less and keep busy, you are destined to lose weight. It's really not that complicated, yet millions are continually seeking an easier way. You have the ability to move, don't kill yourself by sitting on the couch every night.

Doors open, when you work hard.

Singer and actress, **Reba McEntire**, began to pursue a career in country music in 1974. Unfortunately, her hard honky tonk sound didn't go over very well. Still, she didn't give up. Finally in 1978 one of her songs *Hit Billboards Top Twenty,* it wasn't until 1982 that she had a number one Billboard hit. Today she is known as *"The Queen of Country Music"*, with 31 albums and over 50 million records sold worldwide.

One does not discover new lands without consenting to lose sight of the shore for a very long time.
—Andr Gide

Exercise bands can be used to workout anywhere, whether you are at home, on vacation or a business trip you never have an excuse to skip your workout. If you don't currently own a band you may purchase one for $7-$10 at most retail stores or online. Bands offer great workouts for beginners, intermediate or advanced individuals. You determine the difficulty through the thickness of the band you choose or by adjusting the band position.

DATE

Steps Walked:
Cardio Workout:
Resistance Workout:
Calories Consumed:
Calories Burned:
Difference:
Weight / Body fat:

Eating healthy tastes great!

Asparagus á la King
1 lb fresh asparagus, cut into 1" pieces
4 hard boiled eggs, diced
1/4 cup light butter
1/4 cup wheat flour • 2 cups skim milk
2 cups low fat cheese
pepper and oregano to taste
Cook asparagus until tender, set aside. Melt butter, add flour and milk. Cook over low heat until thickened. Add spices and cheese, stir until cheese melts. Add asparagus and eggs. Cook additional 5 minutes.

Read it, live it, love the results.

If pregnant eat plenty of black eyed peas, cooked spinach, great northern beans and asparagus. These are all excellent sources of folate. Folate, an essential for protein synthesis, is required for a pregnant woman's increasing blood supply and the growth of both maternal and fetal tissues. Studies show that sufficient folate may decrease the risk of having a child with a brain or spinal cord defect.

Write it down & get it done.

1
2
3
4
5
6
7
8
9
10

leg extension with band

Sit tall, abs in, shoulders back and chest out with hands in lap or holding sides of a chair. With band wrapped through chair legs, place handle of band on feet. Raise legs straight out front. Hold for 2-3 counts, then lower and repeat 10-15 times. You may also perform this exercise with one leg at a time.

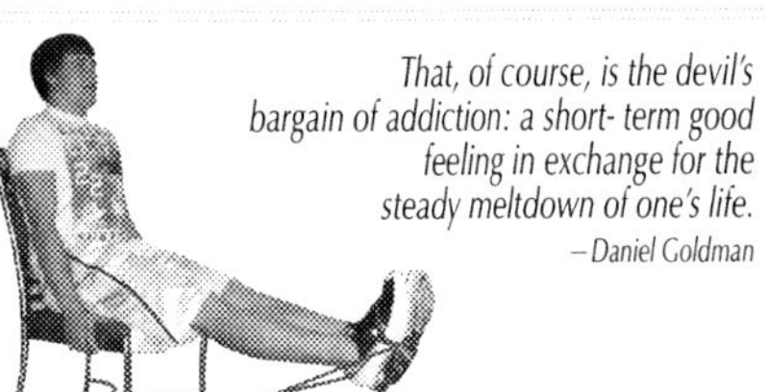

That, of course, is the devil's bargain of addiction: a short- term good feeling in exchange for the steady meltdown of one's life.
– Daniel Goldman

DATE

Steps Walked:
Cardio Workout:
Strength Training:
Calories Consumed:
Calories Burned:
Difference:
Weight / Body fat:

Write it down & get it done.

1
2
3
4
5
6
7
8
9
10

Read it, live it, love the results.

Make eye contact with yourself in the mirror.

Look deep into your soul and discover the person hiding within. The person inside who wants to live a healthy life, who wants to feel energized and excited about life. Now do all you can to bring that person out. Eat healthy, exercise and develop a positive attitude, you'll love yourself more than ever.

Doors open, when you work hard.

Henry Ross Perot, best known for seeking the office of US President 1992 and 1996, began as a salesman for IBM. Supervisors ignored his ideas, despite him being top salesperson. He eventually left IBM to start his own company. He courted large corporations and was refused 88 times before he got his first contract. Today he has an estimated net worth of around five billion dollars. In 2008, he was ranked by Forbes as the 68th richest person in America.

You sit around watching all this stuff happen on TV... and the TV sits and watches us do nothing! The TV must think we're all pretty lame.
– Shannon Wheeler

squats

Stand on the center of the band with feet shoulde-width apart, back straight, shoulders back and chest out, with toes pointed straight ahead or slightly outward. Bend knees and squat down, until thighs are parallel to the floor, keeping your knees behind your toes. Wrap the band around your feet to increase tension. Holding the band, focus your vision straight ahead, then keeping your heels planted firmly on the floor, slowly stand, then lower again.

DATE

Steps Walked:

Cardio Workout:

Strength Training:

Calories Consumed:

Calories Burned:

Difference:

Weight / Body fat:

Eating healthy tastes great!

Banana Flambé

4 bananas, sliced lengthwise
3 tbs light butter
1 tbs orange peel, grated
1 tsp Splenda® brown sugar
10 oz package frozen blueberries,
Thaw & purée with 2 tbs brandy

Melt butter, stir in orange peel and Splenda®. Saute bananas on both sides. Pour blueberry purée over bananas. Heat on low. To serve: Put 2 tbs brandy in ladle, light and pour over bananas, ready to eat when flame dies out.

Read it, live it, love the results.

Don't make celebrations an excuse for eating unhealthy.

Birthdays, promotions and anniversaries have all become excuses to celebrate with large unhealthy meals and desserts. Instead of punishing your body with unhealthy indulgences, prepare healthy foods. It does not take any longer to prepare a healthy meal, than it does an unhealthy meal...and yes, it will still taste great!

Write it down & get it done.

1
2
3
4
5
6
7
8
9
10

lying leg lift with band

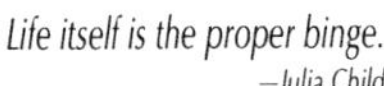

Use a circular band or one which has been tied to create a circle. Placing the band around the lower part of your legs, lie on your right side with the right leg slightly bent to support your body. Supporting yourself with your right elbow, contract your obliques as you lift the left leg as high as possible, pointing your toe towards the ceiling. Hold here for 2-3 counts, lower and repeat. Complete 10-15 repetitions on each side.

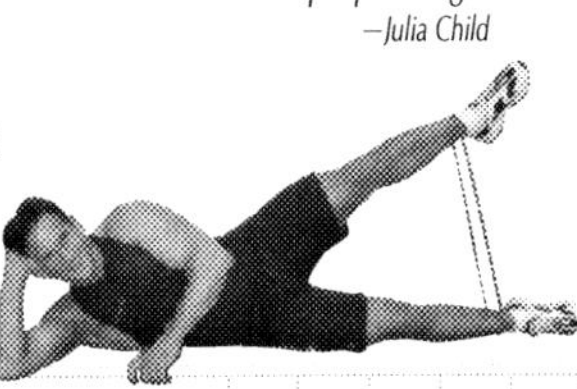

DATE

Steps Walked:

Cardio Workout:

Strength Training:

Calories Consumed:

Calories Burned:

Difference:

Weight / Body fat:

Write it down & get it done.

1
2
3
4
5
6
7
8
9
10

Read it, live it, love the results.

It's up to you to make your life the best it can be.
If you knew you couldn't fail, what would you be doing today?
How would you look?
How would you feel?
Think about your answers.
Now proceed through your life knowing that you can achieve that which you just pictured.
You can make your life anything you want it to be.

Be the change you want to see.

Former quarterback and television sportscaster, **Phil Simms**, spent his professional career with the New York Giants. They made him their first round pick, which surprised many—as most people had never heard of him. When Simms'name was first announced the Giant's fans booed loudly; however, things changed when he won the first five starts of his rookie year. He played his entire professional career with the Giants and was named *Most Valuable Player* of *Super Bowl XXI*.

No trumpets sound when the important decisions of our life are made. Destiny is made known silently.
—*Agnes de Mille*

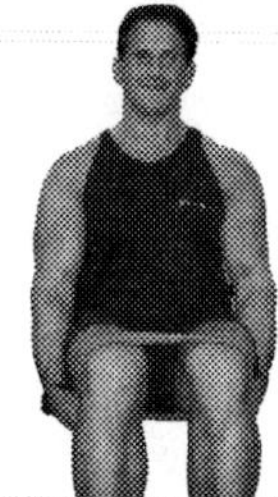

hip adduction with band
Sit tall in chair with abs in, shoulders back and chest out. Wrap a band around your thighs, near the knees, then move the left leg as far out to the left as possible. Hold for2-3 counts, then return to the starting position. Complete 10-15 repetitions on each side.

DATE

Steps Walked:
Cardio Workout:
Resistance Workout:
Calories Consumed:
Calories Burned:
Difference:
Weight / Body fat:

Eating healthy tastes great!

Teriyaki Chicken
8 chicken breasts
1 tbs cornstarch • 1 tbs cold water
1/2 cup Splenda® • pepper to taste
1/2 c soy sauce • 1/4 c cider vinegar
2 tbs minced garlic • 1/2 tsp ginger
Preheat oven to 425°F. Mix all ingredients, except chicken and cook on low, stirring until thick. Brush chicken with sauce and place in nonstick baking dish. Bake 30 minutes, turn pieces over, and bake for another 30 minutes. Brush with sauce every 10 minutes during cooking.

Read it, live it, love the results.

Don't bindge and hang out on the couch when feeling down.
Though eating may make you feel better briefly, when the food is gone, so is the feeling of "happiness." Make it a habit to replace binging with walks or working out, you will feel great while you are doing it, and for hours afterwards. The rewards are incredible.
Use exercise as an anti-depressant and you will find yourself much healthier and happier!

Write it down & get it done.

1
2
3
4
5
6
7
8
9
10

lying hamstring curl with bands

Use a circular band or one which has been tied to create a circle, then attatch the band to a stationary object.Lie on the floor, face down, legs extended out flat, with the other end of the band wrapped around your feet. Keeping your glutes tight, slowly bend your knees bringing the band up towards your glutes. Hold for 2-3 counts then return to the starting position, stopping within inches of the floor.

If you don't like the road you're walking, start paving another one.
– Dolly Parton

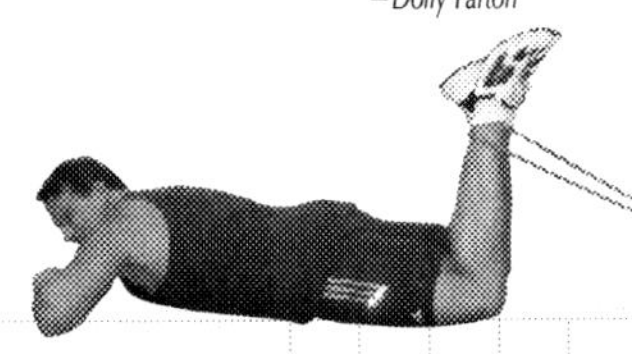

DATE

Steps Walked:
Cardio Workout:
Strength Training:
Calories Consumed:
Calories Burned:
Difference:
Weight / Body fat:

Write it down & get it done.

1
2
3
4
5
6
7
8
9
10

Read it, live it, love the results.

Practice meditation.
As you age the neurons in your brain begin to diminish, reducing your ablity to recall details.
By meditating you are able to improve your memory. Meditation also helps reduce stress while increasing your attention level and ability to remember new information and learn new things.

Without challenge, there is no change.

Country star, **Dolly Parton** began performing as a child, though did not find success until much later when Porter Wagoner asked her to join his country music TV program. She recorded a single with Wagoner that went to the Country Top Ten. This launched a six-year streak of Top Ten singles and a very successful career. She remains one of the most successful country music artists, with 26 number-one singles, and a record 42 Top-10 country albums.

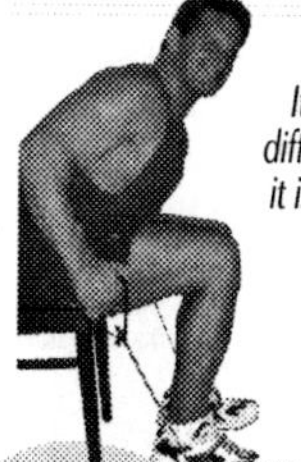

It is not because things are difficult that we do not dare; it is because we do not dare that they are difficult.
– Seneca

seated rows

Sit in a chair with feet flat on the floor, stepping on the center of a band. Bend over, bringing your chest as close as possible to your knees, then grab the bands with palms facing your body. Using your back muscles pull the band up to the side of your chest, squeezing your elbows together behind you. Hold for 2-3 counts, then slowly lower, repeating 10-15 times.

	DATE
Steps Walked:	
Cardio Workout:	
Resistance Workout:	
Calories Consumed:	
Calories Burned:	
Difference:	
Weight / Body fat:	

Eating healthy tastes great!

Spinach Frittata

1 onion • 4 tbs olive oil
1 lb potatos, sliced thin
3 tbs minced garlic
5 cups baby spinach • 8 eggs, beaten
3 tbs Parmesan cheese

Sauté onion, thinly sliced potatoes and minced garlic in 2 tbs olive oil. Once potatoes are done add spinach, cook until wilted. Stir in eggs and 2 tbs oil, cook until nearly done, sprinkle with cheese, broil briefly to brown.

Read it, live it, love the results.

Make healthier choices for breakfast.

Skip the bacon and sausage, enjoy canadian bacon or fat free ham instead. Making small changes to what you eat and drink can save 100 plus calories. Though 100 calories does not sound like a lot, you would have to walk about a mile to burn off those extra 100 calories. Remember, "A calorie NOT consumed, is a calorie you won't have to burn!"

Write it down & get it done.

1
2
3
4
5
6
7
8
9
10

deadlift with band

Stand on the center of a band with feet shoulder-width apart. Squat down and wrap the band around each foot. Holding the band, straighten your legs, while keeping your hands resting on the top of your feet. With your heels planted firmly on the floor, slowly stand, pulling your shoulders back and arching the lower back for a complete lower back contraction. Hold here for 2-3 counts, then return to starting position. Repeat 10-15 times.

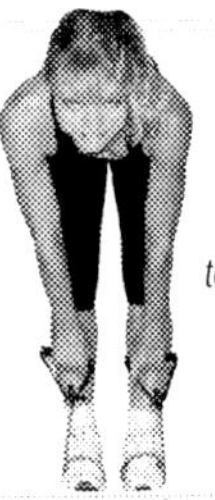

Attempt the impossible in order to improve your work.
– Bette Davis

DATE

Steps Walked:
Cardio Workout:
Strength Training:
Calories Consumed:
Calories Burned:
Difference:
Weight / Body fat:

Write it down & get it done.

1
2
3
4
5
6
7
8
9
10

Read it, live it, love the results.

Walk for at least thirty-minutes, everyday.
The *National Weight Control Registry* shows that walking is one of the main habits of people who successfully keep weight off. You don't even have to do all thirty minutes at once. You can break it up into three ten-minute walks or two fifteen-minute walks. The important thing to remember is that you need to move daily.

Doors open, when you work hard.

Actress **Bette Davis** had a rough beginning, though she never gave up. In failing her first screen test, the head of Universal Studios considered terminating her. Fortunately, the cinematographer told him she had "lovely eyes" and would be suitable for *"The Bad Sister"* part. She went on to become the first actress to receive ten Academy Award nominations and the first woman to receive a *Lifetime Achievement Award* from the *American Film Institute*.

To finish first, you must first finish.
– Rick Mears, Indy Car Driver

seated row

Sit on the floor, with feet out front, knees slightly bent, chest out and abs in, leaning back slightly. With the band wrapped around your feet, hold the band ends with palms facing in. Keeping your elbows in, slowly pull the band towards your rib-cage, contracting the back muscles. Squeeze and hold for 2-3 counts, then slowly return to the starting position, repeat 10-15 times.

DATE

Steps Walked:
Cardio Workout:
Resistance Workout:
Calories Consumed:
Calories Burned:
Difference:
Weight / Body fat:

Eating healthy tastes great!

Italian Chicken and Peas
2 chicken breasts, cooked and diced
2 onions, diced • olive oil
$2^1/_2$ cups low sodium chicken broth
6 oz package frozen peas
$^3/_4$ cup brown rice
4 tbs light butter
$^1/_4$ cup Parmesan cheese
Sauté onions in olive oil. Add remaining ingredients and bring to a boil. Cover and simmer 15-20 minutes or until broth is absorbed. Top with cheese.

Read it, live it, love the results.

Don't Diet!
Though diets often promise the world, many fad diets are detrimental to your health. They can cause discomfort and lead to disappointment when you regain weight soon after you lose it.
Despite what quick weight-loss diet books and magazines may say, the only sensible way to maintain a healthy weight permanently is to eat less and balance the calories from what you eat with the calories you burn.

Write it down & get it done.

1
2
3
4
5
6
7
8
9
10

standing row

Center a band under your left foot, then shift the right foot slightly to the rear. Bend over at your waist keeping your back straight, and abs tight. Holding the band let arms hang straight down with palms facing forward, away from the body. From this position, pull the bands up to chest height, slightly in back of your body, rotating the palms towards your body as you lift. Do not arch your back. Hold up for 2-3 counts, then slowly return to starting position and repeat 10-15 times.

A smile is a curve that sets everything straight.
— Phyllis Diller

DATE

Steps Walked:
Cardio Workout:
Strength Training:
Calories Consumed:
Calories Burned:
Difference:
Weight / Body fat:

Write it down & get it done.

1
2
3
4
5
6
7
8
9
10

Read it, live it, love the results.

Don't ever think you are "too old" to do anything you want! It's never too late to achieve all of that which you desire! There are many seniors who attend college, start new careers and begin working out for the first time. No matter your age, physical ability, or physical activity level, the future is yours. Make it the best it can be, because no matter what, it is going to arrive—be prepared and enjoy!

Your level of success is up to you.

Comedian **Phyllis Diller** did not begin her career until she was 37. She was a frumpy housewife, mother, and advertising copywriter, when her husband pushed her to follow her dreams. San Francisco's famous *Purple Onion Night Club* gave her a 2-week gig, which turned into 87 weeks and jump started her career. She became a *Golden Globe*-nominated *American Comedienne* and is considered to be one of the pioneers of female stand-up comedy.

Many of the things you can count, don't count. Many of the things you can't count, really count.
—Albert Einstein

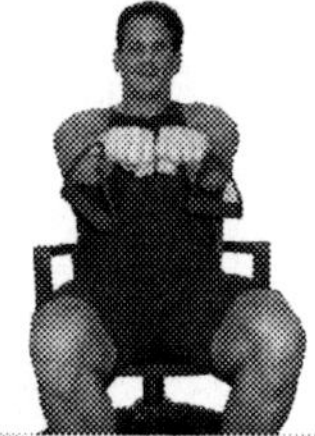

seated bench press with band

Sit tall in a chair, abs in, shoulders back and chest out, with a band wrapped around the back of your chair. Holding the band ends, with palms facing forward, extend arms straight out at shoulder height. Hold here for 2-3 counts, then keeping your back straight, bring the band back until hands are even with your chest. Repeat 10-15 times.

DATE

Steps Walked:
Cardio Workout:
Resistance Workout:
Calories Consumed:
Calories Burned:
Difference:
Weight / Body fat:

Eating healthy tastes great!

Cheese and Broccoli Soup
2 cups low sodium chicken broth
8 cups skim milk • 4 tsp olive oil
8 cups broccoli, chopped
1/2 cup onion, diced
6 tbsp whole wheat flour
4 tsp fresh parsley, chopped
salt and white pepper
6 oz light cheddar cheese
Sauté onion in olive oil. Add flour, mix well. Add remaining ingredients and cook until broccoli is soft. Do not boil.

Read it, live it, love the results.

Eat plenty of fruits and vegetables for strong bones.
Tomatoes, strawberries, cantaloupe, peppers, broccoli, and potatoes are all rich in Vitamin C, a building block of collagen, one of the first elements in bone formation. Some research shows that women who take vitamin C supplements have stronger bones, though it's generally better to get your vitamins from fruits and vegetables.

Write it down & get it done.

1
2
3
4
5
6
7
8
9
10

seated straight arm flye with bands

Sit tall in a chair, abs in, shoulders back and chest out with a band wrapped around the back of the chair. Hold the band ends with palms facing forward and arms extended straight out to sides. Keeping your arms straight, bring hands together straight out in front of your chest. Hold here for 2-3 counts, squeezing the pecs as you squeeze the bands forward. Complete 10-15 repetitions.

A good plan today is better than a perfect plan tomorrow.
– General George S. Patton

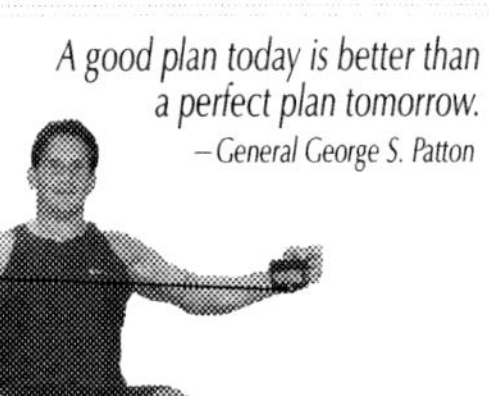

DATE

Steps Walked:
Cardio Workout:
Strength Training
Calories Consumed:
Calories Burned:
Difference:
Weight / Body fat:

Write it down & get it done.

1
2
3
4
5
6
7
8
9
10

Read it, live it, love the results.

Get at least seven to eight hours of sleep each night.
You've seen those who don't get enough sleep—lethargic with dark circles under their eyes. Unfortunately, lack of sleep does more then just add dark circles. Sleep deprive yourself long enough and you will experience dry, dull skin all over your body in addition to reducing your life span.

Doors open when least expected.

Comedian, actor and game show host, **Jeff Foxworthy**, worked in mainframe maintenance at IBM for five years. Then with the urging of co-workers, he entered and won the Great Southeastern Laugh-off at Atlanta's Punch Line comedy club in 1984. It was from this leap of faith that his career took off. Foxworthy became a Grammy-award winning stand-up comedian, best known for his jokes and stories about life as a redneck.

Spectacular achievement is always preceded by spectacular preparation.
– Robert Schuller

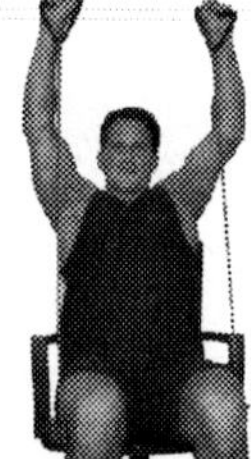

front raise and pullover with bands

Sit on the front edge of a chair with feet flat on the floor, stepping on the center of a band. Holding the band ends, lean back in the chair, resting your hands on your thighs with palms down. Keeping your arms straight, raise them over your head, then lower behind your head as far as possible. Hold here for 2-3 counts then return to starting position. Repeat 10-15 times.

Steps Walked:
Cardio Workout:
Strength Training:
Calories Consumed:
Calories Burned:
Difference:
Weight / Body fat:

DATE

Eating healthy tastes great!

Berry Chicken Salad
1 lb chicken breasts, cut into strips
1 cup fat free French dressing
10 oz pkg mixed salad greens
2 cups sliced strawberries, blueberries and/or raspberries
In skillet, simmer chicken in 1/4 cup of the salad dressing until thoroughly cooked.
Cool. Then in large bowl, toss with greens, berries and remaining dressing.

Read it, live it, love the results.

Eat plenty of fresh vegetables, fruits and whole grains.
Studies show that for maximum anti-aging of your complextion, you should get plenty of vitamins C and E. These two wonder vitamins work well together to restore collagen in your skin, keeping you looking younger and healthier then ever. Of course fresh vegetables, fruits and whole grains are a great source for these vitamins. Your age is up to you.

Write it down & get it done.

1
2
3
4
5
6
7
8
9
10

pushup with band

If you are advanced, perform this pushup on your hands and toes, if not perform on hands and knees. Hands should be at 6-24 inches apart. While in the "down position" place a band across your back, holding the ends in place with hands. Keeping your head in line with the spine, press your body up, straightening your elbows. Hold for 2-3 counts, then lower to starting position. Repeat 10-15 times. Keep elbows out to the sides to stress the pectoral muscles. Keep at sides to work the triceps.

To me, if life boils down to one thing, it's movement. To live is to keep moving.
—Jerry Seinfeld

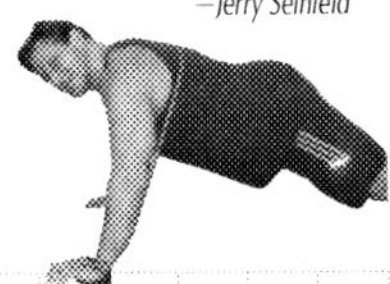

DATE

Steps Walked:
Cardio Workout:
Strength Training:
Calories Consumed:
Calories Burned:
Difference:
Weight / Body fat:

Write it down & get it done.

1
2
3
4
5
6
7
8
9
10

Read it, live it, love the results.

Smile more often.
Smiling does amazing things for your attitude. When you are feeling down, try putting on a smile and you will be amazed at how your spirits are lifted. Not only does a smile put you in a positive state of mind, it also makes you look younger and more attractive. Studies also reveal that smiling may contribute to a measurable reduction in your blood pressure, in addition to releasing endorphins, natural pain killers and serotonin.

Your level of success is up to you.

Comedian, actor and writer, **Jerry Seinfeld** graduated from Queens College, but dreamed of being a comedian. When he first started doing stand-up comedy, his mother and sister said he would never be as funny as his father. Thankfully he didn't let their negativity stand in the way of his dreams. He went on to star as a semi-fictional version of himself in the situation comedy, Seinfeld. He also became a bestselling author.

We make a living by what we get, but we make a life by what we give.
—Sir Winston Churchill

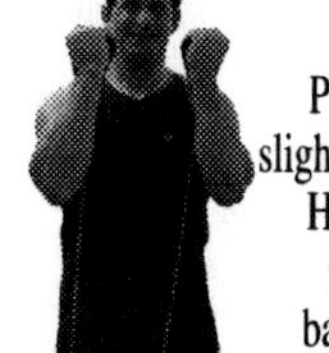

curl with band

Place the center of the band under your feet, then stand with one foot slightly in front of the other, back straight, shoulders back and chest out. Holding the band ends, let your arms hang at sides with palms facing forward. Contract your biceps as you bend your elbows, curling the band up toward your shoulders. Hold here for 2-3 counts, contracting the biceps, then slowly lower to starting position. Repeat 10-15 times.

DATE

Steps Walked:
Cardio Workout:
Resistance Workout:
Calories Consumed:
Calories Burned:
Difference:
Weight / Body fat:

Eating healthy tastes great!

Fiesta Salsa

2 avocados, peeled and diced
1 pint cherry tomatoes, quartered
1 cup frozen corn, thawed
4 oz can green chilies, drained and diced
1 bunch green onions, diced
3 tbs lime juice
1/2 tsp Sweet and Low®
black pepper to taste
Combine all ingredients and chill. Serve with baked tortila chips.

Read it, live it, love the results.

Avocado, the killer of breast cancer cells?

Studies state that a toxin found in the avocado can kill cancer cells. Scientists believe that the toxin has a great effect on the heart muscle tissue as well as on tissues of the lactating mammary gland.
Some considered it the world's healthiest fruit, because of its nutrient contents such as vitamin K, dietary fiber, potassium, folic acid, vitamin B6, vitamin C and copper.

Write it down & get it done.

1
2
3
4
5
6
7
8
9
10

concentration curl

Kneel, placing the right knee on the floor with the left knee bent at a 90-degree angle, foot flat on floor, stepping on a band. Holding the band with the left hand, palm up, lean forward placing the left elbow against the inside hollow of left knee. Drop the forearm down to align with the side of the leg. Contract the bicep, as you slowly raise your hand to the front of your shoulder, hold here for 2-3 counts then slowly return to starting position.

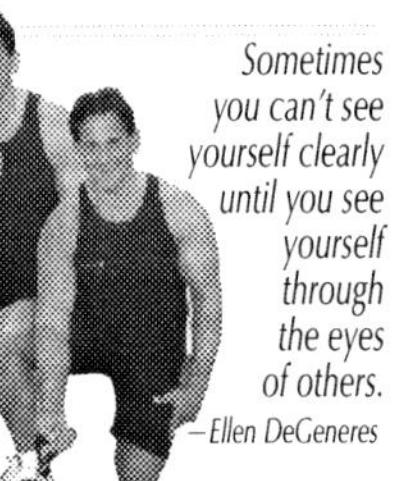

Sometimes you can't see yourself clearly until you see yourself through the eyes of others.
—Ellen DeGeneres

DATE

Steps Walked:

Cardio Workout:

Strength Training:

Calories Consumed:

Calories Burned:

Difference:

Weight / Body fat:

Write it down & get it done.

1
2
3
4
5
6
7
8
9
10

Read it, live it, love the results.

Winners are not born, they are made.

When you see an individual receiving a gold medal you see the result of a lot of hard work. These people don't have special powers nor were they granted special benefits from God. They worked hard for what they wanted. With hard work and desire, you too will be a winner.

Without challenge, there is no change.

Emmy Award-winning American stand-up comedian, **Ellen DeGeneres**, went through much trial and error before finding her dream. She went to college for one semester, did clerical work in a law firm, sold clothes at a chain-store, painted houses, worked as a waitress, hostess and bartended. Finally, she realized she didn't want to "answer to a boss" and became a very successful entrepreneur. Today, she hosts her award winning talk show, *The Ellen DeGeneres Show.*

3-part curls "21's"

Stand on the center of a band with one foot slightly in front of the other, back straight, shoulders back and chest out. Holding the band ends, let arms hang straight down with palms facing forward. Contract your biceps as you curl your hands halfway up, pump twice, then drop back down. Repeat seven times, then without pausing, curl all the way up then halfway down with a 2 count pump at the halfway point. Complete seven repetitions of this movement. Finish off the exercise by performing seven full-range curls.

Steps Walked:
Cardio Workout:
Resistance Workout:
Calories Consumed:
Calories Burned:
Difference:
Weight / Body fat:

DATE

The man who follows the crowd will usually get no further than the crowd. The man who walks alone is likely to find himself in places no one has ever been. – Alan Ashley-Pitt

Eating healthy tastes great!

Cottage Cheese Herbed Onions
2 lbs onions, sliced
1/4 cup light butter
1/4 cup wheat flour • 1/2 cup skim milk
1 1/2 cup low fat cottage cheese
1/2 cup Parmesan cheese
pepper and marjoram to taste
Preheat oven to 375°F.
Melt butter in sauce pan, stir in flour and milk, cook until thick. Add cottage cheese and spices. Place onions in casserole dish, layering with cottage cheese mix. Bake 25 minutes.

Good health is not a privilege, nor can it be bought.
Good health is acquired only through hard work and dedication. Even a man with little money can exercise and eat the right foods. Your health is based upon the decisions you make. When you work hard to create a healthy body you reap the rewards money cannot buy—good health, energy and self-respect.

Write it down & get it done.

1
2
3
4
5
6
7
8
9
10

cross body hammer curl
Stand on the center of a band with one foot slightly in front of the other, back straight, shoulders back and chest out. Holding the band ends, let arms hang at sides with palms facing body. Contract your biceps as you curl the right hand toward the left shoulder. Lower slowly to starting position and repeat with the left hand to the right shoulder. Repeat this alternating count 10-15 times.

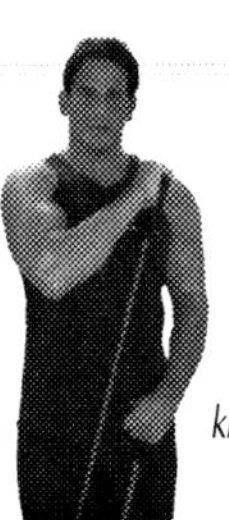

The great and glorious masterpiece of man is to know how to live to purpose.
–Michel de Montaigne

DATE

Steps Walked:
Cardio Workout:
Strength Training:
Calories Consumed:
Calories Burned:
Difference:
Weight / Body fat:

Write it down & get it done.

1
2
3
4
5
6
7
8
9
10

Read it, live it, love the results.

Get started now.
Procrastinate today and you will regret it tomorrow. There's seldom a good reason to put off until tomorrow what you can do today. If you want to lose weight begin today and you will feel better than ever about yourself, today and each day thereafter.

Doors open when least expected.

Actress, **Meg Ryan** had originally attended college to study journalism. However, while acting in television commercials to earn extra money, she was "discovered." Her success led her to drop out of college with just one semester left to graduate. Her "part time" job proved to be a great career move. She has become a Golden Globe-nominated film actress whose lead roles in four 1990s romantic comedies, grossed over $670 million worldwide.

outside curl

Stand on the center of a band with one foot slightly in front of the other, back straight, shoulders back and chest out. Holding band ends, let arms hang at sides with palms facing away from body. Contract your biceps as you bend your elbows, curling your hands up towards your shoulders. Hold here for 2-3 counts, then lower slowly to starting position. Repeat 10-15 times.

Build a dream and the dream will build you.
– Robert Schuller

Steps Walked:
Cardio Workout:
Strength Training:
Calories Consumed:
Calories Burned:
Difference:
Weight / Body fat:

DATE

Eating healthy tastes great!

Spinach Quesadillas
16 oz bag frozen cut leaf spinach
2 cups shredded low fat monterey jack cheese
8 -10" low carb tortillas • salsa
Drain spinach and squeeze between paper towels to remove moisture. On four tortillas, sprinkle 1 cup cheese, layer on spinach, sprinkle remaining cheese, then top with another tortilla. In skillet, cook each for 2-3 minutes on each side, then cut into six wedges. Serve with salsa.

Read it, live it, love the results.

To be successful you must be responsible for yourself.
There is no one forcing you to eat unhealthy foods or to lead a sedentary lifestyle. These are the choices you make. Though you may have many excuses as to why you've made these choices, know that they are still your choices and you have the option to change them. Don't let excusses ruin your health and life.

Write it down & get it done.

1
2
3
4
5
6
7
8
9
10

reverse curl

Stand on the center of a band with one foot in front of the other, back straight, knees slightly bent. Holding the band ends, let arms hang in front of body, with palms facing thighs. Bending your elbows, contract the biceps as you curl your hands toward your shoulders. Hold 2-3 counts, then lower slowly to starting position. Repeat 10-15 times.

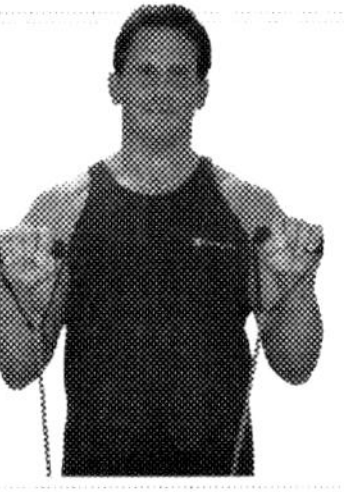

Learn to get in touch with the silence within yourself and know that everything in this life has a purpose.
– Elisabeth Kbler-Ross

DATE

Steps Walked:
Cardio Workout:
Strength Training:
Calories Consumed:
Calories Burned:
Difference:
Weight / Body fat:

Write it down & get it done.

1
2
3
4
5
6
7
8
9
10

Read it, live it, love the results.

Know what you desire and don't let anything stop you. You can go from ordinary to extraordinary, when you believe in yourself and work hard to achieve that which you desire. Your success is based upon a positive attitude and unrelenting drive to conquer anything that gets in the way of reaching your goals.

Doors open when least expected.

Stand-up comedian, television host, and actor, **Howie Mandel** began his comedy career as a result of a dare during a trip to LA, when he and friends attended amateur night at the Comedy Store. A producer in the crowd loved Mandel and hired him to appear on the game-show *Make Me Laugh*. This dare led to a very successful career. Today he is best known as the host of the NBC game show, *Deal or No Deal.*

kickback

Place the band under your feet, then keeping your back straight, bend over with your left leg slightly bent and the right leg shifted backwards. Holding the band ends, bend your elbows 90-degrees and hold them in at your sides. Without moving the upper arm, press the lower arm backwards, until your thumbs are pointing away from your body. Flex your triceps briefly, then return to the starting position and repeat 10-15 times.

Inches make champions.
– Vince Lombardi

Steps Walked:
Cardio Workout:
Resistance Workout:
Calories Consumed:
Calories Burned:
Difference:
Weight / Body fat:

DATE

Eating healthy tastes great!

Grilled Turkey Tenderloins
1 lb turkey tenderloins
1/3 cup mango chutney
2 tbs honey • black pepper to taste
Brush honey over the turkey tenderloins and sprinkle with salt and pepper; place on grill, 4-6" from coals. Cover grill and cook for 20-30 minutes, turning twice, until juices run clear when pricked with a fork. Slice and serve with mango chutney.

Read it, live it, love the results.

Own your body.
You were brought into this world with only one possession you will retain for your entire life—your body. Picture your body as an automobile. Have you allowed it to rust, let the tires bald and the engine go without oil or tune ups? Often people treat material possessions better than they do their own body. Material possessions can be replaced, your body cannot.

Write it down & get it done.

1
2
3
4
5
6
7
8
9
10

reach out

Standing on the center of a band with your right heel, bring your left leg slightly forward to support your lower back. Holding the band ends, place your hands behind your head with the palms facing your head. Raise your hands up and out, then slowly return to starting position. Repeat 10-15 times.

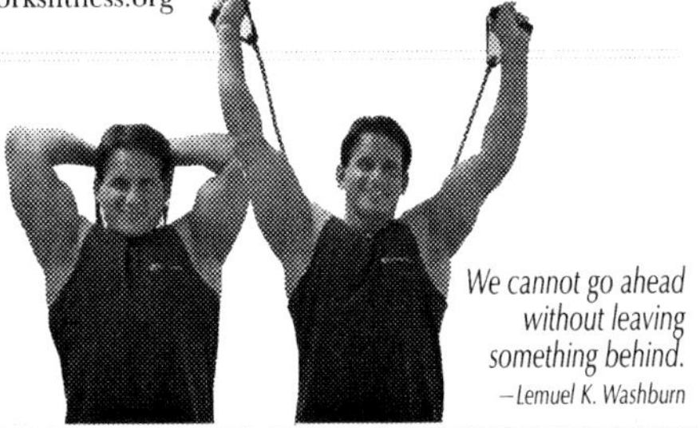

We cannot go ahead without leaving something behind.
—Lemuel K. Washburn

DATE

Steps Walked:
Cardio Workout:
Strength Training:
Calories Consumed:
Calories Burned:
Difference:
Weight / Body fat:

Write it down & get it done.

1
2
3
4
5
6
7
8
9
10

Read it, live it, love the results.

When you believe in yourself you can make anything happen. It's your beliefs that drive your thoughts, your thoughts that drive your feelings, and your feelings that drive your behaviors. When you behave as if you have that which you desire, you will achieve it. Whether it be creating a healthy lifestyle or anything else you desire to achieve.

Doors open, when you work hard.

Emmy Award winning comedian and actor, **Don Rickles**, frustrated with the lack of acting work available for TV, began doing stand-up comedy. By learning to respond to hecklers, he became known as an insult comedian. The audience loved his insults even more than his prepared material. He developed the insults as part of his act and through the years won many awards.

Don't go around saying the world owes you a living. The world owes you nothing. It was here first.
– Mark Twain

overhead extension

Stand with feet shoulder width apart, one foot slightly in front of the other, shoulders back, chest out, abs in with center of band under your right foot. Holding the band ends, extend hands above your head. Bending your elbows, lower your hands behind your head, while keeping the upper arm vertical, with elbows pointing towards the ceiling. Continue down until your biceps and forearms touch, then press your hands back to the starting position, flexing triceps at the top. Repeat10-15 times.

DATE

Steps Walked:
Cardio Workout:
Resistance Workout:
Calories Consumed:
Calories Burned:
Difference:
Weight / Body fat:

Eating healthy tastes great!

Cream of Mushroom Soup
8 cups low sodium chicken broth
1 cup low fat sour cream
6 cups mushrooms, sliced
3/4 cup onion, diced • 3 tbs light butter
3 tbsp wheat flour • 2 tbs sherry
1 tsp basil, thyme and minced garlic
black pepper to taste
Melt butter, whisk in flour until smooth. Add the remaining ingredients, stirring constantly, bring soup to a boil then reduce heat and cook until thickened.

Read it, live it, love the results.

Be responsible for your health.
When at work, if you don't fulfill your responsibilities, you are held accountable. The same applies to your health. When you neglect to take care of yourself, you will be held accountable. Unfortunately, the penalty is generally much worse than that handed out by even the meanest of bosses.

Write it down & get it done.

1
2
3
4
5
6
7
8
9
10

single arm kickback

Place the band under your feet, then keeping your back straight, bend over with your left leg slightly bent and the right leg shifted backwards 15-18 inches. With one end of the band lying on the floor, hold the other with your right hand. Bend your elbow 90-degrees and place at your side, while resting your left hand on your left thigh. Without moving your upper arm, pull the band back until your thumb is pointing away from your body. Hold this position 2-3 counts, then return to starting position. Complete 10-15 repetitions on each side.

DATE

Honesty is the single most important factor in having a direct bearing on the final success of an individual, corporation, or product. –Ed McMahon

Steps Walked:
Cardio Workout:
Strength Training:
Calories Consumed:
Calories Burned:
Difference:
Weight / Body fat:

Write it down & get it done.

1
2
3
4
5
6
7
8
9
10

Read it, live it, love the results.

Don't let today's disappointments discourage you from succeeding tomorrow.
When disappointment crosses your path you have the option to step over it, or allow it to stop you in your tracks. Step over it and continue on your way to success, the choice really is yours.
Only you can stop yourself from succeeding.

Be the change you want to see.

One of the most renowned Jewish victims of the Holocaust, **Anne Frank** is famous for her diary, which documents her experiences hiding during the German occupation of the Netherlands in World War II. Her diary become one of the world's most widely read books, and the basis for several plays and films. Sadly, she didn't survive to benefit from it's success, as she and her sister were captured and placed in a concentration camp where they both died of typhus.

The only true happiness comes from squandering ourselves for a purpose.
—William Cowper

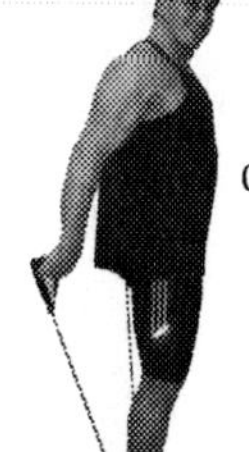

behind back tricep press with band

Stand on the center of a band, with one foot slightly in front of the other, back straight, shoulders back and chest out. With hands behind your back, hold band ends with palms facing in, letting your thumbs rest on your buns. Keeping your arms straight, raise hands as far back and high as possible, squeezing your shoulder blades together while opening your chest. Hold for 2-3 counts, repeat 10-15 times.

	DATE
Steps Walked:	
Cardio Workout:	
Resistance Workout:	
Calories Consumed:	
Calories Burned:	
Difference:	
Weight / Body fat:	

Eating healthy tastes great!

Stuffed Chicken Breasts

4 chicken breasts, with pocket cut
1 cup apples, diced • 1/4 cup raisins
3/4 cup wheat bread crumbs • olive oil
1 tsp Splenda® • 1 onion, minced
3 tbs hot water • pepper to taste

Preheat oven to 375ºF. Sauté onion in olive oil, then add remaining ingredients and mix well. Fill breast with stuffing, fasten with toothpick. Place breasts in baking dish. Pour in 1/2 cup water. Bake covered 45 minutes, uncovered 15 minutes.

Read it, live it, love the results.

Chicken may help you lose weight, keep bones strong and avoid cancer.

Studies show that chicken, which is high in protein—essential in growth and development—plays an important role in assisting overweight and obese people in losing weight. In older people, these proteins help against bone loss. Being a rich source of niacin, a B-vitamin it also protects the body against cancer.

Write it down & get it done.

1
2
3
4
5
6
7
8
9
10

front raise

Place the band under your left foot, shifting the right foot slightly to the rear as you stand with your back straight, shoulders back and chest out. Holding the band ends let your hands rest on your thighs with palms facing body. Keeping your elbows slightly bent and fixed, lift your arms straight out front, parallel to the floor. Hold here for 2-3 counts, then slowly return to the starting position.

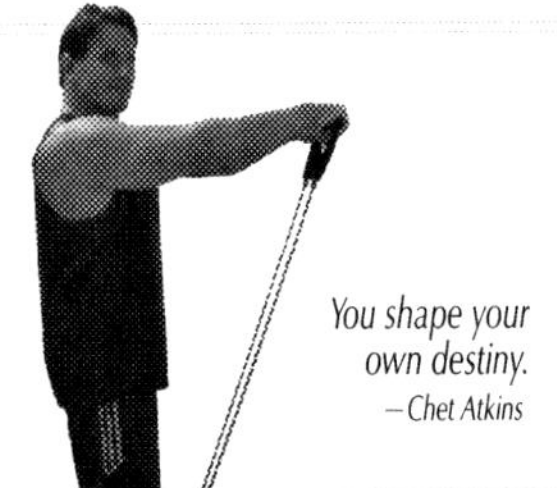

You shape your own destiny.
– Chet Atkins

DATE

Steps Walked:
Cardio Workout:
Strength Training:
Calories Consumed:
Calories Burned:
Difference:
Weight / Body fat:

Write it down & get it done.

1
2
3
4
5
6
7
8
9
10

Read it, live it, love the results.

Focus on living a low stress life. When under mental pressure, adrenaline is released from the adrenal gland telling the body to convert stored sugar from the liver to glucose—preparing your body for the supposed fight-or-flight. Unfortunately, we seldom do either, and the excess blood sugar, that didn't get used, is stored as fat. Letting stress get the best of you time and time again, could lead to an early death. Relax and enjoy life.

Doors open, when you work hard.

County star, **Chet Atkins** was obsessed with the guitar even as a child. His first guitar had a nail for a nut and was so bowed that only the first few frets could be used. He later purchased a semi-acoustic electric guitar and amp but had to travel miles for electricity since they didn't have electric at home. As a result of his dedication and hard work, he is now very successful and holds numerous awards for his work.

lateral raise

Place the band under your left foot, shifting the right foot slightly to the rear as you stand with your back straight, shoulders back and chest out. Holding the band ends, let your hands rest at your sides with palms facing body. Keeping your elbows slightly bent and fixed, lift your arms out to the sides, parallel to the floor. Hold here briefly,then slowly return to starting position. Repeat 10-15 times.

Surviving [life] is the whole point. Quitting it will not make you strong. Surviving it will!
—from Pump Up The Volume

DATE

Steps Walked:
Cardio Workout:
Resistance Workout:
Calories Consumed:
Calories Burned:
Difference:
Weight / Body fat:

Eating healthy tastes great!

Poached Eggs over Spinach & Mushrooms

4 eggs • 1 tsp light vinegar
1 cup onions, diced
2 cups mushrooms, sliced
½ cup tomatoes, diced
3 tbs minced garlic
10 oz package frozen spinach
thawed with excess water removed
black pepper to taste
Sauté vegetables with garlic. Poach eggs and serve on top of vegetables.

Read it, live it, love the results.

Burn more calories than you eat.
If you want to maintain your weight, you must balance calories consumed with calories burned. If you spend more time eating than moving—you will gain weight. However, if you eat less and keep busy, you are destine to lose weight. It's really not that complicated, yet millions are continually seeking an easier way. You have the ability to move, don't kill yourself by sitting on the couch every night.

Write it down & get it done.

1
2
3
4
5
6
7
8
9
10

seated military press
Center the band on the seat of a chair then sit on it, keeping your abs in, shoulders back and chest out. Hold the band ends and bring them up to your shoulders. Tense the shoulder muscles and push straight up, reaching as high as possible. Focus on isolating and contracting the deltoid muscles, hold for 10 counts, lower and repeat 5-10 times.

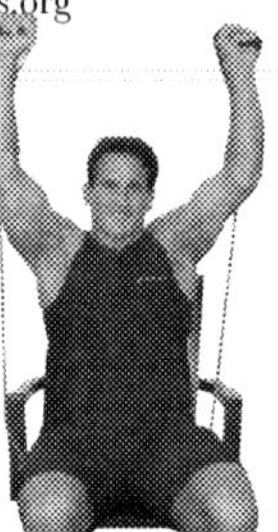

Just because you can't do everything doesn't mean you shouldn't do something.
– Earl Nightengale

DATE

Steps Walked:
Cardio Workout:
Strength Training:
Calories Consumed:
Calories Burned:
Difference:
Weight / Body fat:

Write it down & get it done.

1
2
3
4
5
6
7
8
9
10

Read it, live it, love the results.

Keep your body and mind active. A recent study performed at Albert Einstein College of Medicine, revealed that people who danced four or more times a week had a seventy-six percent lower dementia risk than people who rarely or never danced. Experts feel this is because, *"Dancing involves both mental and physical effort."* Other studies show that gardening and odd jobs that require thought may also reduce dementia risk.

Doors open when least expected.

Actor **Burt Reynolds** went to college on a football scholarship, unfortunately, torn knee cartilage and a car accident ended his football career. With football behind him, an instructor pushed Reynolds to try out for a play. He was cast in the lead and won a Drama Award for his performance. This led to a remarkable career whereas he was the number-one box-office attraction for five years in a row from 1978 to 1982, becoming one of America's most recognizable personalities.

What the mind can conceive and believe, it can achieve.
—Napoleon Hill

shoulder press

Place the band under your left foot, shifting the right foot slightly to the rear as you stand with your back straight, shoulders back and chest out. Holding the band ends, bend elbows to 90-degrees, placing them at your sides with palms facing body. Keeping the arms at the 90-degree angle, slowly raise straight out to sides, until arms are parallel to floor. Hold for 2-3 counts, then lower slowly. Repeat 10-15 times.

	DATE
Steps Walked:	
Cardio Workout:	
Strength Training:	
Calories Consumed:	
Calories Burned:	
Difference:	
Weight / Body fat:	

Eating healthy tastes great!

Loaded Tuna Salad
12 oz can solid white tuna, packed in water, drained
11 oz can mandarin oranges, drained
1 cup mushrooms, sliced
1/2 cup onion, diced
14 oz can artichoke hearts, drained
1 cup water chestnuts, drained and sliced
1/4 cup fat free mayonnaise
1/4 cup fat free plain yogurt
1 tbs lemon juice • 1 tsp Splenda®
Combine all ingredients and chill. Serve over bed of baby spinach.

Read it, live it, love the results.

Eliminate trans fats from your diet. Unlike other dietary fats, trans fats are extremely dangerous to your health, increasing your risk of coronary heart disease and raising your "bad" LDL cholesterol levels, increasing your risk of death. These fats are found in many processed foods, such as cookies, crackers and snack foods. Read the nutritional labels and know what you are eating. You are responsible for your body, don't ever think differently.

Write it down & get it done.

1
2
3
4
5
6
7
8
9
10

arnold press

Place the band under the ball of your right foot, shifting the left foot slightly to the rear as you stand with your back straight, shoulders back and chest out. Hold the band ends at chest level with palms facing chest. Rotate your palms as you press your hands up, when arms are fully extended palms will be facing out. Lower slowly, with reverse rotation to starting position. Repeat 10-15 times.

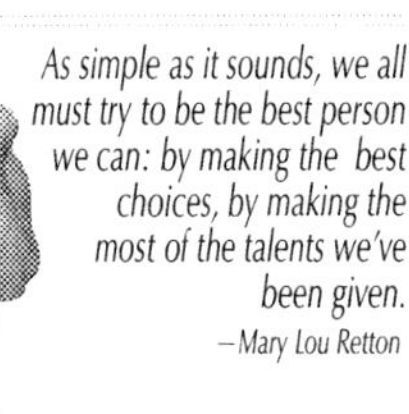

As simple as it sounds, we all must try to be the best person we can: by making the best choices, by making the most of the talents we've been given.
–Mary Lou Retton

DATE

Steps Walked:
Cardio Workout:
Strength Training:
Calories Consumed:
Calories Burned:
Difference:
Weight / Body fat:

Write it down & get it done.

1
2
3
4
5
6
7
8
9
10

Read it, live it, love the results.

It is up to you to choose the right roads.
We are all on the same trip, we simply take different roads to get there. Don't pass by those roads that take you uphill, it's these roads that will get you to higher grounds. Choosing the easier downhill paths lead nowhere but down.

Life's tough, get over it, she did!

American gymnast **Mary Lou Retton** was the first female gymnast outside Eastern Europe to win the *Olympic All-Around* title. Retton was born with hip dysplasia and had a hip replacement, however she never let this interfere with her dream of being the best gymnast possible. In 1997, Retton was inducted into the *International Gymnastics Hall of Fame*. In 1985 she retired from gymnastics after winning her third *American Cup* title.

Go as far as you can see, when you get there you'll see further. —Latin proverb

front to back press

Stand on the center of a band with feet shoulder-width apart, shoulders back, chest out and abs in. Hold band ends with an overhand grip and lift them to shoulder height, keeping elbows pointing down to your sides. Press hands to arm's length overhead, then lower them behind your head to your ears. Press back to arm's length overhead and then lower to starting position. Complete 10-15 repetitions.

	DATE
Steps Walked:	
Cardio Workout:	
Resistance Workout:	
Calories Consumed:	
Calories Burned:	
Difference:	
Weight / Body fat:	

Eating healthy tastes great!

Grilled Chicken Breasts

8 chicken breasts • 2 tsp lime juice
1/4 cup olive oil • 2 tbs vinegar
1 tbs Worcestershire sauce
1 packet Splenda® • 2 tbs minced garlic
pepper, tabasco® sauce and paprika
Place chicken in baking dish. Combine remaining ingredients and pour over chicken. Marinate 2 hours. Place breasts on grill. Cook until well done, turn and baste with marinade frequently for 35-40 minutes.

Read it, live it, love the results.

Pace yourself.

It took longer than five days, five weeks or even five months to develop unhealthy habits and gain weight. Don't expect to see instant results. On the average you should lose two pounds a week, and two percent body fat a month. Never give up, the results will come, as long as you are persistent in acheiving your goals. You were given this one body to care for—make it your top priority.

Write it down & get it done.

1
2
3
4
5
6
7
8
9
10

using the ball

Using the ball is a great way to get an effective workout. As using it to perform exercises increases your core stability, giving you greater balance and coordination. The ball is perfect in supporting the curvature of the back and giving a full range of flexible motions which help define and shape even the most difficult abdominal muscles. When you mix up your workouts by adding in the ball exercises, you will love the results.

I don't believe in circumstances. The people who get on in this world are the people who get up and look for circumstances they want.
–George Bernard Shaw

DATE

Steps Walked:
Cardio Workout:
Strength Training:
Calories Consumed:
Calories Burned:
Difference:
Weight / Body fat:

Write it down & get it done.

1
2
3
4
5
6
7
8
9
10

Read it, live it, love the results.

Instill a sense of fear in yourself. Fear is one of the strongest motivators in the human psyche, and it may be the motivation you need. Educate yourself on the results of NOT leading a healthy lifestyle. Know that when you eat unhealthy you will suffer the consequences of high blood pressure, heart disease, diabetes, high cholesterol, and ultimately an untimely death.

Your level of success is up to you.

One of my favorite motivational speakers **Brian Tracy**, worked as a laborer on a tramp steamer for eight years, after dropping out of high school. When this job ended he went into sales–where he struggled. In an effort to succeed he worked with other successful salesmen and emulated them. By the end of his first year, he became the top salesman. After his second year, he became Vice President in charge of ninty-five people. At the time, he was only 25 years old!

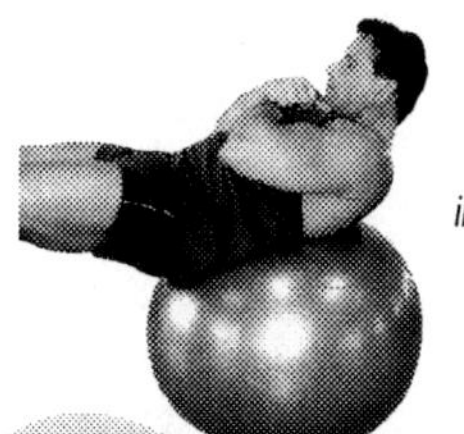

You will recognize your own path when you come upon it, because you will suddenly have all the energy and imagination you will ever need.
—Jerry Gillies

ball crunch

Lie face up on a ball, with your lower back pressed into the ball. Place your your arms over your chest or rest your fingertips near your ears. Contracting your abs, curl your upper body up, while keeping the ball stable. Hold for 2-3 counts then slowly lower and repeat 10-15 times.

DATE

Steps Walked:
Cardio Workout:
Resistance Workout:
Calories Consumed:
Calories Burned:
Difference:
Weight / Body fat:

Eating healthy tastes great!

Incredible Stuffed Peppers
1 lb lean ground turkey
6 green peppers, halved
16 oz can kidney beans, drained
8 oz low fat cheese • 2 tbs olive oil
4 tbs minced garlic • 4 tbs ketchup
1 tsp Worcestershire® sauce
pepper to taste // Preheat oven to 350°F. Panbroil peppers for five minutes, drain. Sauté turkey and onion in olive oil, remove from heat. Stir in remaining ingredients. Fill peppers with the mixture. Bake 30 minutes.

Read it, live it, love the results.

Eat a diet rich in vitamins C and E. Studies show that Vitamins E and C help fight free radical damage to your body. Free radicals are the by products of everyday chemical reactions in your body, which can do harm to your cells. As you age, your body's ability to fight these free radicals, which have been implicated in more than twenty age-related diseases, diminishes.

Write it down & get it done.

1
2
3
4
5
6
7
8
9
10

ball pass

Lie face up on the floor, legs straight out, hands extended straight behind your head, holding a ball. Keeping your legs straight, lift the ball above your head, while simultaneously bringing your legs straight up to grab it. Once between legs, slowly return the hands and legs to the floor without touching the floor. Repeat the action, bringing the feet up with the ball, then grabbing it with your hands. Continue passing the ball 10-15 times.

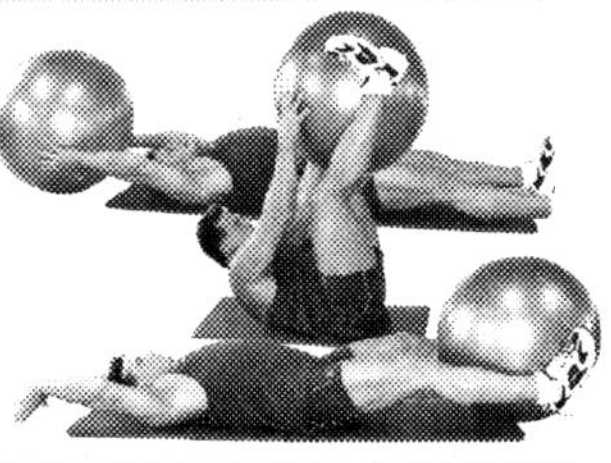

DATE

Enthusiasm is excitement with inspiration, motivation, and a pinch of creativity.
– Bo Bennett

Steps Walked:
Cardio Workout:
Strength Training:
Calories Consumed:
Calories Burned:
Difference:
Weight / Body fat:

Write it down & get it done.

1
2
3
4
5
6
7
8
9
10

Read it, live it, love the results.

Live for today, but make sure the choices you make don't destroy your tomorrows.
Ask yourself how the decisions you make now will affect you one day, one week or even one year from now. It's these decisions that shape your life for the good or bad.

Be the change you want to see.

The Queen of Rock & Roll, **Tina Turner**, left her husband Ike Turner after a horrible beating in Dallas, the Fourth of July weekend in 1976. With just thirty-six cents, a gas-station credit card and a strong will to succeed, she spent the next few months staying with friends, hiding from Ike. Eventually she was back on her feet and more successful than ever, becoming one of the most successful female rock artist ever.

I'd rather attempt to do something great and fail than to attempt to do nothing and succeed.
–Dr. Robert Schuller

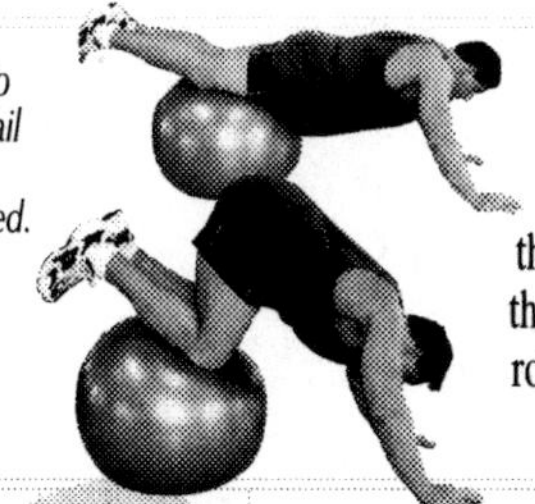

jackknife on ball

Lie face down on a ball, rolling yourself forward until knees are rested on the ball and your palms are flat on the floor, with your body parallel to the floor. Balancing the ball with your legs, bring your knees into your chest, rolling the ball forward. Hold for 2-3 counts, then return to starting position. Repeat 10-15 times.

DATE

Steps Walked:
Cardio Workout:
Strength Training:
Calories Consumed:
Calories Burned:
Difference:
Weight / Body fat:

Eating healthy tastes great!

Low Fat Tuna Salad
32 ozs of water-packed tuna, drained
2 cups baby spinach, chopped
2 tbs onion, finely chopped
1/2 cup tomatoes, diced
1/2 cup dill pickles, finely chopped
1/2 cup celery, diced
1/4 cup cucumber, diced
1 cup fat free mayonnaise
1 tbs dijon mustard and minced garlic
1 tsp oregano and basil
Combine ingredients and chill.
Serve over a bed of spinach.

Read it, live it, love the results.

For a healthy heart and attitude enjoy the great taste of fish,
Studies indicate that the omega-3's in fish are among the most heart healthy nutrients available to us. In addition to lowering your risk of heart disease, the number one killer of Americans, omega-3's also help lower blood pressure, improve mood and feed your brain. All of which are important in increasing your life span, and ensuring a healthy, happy life.

Write it down & get it done.

1
2
3
4
5
6
7
8
9
10

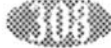

the rolling ball

Kneel on the floor with a ball in front of you with elbows and forearms on top of the ball. Tightening your abs, slowly roll forward, pushing the ball as far away as possible without straining your lower back. Hold here for 2-3 counts then return to starting position. Repeat 10-15 times. To intensify this exercise you may place your fingertips on the ball when rolling out, instead of your elbows.

Winning is not everything, but the effort to win is.
—Zig Ziglar

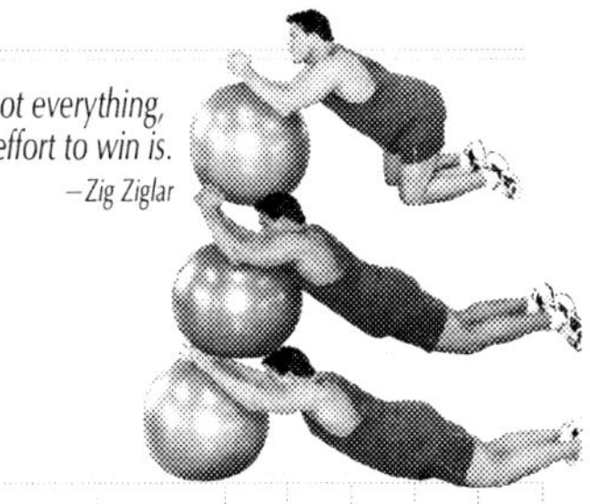

DATE

Steps Walked:
Cardio Workout:
Resistance Workout:
Calories Consumed:
Calories Burned:
Difference:
Weight / Body fat:

Write it down & get it done.

1
2
3
4
5
6
7
8
9
10

Read it, live it, love the results.

Learn from your failures, don't become disheartened by them. Many never make an attempt to create a healthy lifestyle only because they fear failure. However, failure breeds success. The best companies embrace mistakes and learn from them. When you make an attempt to reach a goal without success, don't give up, simply try something different. Only those who give up, become failures.

Doors open, when you work hard.

The first female solo artist inducted to the Country Music Hall of Fame, **Patsy Cline**, had suffered from a serious illness as a child which caused her to have a throat infection. According to Cline, this resulted in her gift of "a voice that boomed like Kate Smith's." As a country music singer, she has been considered one of the most influential, successful, revered, and acclaimed female vocalists of the 20th century.

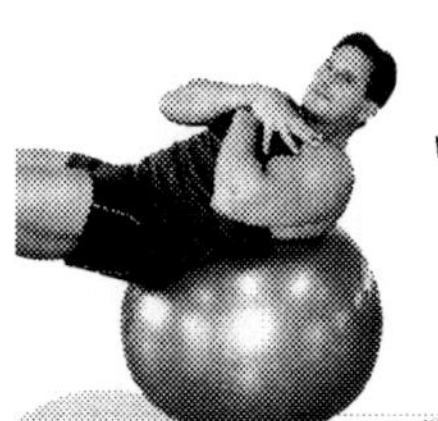

Show me someone who has done something worthwhile, and I'll show you someone who has overcome adversity.
—Lou Holtz

oblique crunch

Lie face up on a ball, with your lower back pressed into the ball. Place your your arms over your chest or rest your fingertips near your ears. Contracting your abs, curl your upper body up, twisting to the right, while keeping the ball stable. Hold for 2-3 counts then lower slowly and repeat 10-15 times, then complete a set to the left.

	DATE
Steps Walked:	
Cardio Workout:	
Strength Training:	
Calories Consumed:	
Calories Burned:	
Difference:	
Weight / Body fat:	

Eating healthy tastes great!

Glazed Chicken Breasts
4 chicken breasts
1/4 cup Dijon mustard
1/4 cup green onions, finely chopped
1 tsp rosemary leaves, dried
2 tbs minced garlic
1/4 cup sugar-free orange marmalade
Preheat oven to 350°F. Combine mustard, green onions and spices and spread over breasts, top with orange marmalade, spread evenly. Bake 40-50 minutes until chicken is cooked through.

Read it, live it, love the results.

Enjoy meat and concord grapes with each meal for a healthy liver.
A great old-time remedy that may make you feel better. Most people eat too many starches *(breads, pastas rices)*, as a result the liver is overworked, using a considerable amount of digestive juices to break down these starches. Animal protein does not tax the liver for its digestion, and the acid in the grape juice makes the meat even easier to digest. Treat your body well, and it will treat you well!

Write it down & get it done.

1
2
3
4
5
6
7
8
9
10

the balance act

Cut not the wings of your dreams for they are the heartbeat and the freedom of your soul –Flavia

Lie face down on a ball, balancing on your hips and lower belly. Place your palms on the floor while extending your feet straight out back, keeping your body in a flat plank position. Hold for 20-30 counts, lower and repeat, this time extending the right arm straight out. Hold here for 20-30 counts, then repeat with left.

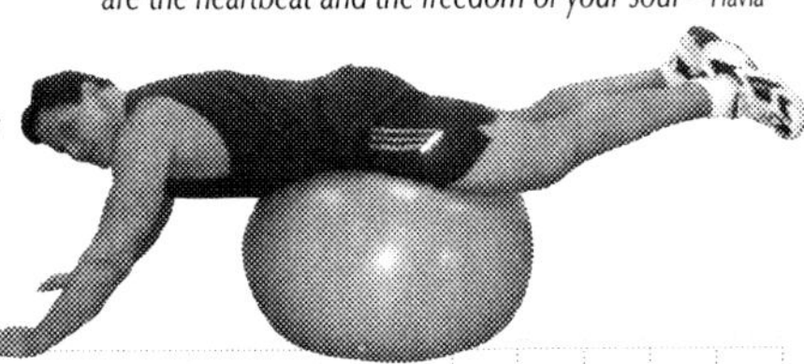

DATE

Steps Walked:

Cardio Workout:

Strength Training:

Calories Consumed:

Calories Burned:

Difference:

Weight / Body fat:

Write it down & get it done.

1
2
3
4
5
6
7
8
9
10

Read it, live it, love the results.

To succeed you must have a positive attitude.
Those with a positive attitude are optimistic, enthusiastic, believe in themselves, have integrity, are courageous and confident in themselves and show extreme determination. Master these qualities, and you will become the master of your life. Positive thinkers are also patient, calm and focused.

Your level of success is up to you.

Golden Globe winning actor **Don Johnson**, famous for his role on Miami Vice, struggled for years trying to establish himself as an accomplished actor. It wasn't until after a long string of failed pilot movies which were never followed by an actual TV series that he landed the starring role on Miami Vice. In addition to being an actor, he is also a successful singer, songwriter, producer, and director.

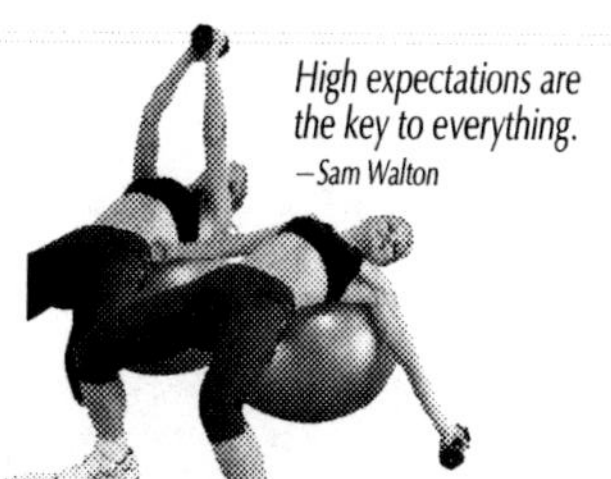

dumbbell pass

Lie face up on a ball in the "table top" position, with your shoulders resting on the ball and hands straight up holding a dumbbell. Keeping your glutes and abs tight and your arms straight, take the dumbbell in the right hand and slowly lower to the right, until it touches the floor, then raise to starting position, pass to the left and lower to the left. Continue passing the dumbbell, 10-15 times.

DATE

Steps Walked:

Cardio Workout:

Resistance Workout:

Calories Consumed:

Calories Burned:

Difference:

Weight / Body fat:

Eating healthy tastes great!

Fruity Chicken Spinach Salad

1/2 cup cooked chicken, chopped
4 cups baby spinach
2 tbs olive oil
1 tbs red wine vinegar
1 pear, thinly sliced
1/2 cup dried cranberries
1/2 cup walnut pieces
1/2 cup red onion, thinly sliced
black pepper to taste
Whisk oil, vinegar, salt & pepper. Add remaining ingredients, toss well and serve chilled.

Read it, live it, love the results.

Reduce your risk of heart disease by adding walnuts to your diet.

Studies show that walnuts are one of the best plant sources of protein available, in addition to being rich in fiber, B vitamins, magnesium, omega-3 fatty acids and antioxidants such as vitamin E. Incorporating them into your diet reduces your risk of heart disease by improving blood vessel elasticity and plaque accumulation. Walnuts also help lower LDL cholesterol and the C-Reactive Protein.

Write it down & get it done.

1
2
3
4
5
6
7
8
9
10

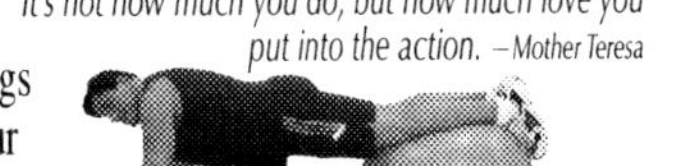

leg rolls on ball

Lie face down on a ball, rolling yourself forward until your lower legs and feet are resting on the ball with your palms flat on the floor. Your body should be parallel to the floor. Slowly roll the ball to the right, engaging your obliques as your twist your body, until the right leg comes off the ball. Hold here for 2-3 counts, then return to starting position, and roll to the left. Complete 10-15 repetitions of this alternating movement.

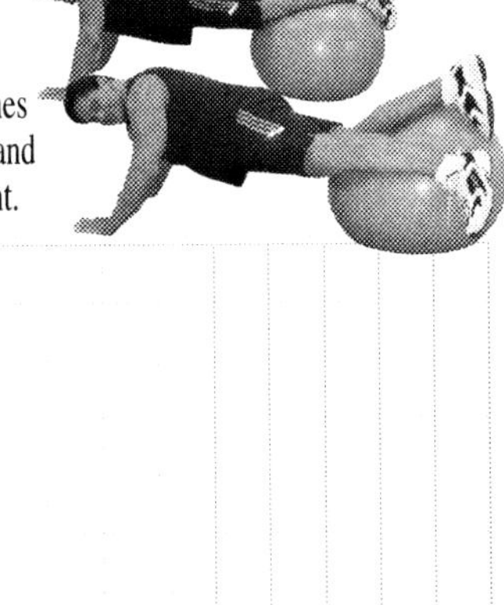

DATE

Steps Walked:
Cardio Workout:
Strength Training:
Calories Consumed:
Calories Burned:
Difference:
Weight / Body fat:

Write it down & get it done.

1
2
3
4
5
6
7
8
9
10

Read it, live it, love the results.

Don't expect results without putting forth an honest effort.
You reap what you sow, more than you sow, later than you sow.
When you choose to lead a healthy lifestyle don't expect immediate results, the results will come over time giving you a reward money can't buy. On the other hand, if you choose to lead an unhealthy lifestyle, you will *"reap"* many things you don't desire. Your choices determine what you *"reap."*

Doors open, when you work hard.

The lead singer of Led Zepplin, **Robert Plant**, had various jobs while pursuing his music career, including working for a construction company and Woolworths. Musically, he cut three obscure singles and sang with a variety of bands wihtout success. Eventually he launched Led Zepplin, one of the first heavy metal bands in history.

In all human affairs there are efforts, and there are results, and the strength of the effort is the measure of the result.
—James Allen

squat with ball

Stand with a ball placed between your lower back and the wall. Position feet shoulder-width apart, shoulders back and chest out. Focusing your vision straight ahead, with your heels planted firmly on the floor, squat down, letting the ball roll along your back as you lower your body. Keeping your knees behind your toes, stop when your thighs are parallel with the floor. Hold for 2-3 counts, then return to starting position. Repeat 10-15 times.

DATE

Steps Walked:
Cardio Workout:
Strength Training:
Calories Consumed:
Calories Burned:
Difference:
Weight / Body fat:

Eating healthy tastes great!

Creamed Chicken
6 chicken breasts, diced
olive oil
1/3 cup light butter
1/3 cup wheat flour
1 cup low sodium chicken broth
1 1/2 cups fat free sour cream
Sauté chicken in olive oil. Melt butter, remove from heat and stir in remaining ingredients.
Return to heat and cook additional 10 minutes.

Read it, live it, love the results.

Eat nutrient dense foods, low in calories.
Some experts believe that calorie restriction may be a strategy in extending your life span. Studies on rodents, fish, fruit flies, worms and monkeys indicate eating less increases life spans. In humans, calorie restriction has been shown to lower cholesterol, fasting glucose and blood pressure. Though you must make sure you get sufficient vitamins, minerals and nutrients.

Write it down & get it done.

1
2
3
4
5
6
7
8
9
10

elbow to knee crunch

Kneel on the floor with a ball positioned to your right. Lean on the ball, extending your left leg out straight, with your left arm extended up and back. Contract your obliques as you bring your left knee to your left elbow. Hold for 2-3 counts, return to the starting position. Complete 10-15 repetitions on each side.

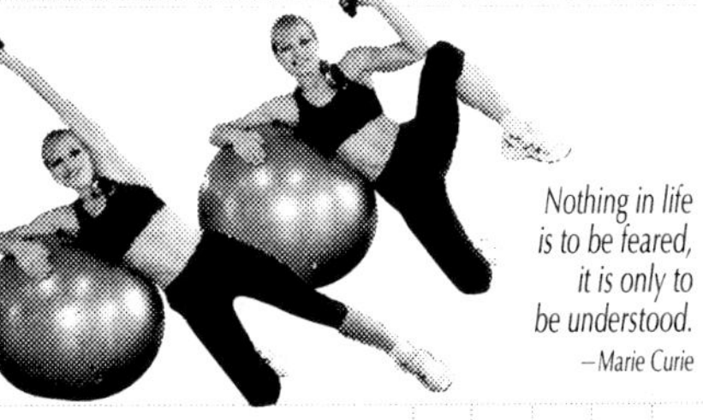

Nothing in life is to be feared, it is only to be understood.
—Marie Curie

DATE

Steps Walked:
Cardio Workout:
Strength Training:
Calories Consumed:
Calories Burned:
Difference:
Weight / Body fat:

Write it down & get it done.

1
2
3
4
5
6
7
8
9
10

Read it, live it, love the results.

Keep your thoughts positive. When you continually think negative thoughts you will strip yourself of strength and confidence. Be aware of what you say and think to yourself. Each time a negative thought enters your mind, stop and replace it with a strong, positive and empowering thought.

Your level of success is up to you.

Rock star **Roger Daltrey**, best known as the founder and lead singer of English rock band *The Who*, made his first guitar from a block of wood. He formed a skiffle band called The Detours, and when his father bought him an Epiphone guitar in 1959, he became the lead guitarist for the band. It was the beginning of his musical career. In addition to music and acting, Daltrey has acted as producer on several films.

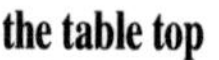

You can't have a better tomorrow if you are thinking about yesterday all the time. –Charles F. Kettering

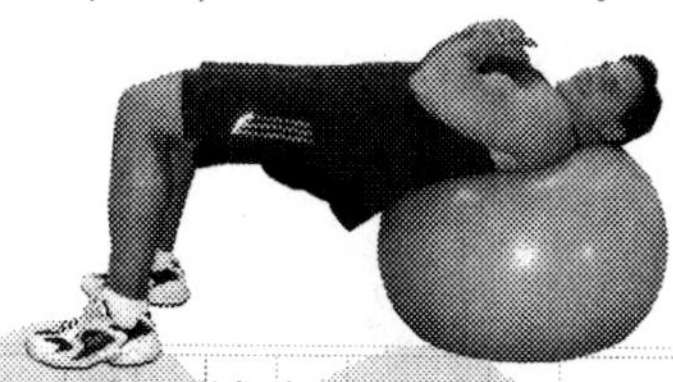

the table top

Sit on the floor with your upper back pressed into a ball. Squeezing your glutes and pressing through your heels, bring yourself up into a "table top" position, with your head, neck and shoulders resting on the ball. Hold here for 20-30 counts, slowly lower to starting position, and repeat 5-10 times. You may place a dumbbell on your pelvis for added resistance.

	DATE
Steps Walked:	
Cardio Workout:	
Resistance Workout:	
Calories Consumed:	
Calories Burned:	
Difference:	
Weight / Body fat:	

Eating healthy tastes great!

Chicken Cacciatore

6 chicken breasts, diced
olive oil
1 onion, sliced
1 green pepper, diced
3-16oz cans canned tomatoes
pepper, oregeno, basil
and thyme to taste

Sauté chicken in olive oil. Add remaining ingredients, reduce heat, cover and cook 45-50 minutes.

Read it, live it, love the results.

Reduce your sugar intake.

When insulin levels are high the amount of fat your body is able to burn is decreased, therefore making it harder to lose weight. In addition, high insulin levels also increase inflammation, which contributes to chronic pain conditions. If you currently suffer from joint pain of any kind, cut back on your sugar intake and you will be amazed at the reduction of your pain.

Write it down & get it done.

1
2
3
4
5
6
7
8
9
10

pelvic lift rolls

Lie on the floor, face up with heels on a ball. Extend your arms at your sides with palms down or locked together under your buttocks. Pressing your heels into the ball, lift your hips towards the ceiling as you "pull" the ball in towards your buns. Push the ball back to starting position and repeat 10-15 times.

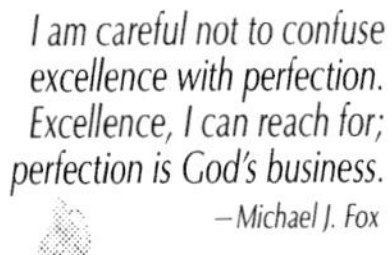

I am careful not to confuse excellence with perfection. Excellence, I can reach for; perfection is God's business.
— Michael J. Fox

DATE

Steps Walked:
Cardio Workout:
Strength Training:
Calories Consumed:
Calories Burned:
Difference:
Weight / Body fat:

Write it down & get it done.

1
2
3
4
5
6
7
8
9
10

Read it, live it, love the results.

Believe in yourself.
When you believe you can do something, you will be able to do so. Your positive beliefs are the key to changing your behaviors. When you think positive thoughts powerful messages are sent to your brain, affecting your actions and creating positive outcomes. On the flip side, if you send negative messages to your brain you will create negative outcomes. Control your thoughts and you'll control your future.

Doors open, when you work hard.

Actor **Michael J. Fox**, the star of *Family Ties*, nearly missed getting the part. His first audition didn't go well, however the casting director pushed for him. The NBC executive finally gave in, commenting, *"Go ahead if you insist. But I'm telling you, this is not the kind of face you'll ever see on a lunch box"*. A few years later, after *Back to the Future* opened to big success, Fox's picture appeared on a lunch box.

Although the world is full of suffering, it is full also of the overcoming of it.
—Helen Keller

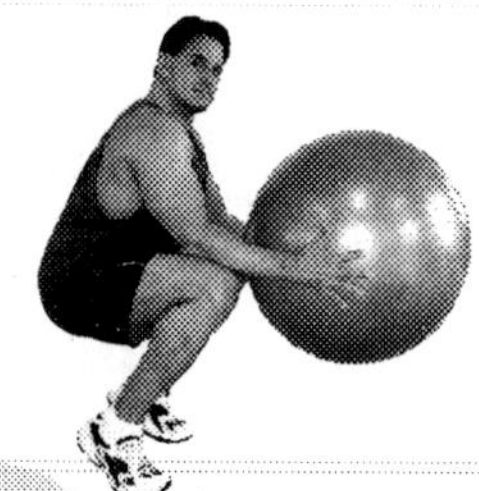

squatting calf raises
Stand with feet shoulder-width apart, holding a ball at chest height, then sit back into a squatting position, with your thighs parallel to the floor. Holding this position, raise up on your toes and hold for 2-3 counts, completing 20-30 repetitions.

	DATE						
Steps Walked:							
Cardio Workout:							
Resistance Workout:							
Calories Consumed:							
Calories Burned:							
Difference:							
Weight / Body fat:							

Eating healthy tastes great!

Low-Fat Blueberry Bran Muffins
1 cup blueberries • 1 1/2 cups wheat bran
1 cup skim milk • 1/2 tsp vanilla extract
1/2 cup unsweetened applesauce
1 egg • 1/3 cup Splenda® brown sugar
1/2 cup flour • 1/2 cup whole wheat flour
1 tsp baking soda • 1 tsp baking powder
Preheat oven to 375°F.
Mix bran and milk, let stand for 10 minutes. Combine with remaining ingredients. Pour into greased muffin pan. Bake 15 to 20 minutes.

Read it, live it, love the results.

Don't forget the blueberries!
Blueberries are loaded with antioxidants, which destroy free radicals. Studies show that a blueberry-rich diet improves memory and motor skills and reverses age-related declines in balance and coordination. Blueberries may also lower blood pressure, this is important since elevated blood pressure can damage delicate blood vessels in the brain and can lead to strokes.

Write it down & get it done.

1
2
3
4
5
6
7
8
9
10

standing calf

Stand with feet shoulder-width apart 24-36 inches from a wall. Place a ball against the wall at chest height. Leaning into the wall, lift your right foot and support your weight with the right. Raise up on the toes of your right foot and hold for 2-3 counts. Lower to floor, then raise again. Repeat 20-30 calf raises on each leg. Once you complete single calf raises on each leg, perform a set using both legs.

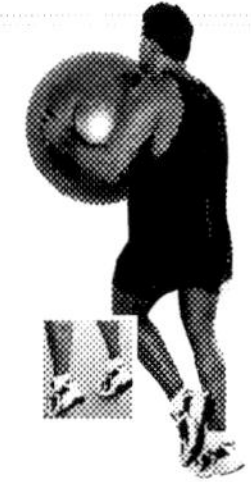

Give a man health and a course to steer; and he'll never stop to trouble about whether he's happy or not.
– George Bernard Shaw

DATE

Steps Walked:
Cardio Workout:
Resistance Workout:
Calories Consumed:
Calories Burned:
Difference:
Weight / Body fat:

Write it down & get it done.

1
2
3
4
5
6
7
8
9
10

Read it, live it, love the results.

Faith is the starting point for that which you desire—know it, believe it and embrace it.
It's faith that will get you through the tough times and bring to you all of that which you desire. The formula is simple. You take that which you desire, plant it as you would a seed, then nourish it. The more you nourish the desire, the stronger it will grow, eventually becoming a reality. It's up to you to make your dreams come true.

Doors open, when you work hard.

Conservative political commentator, **Rush Limbaugh**, always had a love for radio. His father and mother wanted him to attend college, so he enrolled at Southeast Missouri State, however, dropped out after about a year, according to his mother, "*he flunked everything, even a modern ballroom dancing class*". As she told a reporter in 1992, "*He just didn't seem interested in anything except radio.*" It was a dream, he made a reality.

Pay no attention to what the critics say; no statue has ever been erected to a critic.
—Jean Sibelius

back extension

Lie face down on a ball, balancing on your hips and lower belly. Your legs should be extended straight out back with toes on floor, hands behind your head or back. Contract your glutes as you lift your chest off the ball, raising your upper body up until it is in a straight line. Don't lift too far, as this will hurt your lower back. Hold for 2-3 counts, lower and repeat 10-15 times.

	DATE
Steps Walked:	
Cardio Workout:	
Resistance Workout:	
Calories Consumed:	
Calories Burned:	
Difference:	
Weight / Body fat:	

Eating healthy tastes great!

Eggplant and Tomato Casserole
2 medium eggplants, 1/4" slices
1/4 cup onion, diced • 1/4 cup light cheese
2-16oz cans stewed tomatoes
1 tsp Sweet and Low® • 2 tbs wheat flour
paprika, oregano, thyme and pepper
Preheat oven to 350°F
Brown eggplant in skillet with olive oil. Blend flour and liquid from tomatoes, then add rest of ingredients, boil, then simmer 5 minutes. Layer eggplant and sauce in baking pan. Top with cheese. Bake 30 minutes.

Read it, live it, love the results.

Eating watermelon and tomatoes may keep you from getting cancer.
More so than any other fruit or vegetable, watermelon contains the highest level of the antioxidant lycopene. Lycopene plays a key role in disarming free oxygen radicals, which are thought to contribute to the development of many cancers. Other great sources of lycopene include tomatoes, red grapefruits and guavas.

Write it down & get it done.

1
2
3
4
5
6
7
8
9
10

one legged deadlift

Position a ball directly behind you, then place your right leg on the ball, keeping the left knee slightly bent. With shoulders back, chest out and abs in, hold dumbbells against your thighs, palms facing your body. Bend at your hips, dropping the dumbbells down, keeping them close to the leg. Hold for 2-3 counts, then contract your glutes and hamstrings and return to the starting position. Repeat 10-15 times,

We can always redeem the man who aspires and strives.
—Johann Wolfgang von Goethe

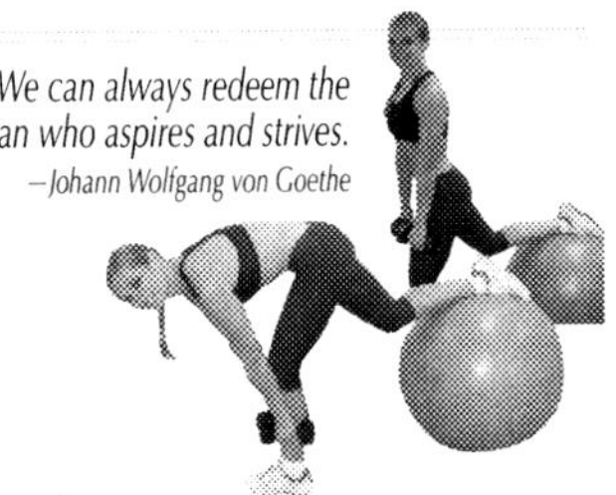

DATE

Steps Walked:

Cardio Workout:

Strength Training:

Calories Consumed:

Calories Burned:

Difference:

Weight / Body fat:

Write it down & get it done.

1
2
3
4
5
6
7
8
9
10

Read it, live it, love the results.

Don't be "tricked" by the ads and stories from people who have "magically" lost weight without diet and exercise.
The people used in commercials to sell diet products are usually paid to endorse that product. In most ads you don't hear the "full" story. Anyone who has lost weight, and kept it off, has more than likely done it as a result of making lifestyle changes, which includes a healthy diet and staying active.

Be the change you want to see.

Artist, **Salvador Dali** came to be regarded as the leader of the surrealist movement. Though being a maverick genius he refused to find comfort within a niche, and would often disagree with his contemporaries, particularly with their political views. He was tried, and expelled from the group as World War II moved through Europe. As the war progressed, Dali and his wife left Europe and moved to America, where he was welcomed with open arms.

Perpetual optimism is a force multiplier.
– Colin Powell

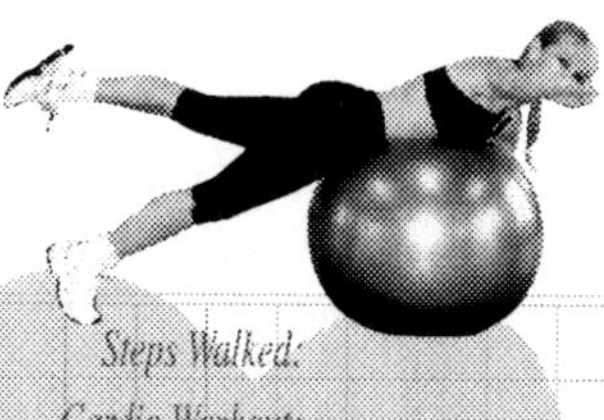

airplane on ball

Lie face down on a ball, balancing on your hips and lower belly. Your legs should be extended straight out back balancing on your toes, with palms flat on the floor. (Holding dumbbells is optional.) Extend the right arm straight out to the side, the left leg straight out back, hold for 10 counts. Return to starting position, repeat 2-5 times, then complete a set on the opposite side.

	DATE
Steps Walked:	
Cardio Workout:	
Strength Training:	
Calories Consumed:	
Calories Burned:	
Difference:	
Weight / Body fat:	

Eating healthy tastes great!

Luscious Almond Mocha
$^{1}/_{2}$ cup Hershey's® special dark Cocoa
$^{1}/_{2}$ cup powdered instant coffee
$^{1}/_{2}$ cup Splenda® • 1 cup hot water
6 cups skim milk • 1 tbs vanilla extract
$^{1}/_{2}$ tsp almond extract
Whisk together first 4 ingredients in pan until smooth. Bring to a boil–boil 2 minutes, whisking constantly. Reduce heat, add milk; Do Not Boil. Stir in extracts. Serve in mug. Garnish with fat free whipped topping.

Read it, live it, love the results.

Try Hot Cocoa to give your brain a boost.
Studies show that the antioxidant content of two tablespoons of pure cocoa powder is "almost two times stronger than red wine, two to three times stronger than green tea and four to five times stronger than that of black tea." The great news is that the antioxidants in hot cocoa protect brain cells from oxidative stress that can lead to Alzheimer's and other disorders.

Write it down & get it done.

1
2
3
4
5
6
7
8
9
10

wall pushup

Stand a few feet from the wall, holding a ball against the wall at eye level. Pressing against the ball with both hands, keep your feet in place, as you slowly lower your body until your chin touches the ball. Hold for 2-3 counts, then push your body back to starting position. Repeat 10-15 times. *To intensify, position the ball against the wall and floor.*

Enthusiasm is the mother of effort, and without it nothing great was ever achieved.
– Ralph Waldo Emerson

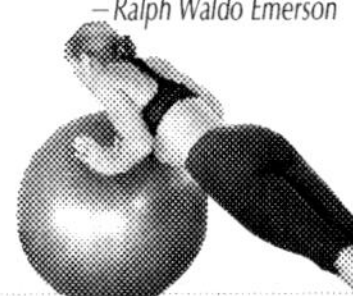

DATE

Steps Walked:
Cardio Workout:
Strength Training:
Calories Consumed:
Calories Burned:
Difference:
Weight / Body fat:

Write it down & get it done.

1
2
3
4
5
6
7
8
9
10

Read it, live it, love the results.

When dining out, bring leftovers home.
Many people are overweight simply because they eat too much. Monitor your portion sizes and you will begin to drop clothes sizes. A portion of meat should be about the size of a deck of cards, a portion of rice or pasta about the size of your fist. Most restaurants double or triple these amounts, so even with healthy foods you often consume too many calories.

Be the change you want to see.

Leader of the Transcendentalist movement in the early 19th century, **Ralph Waldo Emerson**, was called *"a rather dull scholar"* by his father. This changed after his father's death. At the age of 9 he went to the Boston Latin School, then, at 14, he received a scholarship for Harvard College. Here, he was appointed the Freshman's President. Emerson was considered one of the great orators of the time.

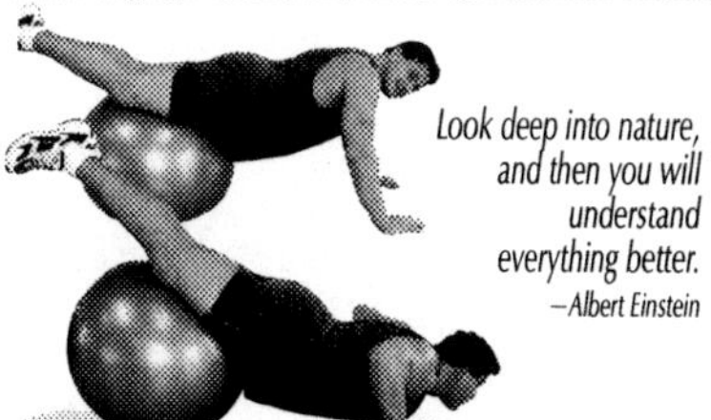

Look deep into nature, and then you will understand everything better.
—Albert Einstein

decline ball pushup
Lie face down on a ball, rolling yourself forward until your knees are rested on ball and your palms are flat on the floor, with your body parallel to the floor. Balancing the ball with your legs, lower your upper body, bringing your nose to within inches of the floor. Hold here for 2-3 counts then return to the starting position. Repeat 10-15 times.

Steps Walked:
Cardio Workout:
Strength Training:
Calories Consumed:
Calories Burned:
Difference:
Weight / Body fat:

DATE

Eating healthy tastes great!

Vanilla Fruit Salad
16 oz can fruit cocktail, with juice
6 oz can mandarin oranges, drained
16 oz can pears, with juice
16 oz can crushed pineapple, with juice
2 bananas, sliced
1 cup concord grapes, halved
2 small boxes instant fat free vanilla pudding

(Use canned fruits with no sugars added)
Mix all ingredients and chill.

Read it, live it, love the results.

The Concord Grape has been a natural remedy for years.
Grapes have been symbolic for thousands of years. From passages in the Bible to natural cures for our grandparents, grapes contain incredible nutritional values. They are a source of; Vitamins A, B1, B6, B12 and C. They also contain Calcium, Phosphoros, Iron, Copper, Potassium and Niacin. Enjoy them throughout the day for a healthy, happy body!

Write it down & get it done.

1
2
3
4
5
6
7
8
9
10

bench press on ball

Lie on ball, face up with your body parallel to the floor. Feet flat on the floor with shoulders and upper back resting on the ball. Holding a dumbbell in each hand, extend arms straight up with palms facing feet. Keeping your shoulders pressed into the ball and your back flat, lower dumbbells until they are chest level, just above the shoulders. Hold for 2-3 counts, then return to starting position, pressing the ends of the dumbbells together once they reach the top. You should be able to feel your chest rise. Complete 10-15 repetitions.

DATE
Concentrate all your thoughts upon the work at hand.
The sun's rays do not burn until brought to a focus.
–Alexander Graham Bell
Steps Walked:
Cardio Workout:
Strength Training:
Calories Consumed:
Calories Burned:
Difference:
Weight / Body fat:

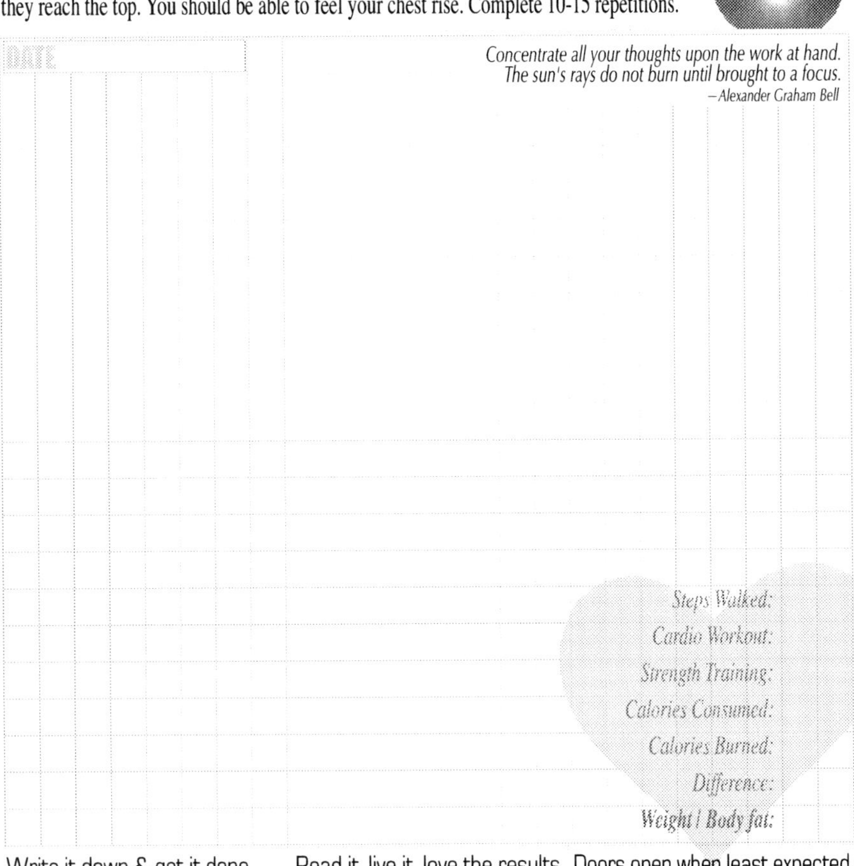

Write it down & get it done.

1
2
3
4
5
6
7
8
9
10

Read it, live it, love the results.

Read about the success of others.

You can find strong inspiration through real life success stories. Relate with the individuals and understand what they went through to achieve their goals. You will be amazed at the hurdles many people have had to overcome to become the success they are today.

Doors open when least expected.

Inventor, **Alexander Graham Bell**, who is widely credited with the invention of the telephone, didn't do well in high school. His school record was marked by absenteeism and lacklustre grades. It wasn't until Bell left school and was sent to London to live with his grandfather that he developed a love of learning. The two of them spent long hours in serious discussion and study. Thanks to a caring grandfather, Bell went on to become quite successful.

Get happiness out of your work or you may never know what happiness is.
—Elbert Hubbard

preacher curl

Kneel on the floor in front of your ball, holding dumbbells, with your elbows resting on the ball. Focusing on your biceps, drop the dumbbells straight down, extending as far as possible, then slowly return to starting position. Repeat 10-15 times.

Steps Walked:
Cardio Workout:
Resistance Workout:
Calories Consumed:
Calories Burned:
Difference:
Weight / Body fat:

DATE

Eating healthy tastes great!

Shrimp and Green Bean Delight
1 lb shrimp, peeled and deveined
4 cups green beans, trimmed
3 tbs olive oil
1/4 cup minced garlic
2 tsp paprika
2-16 oz cans large butter beans
1/4 cup red-wine vinegar
black pepper to taste

Steam green beans, then sauté with remaining ingredients in olive oil.

Read it, live it, love the results.

Suffering from PMS? It may be a good time to enjoy some shrimp!
Shrimp is an excellent source of Omega-3 fatty acids which has been shown to ease the symptoms of premenstrual syndrome, avoid blood clots, prevent the development of rheumatoid arthritis, slows the growth of cancerous tumors, and helps prevent Alzheimer's disease.It is also an excellent source of selenium, which neutralizes free radicals.

Write it down & get it done.

1
2
3
4
5
6
7
8
9
10

decline curls on ball

Lie on a ball face up, holding dumbbells, with knees bent and feet flat on the floor. Position arms at sides with palms facing up. Press your elbows into the ball, while keeping the dumbbells suspended just above the floor. Holding the elbows steady, curl the dumbbells toward your shoulders, hold 2-3 counts then slowly return to starting position. Repeat 10-15 times.

The significance of a man is not in what he attains but in what he longs to attain.
– Kahlil Gibran

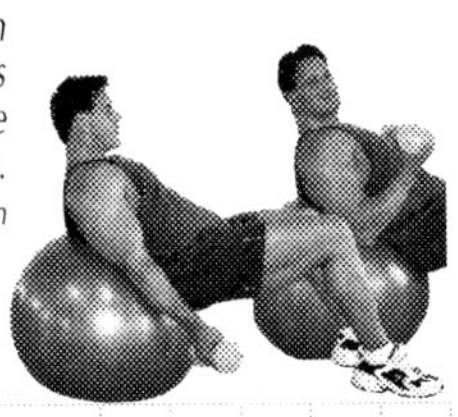

DATE

Steps Walked:
Cardio Workout:
Strength Training:
Calories Consumed:
Calories Burned:
Difference:
Weight / Body fat:

Write it down & get it done.

1
2
3
4
5
6
7
8
9
10

Read it, live it, love the results.

Use your time wisely.
No matter how wealthy or famous you are, 24 hours a day is all you are going to receive. The key is to manage this 24 hours wisely and to get as much as possible out of each day. Organization and time management is key to reaching your goals, utilize each minute and hour to your advantage.

Without challenge, there is no change.

Football coach **Vince Lombardi** had originally considered becoming a Catholic Priest. At the age of 15, he entered Cathedral Prep, a 6-year program to become a Priest. After 4 years, he decided not to pursue this path and transferred to the St. Francis Prep, where he was a standout on the football team, an activity that was discouraged at the seminary. Today, Vince Lombardi has become virtually synonymous with the National Football League.

We make a living by what we get, but we make a life by what we give.
– Sir Winston Churchill

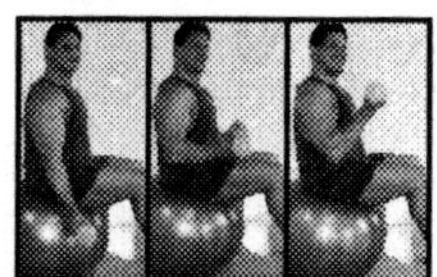

21's

Sit tall on a ball with shoulders back, chest out and abs in. Holding dumbbells, let arms hang straight down with palms facing forward. Contract your biceps as you curl the dumbbells halfway up, pump twice, then drop back down. Repeat seven times, then without pausing, curl the dumbbells all the way up then halfway down with a 2 count pump at the halfway point. Complete seven repetitions of this movement. Then complete the exercise by performing seven full dumbbell curls.

DATE

Steps Walked:
Cardio Workout:
Strength Training:
Calories Consumed:
Calories Burned:
Difference:
Weight / Body fat:

Eating healthy tastes great!

Spicy Pumpkin Pudding
1 cup evaporated skim milk
1 cup pumpkin puree • 3 eggs
1/3 cup apple butter • 1 tsp vanilla
1/2 tsp ground cinnamon

Combine pumpkin puree, eggs, apple butter, vanilla and cinnamon, then whisk. Microwave milk for one minute then add to mix and stir well. Microwave for 8 minutes. Rotate during cooking. Serve warm or refrigerate.

Read it, live it, love the results.

If you desire to be healthy and fit, you will be healthy and fit.
Ralf Waldo Emerson once stated, *"There's nothing capricious in nature, and the implanting of a desire indicates that its gratification is in the constitution of the creature that feels it."* In other words, you desire only those things which you can achieve. Have the desire and you can change your life.

Write it down & get it done.

1
2
3
4
5
6
7
8
9
10

overhead extension
Sit tall on a ball with shoulders back, chest out and abs in. Hold a single heavy dumbbell using both hands as pictured. Press the dumbbell overhead so the arms are fully extended with your palms facing up. Bend the elbows and lower the dumbbell, while keeping your upper arms vertical, back straight, head up and elbows pointing towards the ceiling. Continue down until your biceps and forearms touch. Lift dumbbell back to starting position and repeat 10-15 times.

Thou, O God, dost sell us all good things at the price of labor.
— Leonardo Da Vinci

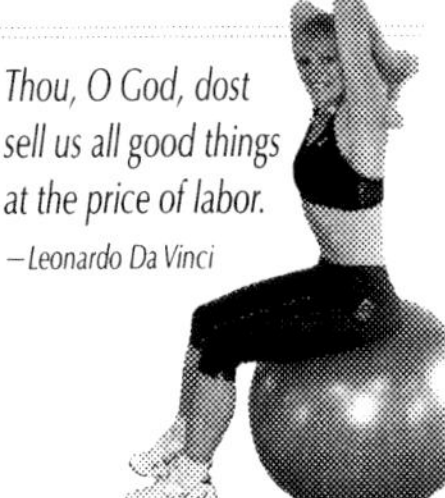

DATE

Steps Walked:
Cardio Workout:
Strength Training:
Calories Consumed:
Calories Burned:
Difference:
Weight / Body fat:

Write it down & get it done.

1
2
3
4
5
6
7
8
9
10

Read it, live it, love the results.

Stay healthy by staying busy.
Keep your mind off food by doing something that's not conductive to eating. When at home don't sit around watching television and playing video games. Instead, create projects for yourself. Do yard work, clean closets, paint a room or two, help a neighbor or friend. There is always something to do! You will love the results and feel better about yourself – mentally and physically.

Success is the reward of hard work.

Actor, comedian and television personality, **David Spade,** began doing stand up comedy when in college. He performed at the Farce Side Comedy Hour, on numerous occasions. Then the mid-80's he also did standup in the Monday night comedy show at Greesy Tony's Pizza. Before finding real success as a comedian, Spade paid the bills by working as a busboy, a valet parker, a skee ball championship competitor and a skateboard shop employee.

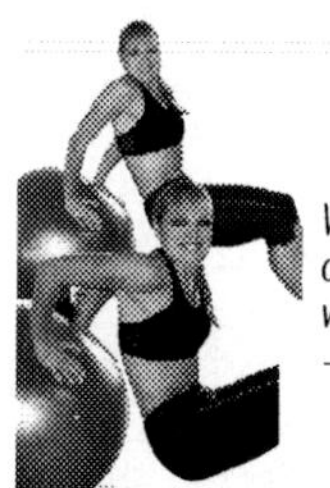

Why not go out on a limb? That's where the fruit is.
—Will Rogers

dips on ball

Place a ball against the wall, then with your back to the ball, place your hands on the ball and extend your legs out, placing your weight the heels. Keeping your legs together and your hands about shoulder width apart, bend your elbows, slowly lowering your body as far as comfortable. Hold this position for 2-3 counts, then return to the starting position. Complete 10-15 repetitions.

DATE

Steps Walked:
Cardio Workout:
Resistance Workout:
Calories Consumed:
Calories Burned:
Difference:
Weight / Body fat:

Eating healthy tastes great!

Chicken and Vegetable Soup
3 chicken breasts, cooked and diced
2-16oz cans crushed tomatoes
6 cups low sodium chicken broth
2 cups onions, diced • olive oil
1 cup red and green peppers, diced
1 cup celery, diced • 2 cups frozen corn
8 oz taco sauce • 2 tsp chili powder
2 tbs minced garlic • black pepper to taste
Sauté onions and peppers. Add remaining ingredients, bring to a boil, reduce heat and simmer 25-30 minutes.

Read it, live it, love the results.

Take some of the load off your kidneys and feel great!
Kidneys collect waste products from the blood and filter these out of the body through urine. When we make the kidneys work over time it takes a toll on our overall health. Watch for foods with the following chemicals. When eaten on a regular basis these chemicals can cause major problems; Sodium nitrate and nitrite, Monosodium glutamate, Benzoate of soda, BHA, BHT and Sulpher dioxide.

Write it down & get it done.

1
2
3
4
5
6
7
8
9
10

lying dumbbell tricep extension behind head

Lie on a ball, face up with your feet flat on the floor and your shoulders and upper back resting on the ball. Extend arms straight up, holding a dumbbell as pictured. While keeping the upper arms and elbows completely still, lower the dumbbell until it is behind your head. Be sure your elbows don't flare outward. Hold for 2-3 counts, then return to starting position, flexing the triceps as you reach the top. Complete 10-15 repetitions.

The most profound relationship we will ever have is the one with ourselves.
–Shirley MacLaine

DATE

Steps Walked:
Cardio Workout:
Strength Training:
Calories Consumed:
Calories Burned:
Difference:
Weight / Body fat:

Write it down & get it done.

1
2
3
4
5
6
7
8
9
10

Read it, live it, love the results.

Get excited about what your future holds, for it's everything you ever wanted.
Imagine yourself living your ideal life and do what it takes to make it happen. Only you can hold yourself back from achieving the future you desire, it really is up to you. No one can do it for you.

Doors open, when you work hard.

Actress **Shirley MacLean's** childhood dream was to be a ballerina. She took ballet classes throughout her youth, never missing one. She was so determined, that once she broke her ankle just before going on stage, yet she performed. It wasn't until after the show that she called for an ambulance.
Her determination and belief in herself made her the star she is today.

It is necessary to try to surpass oneself always; this occupation ought to last as long as life.
—Christina, Queen of Sweden

bent over lateral raise

Sit on a ball with feet flat on the floor, bent over at your waist, with your chest as close as possible to your thighs. With a dumbbell in each hand, let arms hang down at side with palms facing in. Raise dumbbells laterally until your arms are parallel to the floor. Hold for 2-3 counts, then slowly lower to starting position. Repeat 10-15 times.

DATE	
Steps Walked:	
Cardio Workout:	
Resistance Workout:	
Calories Consumed:	
Calories Burned:	
Difference:	
Weight / Body fat:	

Eating healthy tastes great!

Green Chicken Soup
3 chicken breasts, Sautéd and diced
10 cups chicken broth
1 onion, diced • 1 zucchini, sliced
3 celery stalks, chopped
1 cup broccoli, chopped
3 cups baby spinach
15 oz can green beans
2 tbs minced garlic
pepper, basil and parsley to taste
Place all ingredients in large pot and cook for 25-30 minutes.

Eat plenty of fiber-filled greens.
Greens are a nutritious source of antioxidants, which aide your body in resisting cancer, slowing the aging process and reducing risks of other illnesses. The most nutritious and fiber-filled greens include kale (ranked highest), mustard greens, broccoli, bok choy, swiss chard and spinach.

Write it down & get it done.

1
2
3
4
5
6
7
8
9
10

around the world
Sit tall on a ball with shoulders back, chest out, abs in and feet flat on the floor. Holding dumbbells, rest hands on your upper thighs with palms up and elbows slightly bent. Move the dumbbells up and around as if you are drawing an angel in the snow, bringing them behind your head so they touch. Return to starting position and repeat 10-15 times.

Success is the ability to go from one failure to another with no loss of enthusiasm.
—Winston Churchill

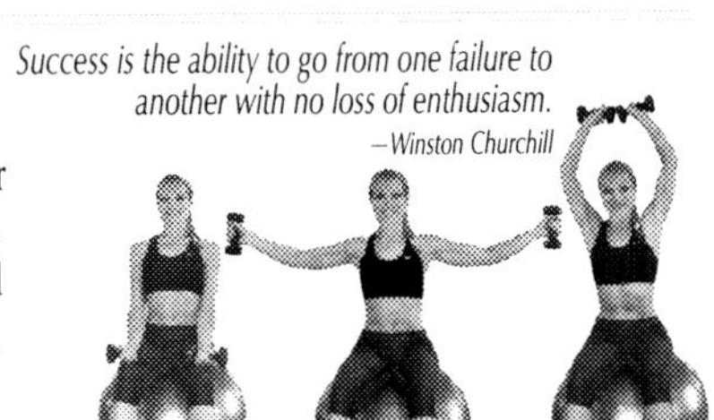

DATE

Steps Walked:
Cardio Workout:
Strength Training:
Calories Consumed:
Calories Burned:
Difference:
Weight / Body fat:

Write it down & get it done.

1
2
3
4
5
6
7
8
9
10

Read it, live it, love the results.

Take time to "hang out" if you suffer from back pain.
Studies show that hanging from a bar or beam with the body fully stretched, for sixty-seconds, can help ease back and shoulder pain. Perform this stretch twice in the morning and twice in the evening. Bars, which can be placed in your door frame, may be purchased at nearly any sporting goods store or online.

Doors open, when you work hard.

Comedian, political commentator, actor, sports commentator, and television and radio personality, **Dennis Miller**, "broke" into comedy in 1979 when he won $500 as a runner-up in Playboy magazine's first annual humor competition. Miller's really big break came in 1985, when he was discovered at The Comedy Store. From here he landed a spot on Saturday Night Live, where he was drafted to read the news.

A man is what he thinks about all day long.
– Ralph Waldo Emerson

Office exercises are a great way to burn calories and build muscle while you work. They are essential if you are not able to fit a regular workout into your day, which can be challenging, especially for those with children. The exercises listed in this section are designed to give you a full body workout using your body weight as opposed to dumbbells or other equipment, making it possible for you to do them anywhere. You may also want to consider doing some of the Band Exercises at your desk.

Steps Walked:
Cardio Workout:
Resistance Workout:
Calories Consumed:
Calories Burned:
Difference:
Weight / Body fat:

DATE

Eating healthy tastes great!

Health Boosting Brownies
4 eggs • 1/2 cup cocoa
1 stick light butter • 1 tbs vanilla
2 cups erythritol (powdered)
4 oz unsweetened chocolate, melted
2 cups flax seed meal • 1 tsp sea salt
1 tbs baking powder • 1 cup walnuts
1/3 cup fat free cream cheese
2/3 cup water • 1 cup Splenda®
Preheat oven to 350°F and grease a 9X13 pan. Combine all ingredients, pour into baking pan and bake for 35 to 40 minutes until top springs back.

Read it, live it, love the results.

Add flaxseeds to your diet.
The seeds and oil of the flax plant contain alpha-linolenic acid, an essential omega-3 fatty acid which appears to be beneficial for heart disease. Flaxseeds are also a great source of fiber, which helps lower cholesterol and prevent constipation. In addition, studies show flaxseeds may protect against cancer.

Write it down & get it done.

1
2
3
4
5
6
7
8
9
10

dumbbell hooks
Sit tall on a ball with shoulders back, chest out and abs in. With a dumbbell in each hand, position hands near your chin. Start with the right hand, punching out diagonally, bringing the dumbbell around at torso level in front of the left ribs, pull back and repeat. Your body should twist with the movement, working the obliques. Complete 25-50 punches with the right, then complete a set with your left.

I am certain of nothing but the holiness of the heart's affections, and the truth of imagination.
—John Keats

DATE

Steps Walked:
Cardio Workout:
Strength Training:
Calories Consumed:
Calories Burned:
Difference:
Weight / Body fat:

Write it down & get it done.

1
2
3
4
5
6
7
8
9
10

Read it, live it, love the results.

You can't become the person you want to be, unless you know who that person is.
Choose two people you admire most, then list the respected qualities of each. Creating a list of these qualities targets the qualities you would most like to see in yourself, strive to achieve these.

Without challenge, there is no change.

Romantic novelist and author of mainstream dramas, **Danielle Steel**, who was married four times, drew upon her own personal romantic difficulties to become the eighth best selling writer of all time. Steel wrote Passion's Promise, about a socialite who falls in love with an ex-con, after the demise of her second marriage. Shortly after her third divorce, Steel released Remembrance, in which the husband is a heroin addict.

Nobody knows what is the best s/he can do.
–Arturo Toscanini

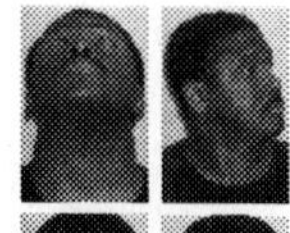

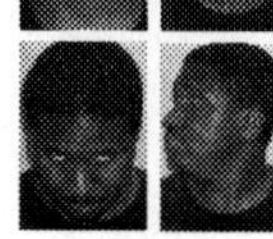

stress relief

If stress, anxiety or poor posture are causing pain or headaches, use this stretch to release the tension. Sit tall in a chair looking forward with head upright, shoulders down and relaxed. Begin with your chin in your chest. Slowly rotate your head to the right, completing five full rotations without straining the neck. Relax, then rotate in the opposite direction five more times. Keep your shoulders down as you perform this exercise.

DATE

Steps Walked:
Cardio Workout:
Strength Training:
Calories Consumed:
Calories Burned:
Difference:
Weight / Body fat:

Eating healthy tastes great!

Pumpkin Pudding

15 oz can of pumpkin
2 boxes instant sugar free vanilla pudding
1 cup skim milk
1 cup light or fat-free cool whip

Mix all ingredients, refrigerate to chill. It's like pumkin pie without the calories!

Read it, live it, love the results.

Drink skim or 1% milk instead of whole milk.

Making small changes in what you eat and drink can save over one hundred calories in some instances. These calories add up quickly especially when added up over the entire day, week and month. If you want to keep your weight down, choose the lowfat or nonfat versions of foods and watch the calories.

Write it down & get it done.

1
2
3
4
5
6
7
8
9
10

reduce stiffness and soreness

Sit tall in a chair looking straight ahead with head upright and shoulders down. Perform the following stretches, holding each for 10-15 counts. (1) Press right palm against your forehead, maintaining pressure as you push forward with your head. (2) Interlock your fingers behind your head, pressing backwards, as you resist with the hands. (3) Place the right hand against the right side of your head, pressing your head into your hand. Repeat on left.

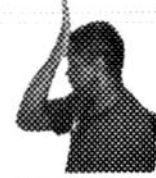
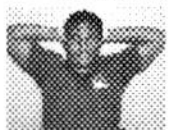
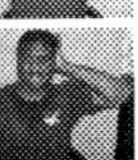

I believe in prayer and in strong belief.
– Tina Turner

DATE

Steps Walked:
Cardio Workout:
Strength Training:
Calories Consumed:
Calories Burned:
Difference:
Weight / Body fat:

Write it down & get it done.

1
2
3
4
5
6
7
8
9
10

Read it, live it, love the results.

Don't compare yourself to models.
It shouldn't be your goal to look like the picture perfect models you see in magazines. Most of them don't even look like their picture-perfect photos, without the help of photo manipulation programs. Focus on creating a healthy body, inside and out without comparing yourself to anyone.

Life's tough, get over it, he did!

One of the principal poets of the English Romantic movement, **John Keats**, received constant critical attacks from the periodicals of his day, however, this did not stop him from writing. Today, Keats's poetry remains among the most popular in English literature. His letters, which expound on his aesthetic theory of "negative capability", are among the most celebrated by any writer.

If you think education is expensive, try ignorance.
– Derek Bok

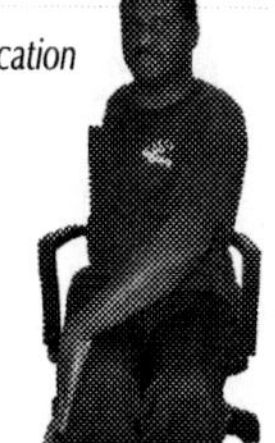

upper body stretch

To begin, sit tall in your chair then reach up with both arms, stretching as high as possible without lifting from your chair. Hold here for 10 counts, then reach up higher with the right arm, holding for another 10 counts. Repeat with the left arm. Next, place your left hand on your right leg and pull slightly as you twist your body to the right. Turn your head to look behind you. Hold for 10-30 counts then repeat on the left side.

	DATE
Steps Walked:	
Cardio Workout:	
Strength Training:	
Calories Consumed:	
Calories Burned:	
Difference:	
Weight / Body fat:	

Eating healthy tastes great!

Apple Sausage
1 lb lean ground turkey
1 tsp sage
1 tsp rosemary
1/2 cup apple, finely diced

Combine all ingredients and shape into breakfast sausage patties. Cook in skillet over medium heat for 4 to 5 minutes on each side until meat is cooked through.

Read it, live it, love the results.

Visit a salad bar for lunch and/or dinner.
Studies show that individuals who eat salads on a regular basis have higher blood levels of lycopene, alpha and beta carotene, folate, and vitamins C, E, and B6 than people who don't dine on salads. The salad bar could be your answer to fighting cancers, building bones and reducing your chance of a stroke, visit one today!

Write it down & get it done.

1
2
3
4
5
6
7
8
9
10

hamstring & lowerback stretch

With your chair two to three feet from your desk, place your right heel on the desk with toes pointed away from your body, your left foot should be flat on the floor. Bending from the waist, reach up as high as possible on your leg. Flex your foot, bringing toes towards your body, hold here for 10-15 counts. Repeat with the other leg.

Along with success comes a reputation for wisdom.
– Euripides

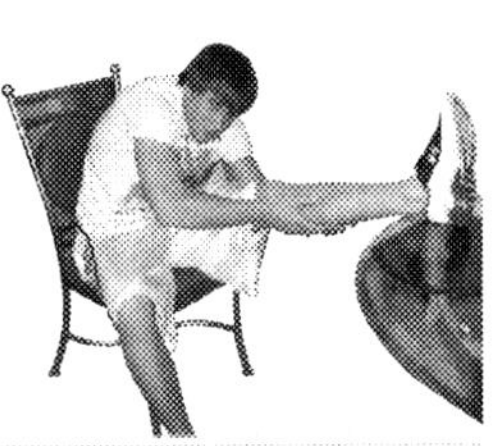

DATE

Steps Walked:
Cardio Workout:
Strength Training:
Calories Consumed:
Calories Burned:
Difference:
Weight / Body fat:

Write it down & get it done.

1
2
3
4
5
6
7
8
9
10

Read it, live it, love the results.

Expect great things from youself.

You should expect more from yourself than anyone else. Set your standards high and don't disappoint yourself. If you don't expect great things from yourself why would you expect them from anyone else. This is your one and only life, make it the best it can possibly be!

Doors open when least expected.

Actor, **Johnny Depp**, had dreamed of becoming a *"rock star"*. His mother bought him a guitar when he was twelve, and he played in various garage bands, eventually dropping out of high school to become a rock musician. However, when he was introduced to Nicolas Cage he decided to pursue an acting career. Since then, Depp has become quite successful, winning many awards for his achievements.

Don't worry so much about your self-esteem. Worry more about your character. Integrity is its own reward.
—Laura Schlessinger

push-ups on desk

Standing with feet shoulder-width apart, place your hands on your desk slightly wider than shoulder-width apart. Legs should be stretched straight out behind you as you balance on your toes. Keeping your body straight as a plank, bend your elbows out to the side and drop your chest to the desk top, hold for 2-3 counts, then slowly press back to starting position. Repeat 10-15 times.

DATE

Steps Walked:
Cardio Workout:
Resistance Workout:
Calories Consumed:
Calories Burned:
Difference:
Weight / Body fat:

Eating healthy tastes great!

Grilled Shrimp Kebabs
1 lb shrimp
16 oz can pineapple chunks
1/4 cup soy sauce
4 slices turkey bacon, 2" pieces
Place shrimp and pineapple chunks in bowl, top with soy sauce, let stand for 30 minutes. Place shrimp, pineapple and bacon onto skewers. Place skewers on aluminum foil. Fold up edges and seal. Place packages on grill, turning once. Cook 12-15 minutes until shrimp is completely cooked.

Read it, live it, love the results.

Exercise daily.
The best things in life are FREE. To maintain a healthy young body—move and stay active, this can be done without spending a dime. Walk daily, climb stairs and perform weight bearing exercises. Exercise strengthens bones, tones muscles, improves flexibility, increases circulation, lowers blood pressure, controls blood sugar, and improves the function of your heart, lungs and brain, all and all it keeps you young.

Write it down & get it done.

1
2
3
4
5
6
7
8
9
10

bun firmers
This is an exercise which can be performed anywhere you are seated—home, office or car. Simply tighten your glutes and abs and hold for 7-10 counts before releasing.

kegels
Women may also perform kegels. Sitting tall, tighten and hold the pelvic floor muscles—those which control the flow of urine. Hold for 10-15 counts, repeating periodically throughout the day.

Action springs not from thought, but from a readiness for responsibility.
—Dietrich Bonhoeffer

DATE

Steps Walked:
Cardio Workout:
Strength Training:
Calories Consumed:
Calories Burned:
Difference:
Weight / Body fat:

Write it down & get it done.

1
2
3
4
5
6
7
8
9
10

Read it, live it, love the results.

Your dreams and desires are yours, and it's your responsibility to make them a reality.
Don't look for a hand out, don't expect others to be responsible for helping you to achieve that which you desire, take responsibility for yourself and make it happen. Success is a result of hard work, not passing blame.

Doors open, when you work hard.

TV personality, celebrity chef and author, **Rachael Ray**, credits the concept of 30-Minute Meals to her experience working at a store. Here, she taught a course, showing people how to make meals in less than thirty minutes. With the success of these classes, she earned a weekly segment on the local TV network. This, along with a public radio appearance and the publication of her first book, led to a Today show spot and her first Food Network contract in 2001.

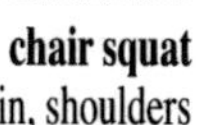

at your desk

chair squat

Sit tall in a chair with abs in, shoulders back and chest out with hands resting in lap, feet flat on floor. Press through your heels as you lift your buns 2-3 inches from the chair. Hold this position 10-15 counts. Repeat 5-10 times.

In absence of clearly defined goals, we become strangely loyal to performing daily acts of trivia.
—author unknown

	DATE
Steps Walked:	
Cardio Workout:	
Resistance Workout:	
Calories Consumed:	
Calories Burned:	
Difference:	
Weight / Body fat:	

Eating healthy tastes great!

Shish Kebab on the BBQ Pit

4 chicken breasts, cut into cubes
6 small onions, cut in half
12 cherry tomatoes • 6 oz mushrooms
3/4 cup olive oil • 1/2 cup sweet white wine
1 tbs lemon juice • 2 tbs minced garlic
black pepper to taste

Combine last six ingredients, mix well, then add chicken. Cover and marinate overnight. On 6 long skewers, alternate chicken, onion, tomatoes and mushrooms. Place on BBQ pit, turn and baste with marinade frequently.

Read it, live it, love the results.

Learn everything you can about health and fitness.

The more you know, the more you'll focus on taking care of yourself. Knowledge is one of the most empowering tools you can use in creating a healthy life. Knowing the facts increases your confidence, resolves fear and inspires you to take action.

Write it down & get it done.

1
2
3
4
5
6
7
8
9
10

one legged squats

Stand with feet shoulder-width apart, back straight, shoulders back and chest out, with toes pointed straight ahead or slightly outward. Resting your right foot on your left calf, focus your vision straight ahead and squat down and back, as if you are sitting in a chair. Keeping your knee behind your toes, squat down as low as you can, or when your thighs are parallel with the floor. Hold for 2-3 counts, then return to starting position. Repeat 10-15 times.

You see things as they are and ask, "Why?" I dream of things as they never were and ask, "Why not?"
–George Bernard Shaw

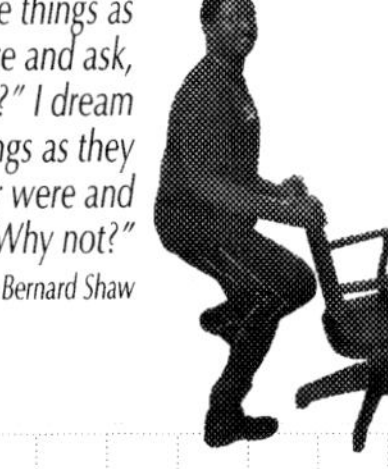

DATE

Steps Walked:

Cardio Workout:

Strength Training:

Calories Consumed:

Calories Burned:

Difference:

Weight / Body fat:

Write it down & get it done.

1
2
3
4
5
6
7
8
9
10

Read it, live it, love the results.

Relax and enjoy life.
Avoiding stress is a great way to increase your life span. Stress, like obesity, contributes to nearly every major disease. Studies indicate that the stress hormone cortisol ages the brain by shrinking the hippocampus, the part of our brain which controls memory and thinking. The increased levels of cortisol also cause weight gain in the stomach and waist area.

Your level of success is up to you

Playwright, **George Bernard Shaw**, spent many hours in the library studying and writing novels when he was young. He earned his allowance by ghost-writing Vandeleur Lee's music column, which appeared in the London Hornet. Unfortunately, his novels were rejected, so his earnings were slim until he became a critic of the arts. Despite rejection, he never gave up.

The biggest mistake people make in life is not trying to make a living at doing what they most enjoy.
—Malcomb Forbes

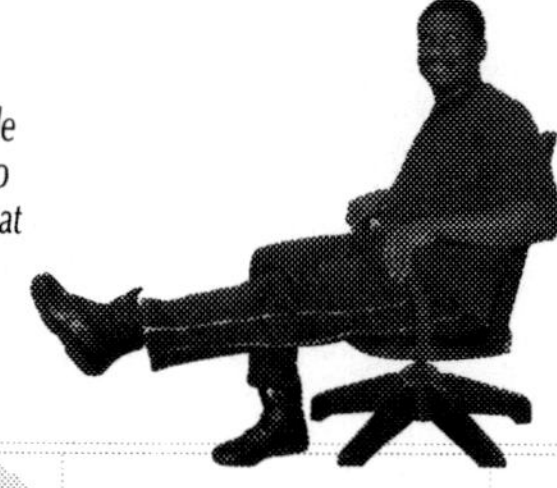

seated single leg lift
Sit tall, abs in, shoulders back and chest out, with feet flat on the floor. Resting your arms on the chair, raise your left leg straight out and hold for 3-5 counts. Lower and repeat 10-15 times. Complete a set with the right leg.

Steps Walked:
Cardio Workout:
Resistance Workout:
Calories Consumed:
Calories Burned:
Difference:
Weight / Body fat:

DATE

Eating healthy tastes great!

French Green Peas
10 oz bag frozen peas
3 slices turkey bacon, cut into pieces
2 onions, sliced thin
$^1/_2$ canned pimiento, cut into strips
3 tbs wheat flour
$1^1/_2$ cup low sodium chicken broth
white pepper and parsley to taste
Blend flour and spices with broth. Cook over medium heat until thick. Add remaining ingredients and cook for 15-20 minutes on low, until peas are tender.

Read it, live it, love the results.

Green Peas can help energize you.
Green peas provide nutrients which help support the energy-producing cells and systems of the body. This makes them an excellent addition to your diet if feeling fatigued and sluggish.
They are also a good source of iron, a mineral necessary for normal blood cell formation and function, whose deficiency results in anemia, fatigue, decreased immune function, and learning problems.

Write it down & get it done.

1
2
3
4
5
6
7
8
9
10

back pull

Sit tall in a chair with abs in, shoulders back and chest out. Place your hands in front of your chest with the right palm facing in and the left palm out. Clasp your fingers, pulling your left arm toward the right side while resisting with the left arm, hold for 2-3 counts. Perform 10-15 repetitions then, repeat on opposite side.

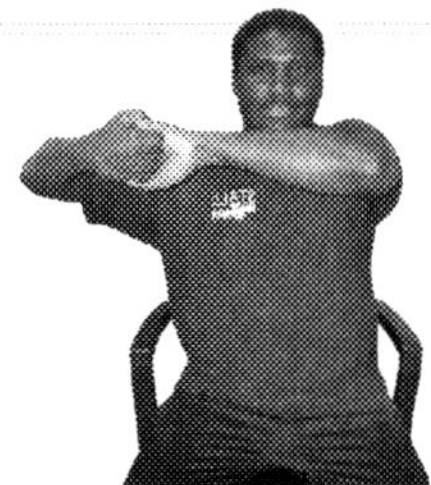

He that is good with a hammer tends to think everything is a nail.
—Abraham Maslow

DATE

Steps Walked:
Cardio Workout:
Strength Training:
Calories Consumed:
Calories Burned:
Difference:
Weight / Body fat:

Write it down & get it done.

1
2
3
4
5
6
7
8
9
10

Read it, live it, love the results.

Working out? Fantastic! Just make sure you don't do the same workout repeatedly.
If you perform the same workout every training session, even for a month, your body will adjust and no longer produce results. I've met many who are dissapointed when their great workout is not longer helping them lose weight—you must change your workout to keep it working.

Doors open, when you work hard.

Talk show host, **Dr. Mehmet Cengiz Oz**, began his TV career by appearing as a health expert on *The Oprah Winfrey Show* for five seasons. *His Transplant!* TV series won both a Freddie and a Silver Telly award. He has also appeared on *Good Morning America, the Today show, Larry King Live and The View,* as well as guest-hosting the *Charlie Rose show.* Today he has his own syndicated daily talk called *The Dr. Oz Show*.

I honestly think it is better to be a failure at something you love than to be a success at something you hate.
— George Burns

knee to chest

Sitting tall in a chair, grab your right knee with both hands and gently pull into your chest until the stretch is felt in your lower back. Hold for 10-30 counts, release, then perform the stretch with left knee.

double Knee to chest

With this exercise you will gently pull both knees into your chest until a stretch is felt in your lower back.

DATE

Steps Walked:
Cardio Workout:
Strength Training:
Calories Consumed:
Calories Burned:
Difference:
Weight / Body fat:

Eating healthy tastes great!

Swiss Breakfast
1 cup Quaker® oats
1/4 tsp cinnamon • 2 tbs raisins
2 tbs sunflower seeds • 1 date, chopped
2 tbs almonds, sliced
2 tbs dried apricots, chopped
1 tbs dried cranberries
Bring 2 cups of water to a boil, then place all ingredients in pot. Simmer uncovered, stirring occasionally until water is absorbed. Cover and let set for about two minutes. Serve with skim milk or soy milk.

Read it, live it, love the results.

Eat unprocessed foods.
Ninety percent of what you eat should be food that could have been hunted, caught, gathered from a garden or plucked from a tree. When we fill our bodies with processed foods the organs are forced to work harder than necessary, this often leads to many health issues. Not feeling well? Eat natural foods and you will be amazed at how quickly your body will respond.

Write it down & get it done.

1
2
3
4
5
6
7
8
9
10

desk push

Sit tall in a chair with abs in, shoulders back and chest out with your feet flat on the floor and palms pressed up against the edge of your desk. Keeping your head straight and elbows tucked into your sides, tighten your back muscles as you firmly press into the desk. Hold for 7-10 counts then release. Repeat 5-10 times.

First of all, I'm happy that I'm healthy.
—Tina Turner

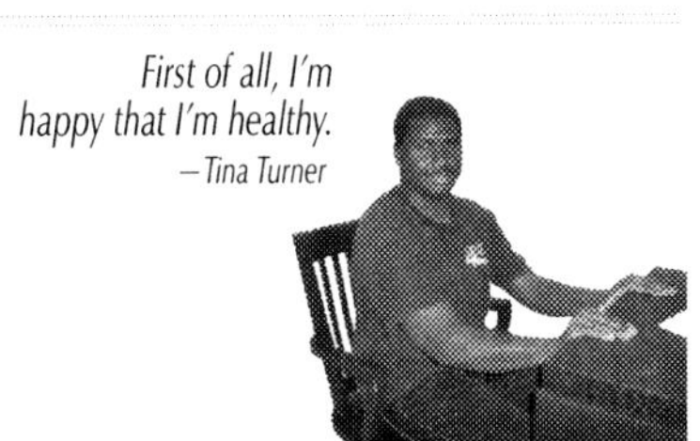

DATE

Steps Walked:
Cardio Workout:
Strength Training:
Calories Consumed:
Calories Burned:
Difference:
Weight / Body fat:

Write it down & get it done.

1
2
3
4
5
6
7
8
9
10

Read it, live it, love the results.

Have faith that you can achieve anything you desire, and you will succeed.

Faith is the visualization of and belief in attainment of your desire. Know your desire and believe you already possess it as you read your *"Desire Statement."* Great runners imagine themselves crossing the finish line before they even begin the race, they have faith they can do it—you must do the same.

Doors open when least expected.

Author and lecturer **Wayne Dyer** spent much of his childhood in an orphanage. This fueled his desire to help others. He first pursued a teaching career, gave motivational lectures and ran a successful private therapy practice. An agent then persuaded him to write a book. He wrote *Your Erroneous Zones.* Initially sales were low so he quit his job and began a publicity tour through the U.S. out of the back of his station wagon—his book then made the best-seller list. It was the first of many.

Do not consider painful what is good for you.
– Euripides

advanced t-pushup on desk

Stand 3-4 feet from a desk, with your hands on the desk shoulder-width apart. Keeping your arms straight hold a plank position. With the abs engaged, rotate your entire body to the right, reaching toward the ceiling with the right hand. With the legs and feet stacked, hold for 2-3 counts, then lift the right leg 12-15 inches and hold for another 2-3 counts, lower, returning your hand to the desk, perform a pushup, bending elbows to 90-degrees. Return to starting position and repeat same movement on the left side. Complete10-15 repetitions.

	DATE
Steps Walked:	
Cardio Workout:	
Strength Training:	
Calories Consumed:	
Calories Burned:	
Difference:	
Weight / Body fat:	

Eating healthy tastes great!

Healthy Collard Greens
3 bunches of fresh collard greens
2 red peppers, diced
4 tbs each; minced garlic, liquid smoke and olive oil
sea salt, garlic powder and cayenne pepper to taste
Cook greens 30-45 minutes on medium until they change color from a bright green, to a paler green. Remove from heat, add spices, olive oil and liquid smoke. Mix well and serve hot.

Read it, live it, love the results.

Collards are great at preventing cancer and age related diseases.
Collards are an excellent source of vitamin A, mostly in the form of beta-carotene, which has been shown to help protect against cancer, heart disease, cataracts, and other diseases of aging through its antioxidant properties. Vitamin A also helps keep the immune system strong. The outer leaves of greens usually contain more beta-carotene than do the inner leaves.

Write it down & get it done.

1
2
3
4
5
6
7
8
9
10

push-ups on desk

Standing with feet shoulder-width apart, place your hands on your desk slightly wider than shoulder-width apart. Legs should be stretched straight out behind you as you balance on your toes. Keeping your body straight as a plank, bend your elbows out to the side and drop your chest to the desk top, hold for 2-3 counts, then slowly press back to starting position. Repeat 10-15 times.

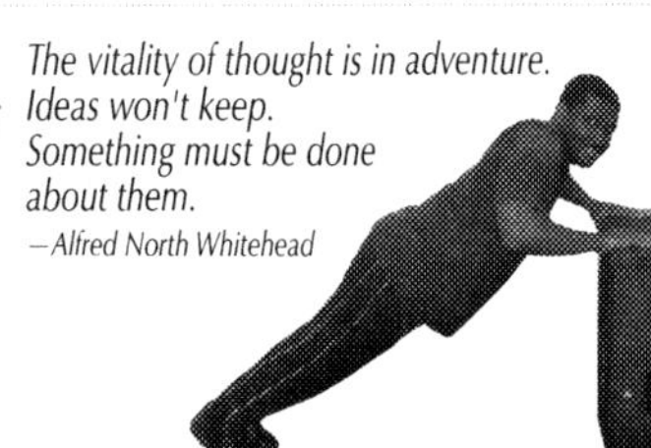

DATE

Steps Walked:

Cardio Workout:

Strength Training:

Calories Consumed:

Calories Burned:

Difference:

Weight / Body fat:

Write it down & get it done.

1
2
3
4
5
6
7
8
9
10

Read it, live it, love the results.

Record that which motivates you. When you come across a quotation that motivates you to achieve your goals, write it down. Put it on your refrigerator, bathroom mirror, computer screen, or any other place where you can view it on a daily basis. Also, be sure to record it in this journal. Whatever you do, don't let it go.

Doors open when least expected.

St. Louis Cardinals manager **Tony La Russa, Jr.**, had actually gone to school to become a lawyer, though shortly before graduating he was offered a position to coach in the minor leagues. He asked one of his professors what he should do, the professor responded; *"Grow up, you're an adult now, you're going to be a lawyer."* We in St. Louis are thankful he chose not to *"grow up"*. Tony also blessed many with his *Tony La Russa's Animal Rescue Foundation. visit: http://www.tlr-arf.org*

When one door of happiness closes, another opens; but often we look so long at the closed door that we do not see the one which has been opened for us.
— Helen Keller

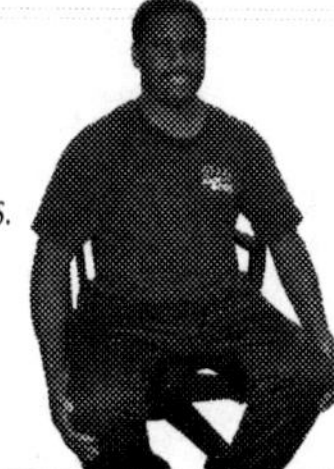

chest press with knees

Sit on the front edge of your chair, with your feet together and knees spread apart. Place hands outside your knees and push inward as you press out with your knees, to resist the inward pushing of your hands. Hold for 10-15 counts, repeat 5 times. This exercise places tension on your pecs.

	DATE
Steps Walked:	
Cardio Workout:	
Resistance Workout:	
Calories Consumed:	
Calories Burned:	
Difference:	
Weight / Body fat:	

Eating healthy tastes great!

Thrifty Man's Lobster

1 lb cod fillets • 2 tbs sea salt
2 tbs white vinegar • water

Place fillets and salt in saucepan, cover with cold water. Bring to boil, lower heat and cook 10 minutes. Drain. Cover again with cold water and white vinegar. Bring to boil. Lower heat and cook 10 minutes more. Drain and serve.

Read it, live it, love the results.

Keep your mind sharp with fish!

Studies have found that, due to the high levels of omega-3 in fish, people who eat at least one fish meal a week are significantly less likely to end up with Alzheimer's disease than those who regularly avoid fish. Studies also show a diet of fish has a positive effect on learning acquisition and memory performance, this is a result of the communication between nerve cells.

Write it down & get it done.

1
2
3
4
5
6
7
8
9
10

isometric curl

Sit tall in your chair with abs in, shoulders back and chest out. Place the palm of your left hand into the palm of your right, interlocking the left pinky with the thumb and forefinger of the right hand. With the right hand positioned at your right side, curl your right arm up, while resisting with the left. Perform 10-15 repetitions, then complete a set on the opposite side.

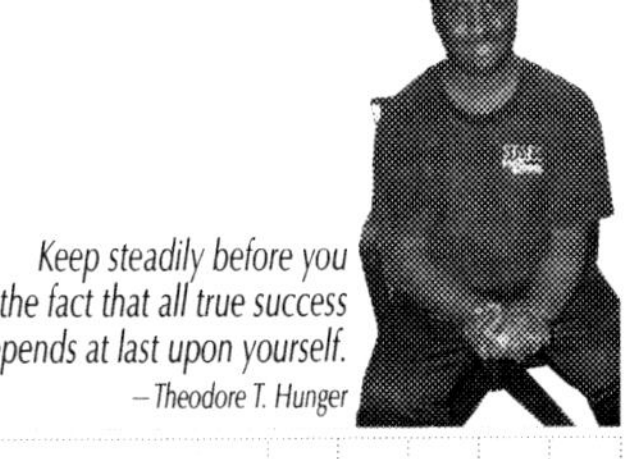

Keep steadily before you the fact that all true success depends at last upon yourself.
– Theodore T. Hunger

DATE

Steps Walked:
Cardio Workout:
Strength Training:
Calories Consumed:
Calories Burned:
Difference:
Weight / Body fat:

Write it down & get it done.

1
2
3
4
5
6
7
8
9
10

Read it, live it, love the results.

Don't deprive yourself of sleep. Experts report that not only does a lack of sleep leave you looking puffy eyed, drinking gallons of coffee and dozing off at afternoon meetings, it steals your youth. When you don't get enough sleep you increase your risk for a variety of major illnesses, including cancer, heart disease, diabetes and obesity.

Your level of success is up to you.

Actress **Michelle Pfeiffer** began her acting career in high school when she worked as Alice in Wonderland at Disneyland. She entered the Miss California competition, though didn't win. However, she never gave up. Eventually she secured small movie and TV roles, it led to her making her mark in Hollywood. In addition to being considered one of the most beautiful women in film, she's also been the recipient of a Golden Globe Award and a BAFTA Award.

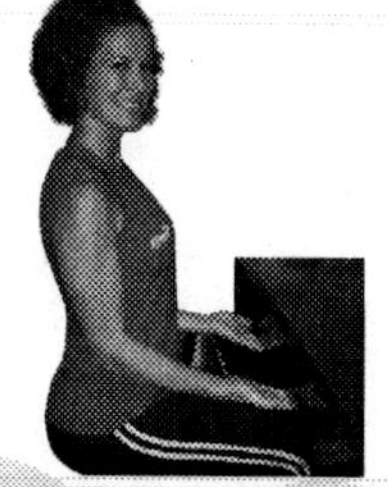

You must be the change you wish to see in the world.
—Mohandas Gandhi

desk lift

Sit tall in your chair with abs in, shoulders back and chest out. Place your hands under your desk with palms up. Keeping elbows at your sides, "lift" up on the desk, flexing your bicep muscles as you do. Hold for 7-10 counts, then release. Repeat 5-10 times.

Steps Walked:
Cardio Workout:
Strength Training:
Calories Consumed:
Calories Burned:
Difference:
Weight / Body fat:

DATE

Eating healthy tastes great!

Szechuan Fish
1 lb cod, cut onto 1½" pieces
2 green onions, diced
4 tbs minced garlic
1 cup fat free chicken stock
3 tbs soy sauce • 1 tbs rice vinegar
1 tbs ginger, grated • 1 tbs sherry wine
½ tsp chili pepper, crushed
In a wok brown the fish on all sides with the green onion and garlic. Combine remaining ingredients and pour over the fish. Cover and cook on low heat for 20 minutes.

Read it, live it, love the results.

Taking fish oil capsules may be the best way to get your Omega-3s.
The American Heart Association recommends eating fish, particularly salmon, herring and other types of fatty fish, at least twice a week. However, you may also take Omega-3 supplements instead. The omega-3 fatty acids in fish oil lower triglycerides, protect the heart and brain, help regulate mood, fight depression and may impact memory and cognition.

Write it down & get it done.

1
2
3
4
5
6
7
8
9
10

isometric concentration curl

Sit on the front edge of a chair with your legs open and feet flat on the floor. Lean forward, placing your right elbow against the inside hollow of your right knee. Pressing your left fist into your right hand, curl the right arm up. Repeat 10-15 times, then complete a set on opposite side. For great results, you must provide as much resistance as possible.

Alone we can do so little; together we can do so much.
—Helen Keller

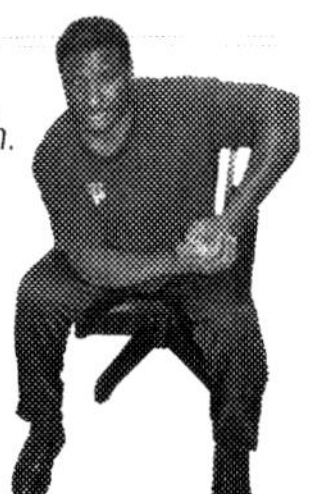

DATE

Steps Walked:
Cardio Workout:
Strength Training:
Calories Consumed:
Calories Burned:
Difference:
Weight / Body fat:

Write it down & get it done.

1
2
3
4
5
6
7
8
9
10

Read it, live it, love the results.

Forbid yourself to be a quitter. As with anything else, the more you do it, the easier it becomes. When you allow yourself to give up, quitting becomes a part of your identity—and the more you do it the easier it becomes. Instead, strive to make success the only acceptable outcome in your life. Make it your identity.

Doors open, when you work hard.

Actress **Betty Grable** had small parts in over 50 Hollywood movies throughout the 1930s before finally gaining national attention. In 1940, she obtained a contract with 20th Century Fox and soon became their top star throughout the decade, becoming one of Hollywood's most popular ladies. Her iconic bathing suit photo made her the number-one pin-up girl of the World War II era. It was later included in *Life 100 Photos that Changed the World.*

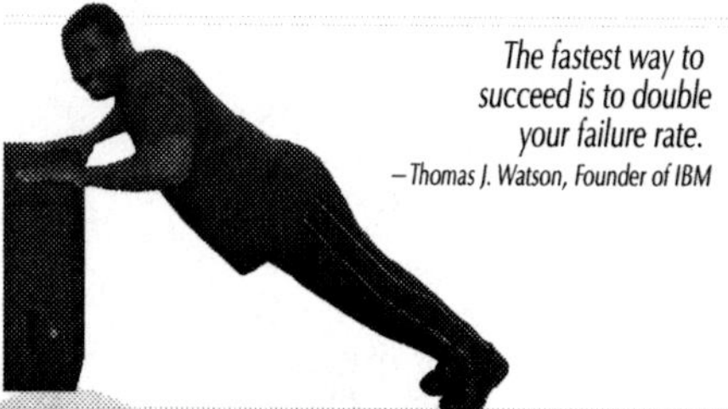

The fastest way to succeed is to double your failure rate.
– Thomas J. Watson, Founder of IBM

plank on desk with elbows in

Stand 3-4 feet from a desk. Place your hands on the desk 5-8 inches apart, then drop your body down into a plank position. Keeping elbows close to your sides, bend them and drop your chest to the desktop. Hold your body in this plank position for 8-10 counts. Repeat 2-3 times.

DATE	
Steps Walked:	
Cardio Workout:	
Resistance Workout:	
Calories Consumed:	
Calories Burned:	
Difference:	
Weight / Body fat:	

Eating healthy tastes great!

Mushy Peas
8 oz frozen peas
1 onion, diced
2 tbs minced garlic
3 tbs low sodium chicken broth
2 tbs sunflower seeds
1 tbs of each, minced; mint, basil, chervil, and parsley
white pepper to taste

Sauté onion in broth.
Add remaining ingredients, sauté then puree in blender. Serve hot.

Try these great foods to rid yourself of nervousness.

If you can be described as *"high strung"* or a *"nervous ninny"* adding more of these foods to your diet should help *"mellow you out"*: Tomatoes, carrots, turnips, leafy green vegetables, kidney beans, dry beans, soy beans lentils, fish, whole grains, nuts, pork and lemon juice.

Write it down & get it done.

1
2
3
4
5
6
7
8
9
10

dips on desk
Position yourself in front of your desk, with hands on the desk about shoulder-width apart. Extend your legs straight out, placing your weight on your heels. Keeping your legs together, bend your elbows slowly lowering your body as far as comfortable. Hold this position for 2-3 counts, then straighten the arms, pushing yourself back to starting position. Repeat 10-15 times.

There is no happiness except in the realization that we have accomplished something.
—Henry Ford

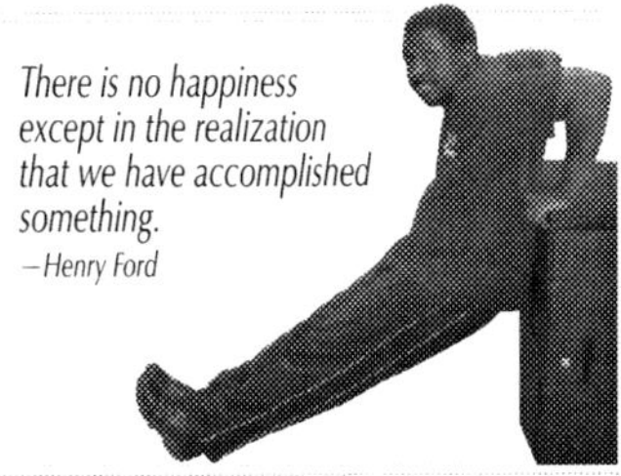

DATE

Steps Walked:
Cardio Workout:
Strength Training:
Calories Consumed:
Calories Burned:
Difference:
Weight / Body fat:

Write it down & get it done.

1
2
3
4
5
6
7
8
9
10

Read it, live it, love the results.

Be grateful for the things you have.
Being alive and able to function on a daily basis is a blessing in itself, anything more is a bonus. Take time each day to reflect on those things you have to be thankful for, such as your home, career, family and friends. You'll soon realize how lucky you truly are.

Life's tough, get over it, she did!

Humanitarian, **Harriet Tubman**, was born into slavery. As a child she was beaten, whipped and suffered a traumatic head injury which caused disabling seizures, headaches, spells of hypersomnia, and powerful visionary and dream activity. She felt these were premonitions from God. After escaping from captivity, she made thirteen missions to rescue over seventy slaves, using the network of antislavery activists and safe houses known as the Underground Railroad.

You miss 100 percent of the shots you never take.
—Wayne Gretzky

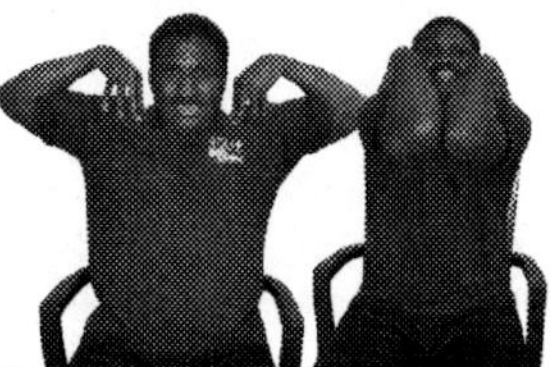

funky chicken

Sit tall, abs in, shoulders back and chest out. Place your fingertips on your shoulders with elbows pointing out to the sides. Push your elbows back as far as possible, hold for2-3 counts then push them forward, touching in front, holding here for 2-3 counts. Complete 10-15 repetitions.

DATE

Steps Walked:
Cardio Workout:
Strength Training:
Calories Consumed:
Calories Burned:
Difference:
Weight / Body fat:

Eating healthy tastes great!

Taco Salad
1 lb lean ground turkey, browned
1 tsp olive oil • 1 onion, diced
3 tbs minced garlic • 1/4 cup tomatoes, diced
14 oz can kidney beans, rinsed
2 tsp cumin and chili powder
1/4 cup chopped fresh cilantro
----
shredded romaine lettuce
low fat sour cream • salsa • light cheese
Brown turkey, then sauté with ingredients above line. Serve over a bed of lettuce, top with cheese, salsa and sour cream.

Read it, live it, love the results.

Cut out sweets and starches.
Give up these drinks and foods and you will see immediate results. Your body will feel better in just a few days!
- Soda and other sweet drinks
- Beer and most mixed drinks
- Cakes, cookies, pies, breads, rolls and pasteries
- Candy
- Ice cream
- Potato chips and similar snacks

Write it down & get it done.

1
2
3
4
5
6
7
8
9
10

body lifts
Sit tall in a chair with abs in, shoulders back and chest out with hands resting on the chair arms. Keeping your feet flat on the floor, slowly lift your buns out of the chair 6-8 inches. Hold here for 2-3 counts, then lower down to within an inch of the seat and hold for another 2-3 counts before returning to the "up" position.
Repeat 10-15 times.

We all do 'do, re, mi,' but you have got to find the other notes yourself.
– Louis Armstrong

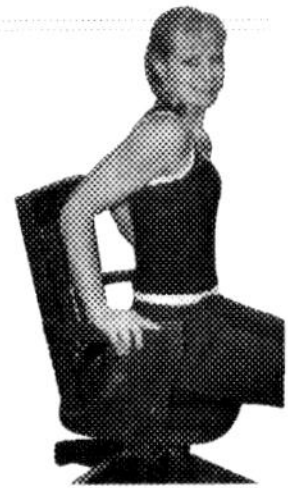

DATE

Steps Walked:
Cardio Workout:
Strength Training:
Calories Consumed:
Calories Burned:
Difference:
Weight / Body fat:

Write it down & get it done.

1
2
3
4
5
6
7
8
9
10

Read it, live it, love the results.

Journal on a daily basis.
Studies completed by scientists at Southern Methodist University and Ohio State University College of Medicine indicate that writing contributes directly to your physical health. Those who wrote thoughtfully and emotionally about traumatic experiences achieved the following results: increased T-cell production, a drop in physician visits, fewer absentee days and generally improved physical health.

Life's tough, get over it, he did!

Jazz artist **Louis Armstrong**, had it rough growing up at the bottom of the social ladder in a highly segregated city. However, instead of seeing his youth as the worst of times, he drew inspiration from it, "Every time I close my eyes blowing that trumpet of mine–I look right in the heart of good old New Orleans... It has given me something to live for." Armstrong was widely regarded as a profound influence on music, perhaps the most important American musician of the 20th century.

There's as much risk in doing nothing as in doing something.
– Trammell Crow

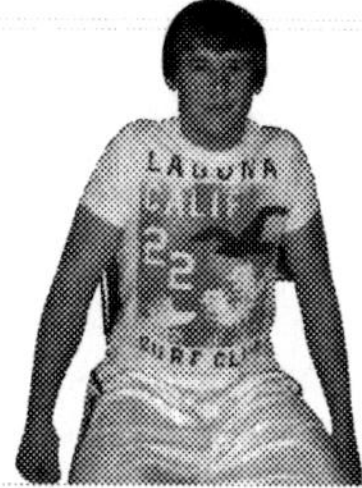

shoulder rolls

Sit tall in a chair with abs in, shoulders back and chest out with feet flat on the floor. Lift your shoulders as high as you can, then rotate in a clockwise motion, completing 5-10 full rotations. Also, complete a set of rotations in the counter-clockwise direction.

DATE

Steps Walked:
Cardio Workout:
Resistance Workout:
Calories Consumed:
Calories Burned:
Difference:
Weight / Body fat:

Eating healthy tastes great!

Salmon Bake
1 1/2 cups cooked brown rice
1 can salmon • 1/4 cup onion, minced
1 egg • 2 egg whites, beaten
2 tbs olive oil
black pepper to taste

Preheat oven to 375°F.
Mix all ingredients and pour into a casserole dish. Spread 2 tbs olive oil on top and bake for 30 minutes.

Read it, live it, love the results.

Avoid simple carbs in the form of white refined, industrial flours and sugars.
Eating white refined foods makes as much sense as smoking cigarettes. These foods have little to no nutritional value, in addition they promote weight gain and aging, which in turn reduces your longevity. It is up to you to make your life the best it can be. Your choices will determine your health.

Write it down & get it done.

1
2
3
4
5
6
7
8
9
10

lateral ift

Sit in a chair, with your weight resting on your left buttock. With the left foot flat on the floor, raise your right foot as high as possible. Hold here for 4-5 counts, then return to the starting position and repeat. Complete 10-15 repetitions on each leg. You may also wear an ankle weight when performing this exercise.

To simply wake up every morning a better person than when I went to bed.
– Sidney Poitier

DATE

Steps Walked:
Cardio Workout:
Strength Training:
Calories Consumed:
Calories Burned:
Difference:
Weight / Body fat:

Write it down & get it done.

1
2
3
4
5
6
7
8
9
10

Read it, live it, love the results.

Research your family medical history and keep track of diseases which run in the family. Studies show that many diseases are hereditary. However, simply because you are at risk for a disease does not mean you will develop that disease, especially if you take the necessary preventive steps to avoid it.

Doors open, when you work hard.

Actor, film director, author, and diplomat, **Sidney Poitier**, was not born a "natural." In his first attempt at theater, he was rejected by audiences. Determined, he spent the next six months dedicating himself to achieving theatrical success. His second attempt at the theater landed him a leading role in a Broadway production for which he received excellent reviews. Poitier went on to have a very successful career winning many awards.

seated abdominal leg pull ins

Sit tall in a chair with abs in, shoulders back and chest out with your legs straight out. Hold the sides of your chair as you lean back. Contract your abdominal muscles as you bring your knees into your chest. Hold here for 2-3 counts, then return to starting position and repeat 10-15 times.

You have to think anyway, so why not think big?
– Donald Trump

Steps Walked:
Cardio Workout:
Resistance Workout:
Calories Consumed:
Calories Burned:
Difference:
Weight / Body fat:

DATE

Eating healthy tastes great!

Baked Bean Burgers
2 16oz cans black beans
2/3 cup ground sunflower seeds
1/4 cup onion, diced • 1/2 cup wheat germ
2 tbs olive oil • 3 to 4 tbs catsup
chili powder to taste
Preheat oven to 350ºF. Combine all the ingredients. Form into 8 patties and place on a lightly oiled baking sheet. Bake for 15 to 20 minutes. If desired, place a slice of light cheese on each and broil to melt before serving.

Read it, live it, love the results.

Eat a diet rich in fiber to reduce your risk of having a "coronary".
Studies show that eating a fiber rich diet makes you feel fuller and decreases your risk of coronary artery disease. Enjoy these fiber rich foods for a healthy life; beans, raspberries, blackberries, strawberries, rye broccoli, green beans, kale, apples, spinach, beets, collard greens, swiss chard, turnip greens, almonds, peanuts, brazil nuts, walnuts, cherries and brussel sprouts.

Write it down & get it done.

1
2
3
4
5
6
7
8
9
10

hip drop with desk

Stand 3-4 feet from a desk with your hands on the desk shoulder-width apart. Drop your body down into a plank position, keeping arms straight, then with your abs engaged, rotate your entire body to the right, placing your right hand on your hip as you stack your legs and feet. Hold here for 10 counts, then lower the hip 3-6 inches, hold for 2-3 counts then return to the starting position. Repeat 10-15 times, then complete a set on the opposite side.

I never had a chance to play with dolls like other kids. I started working when I was six years old.
– Billie Holiday

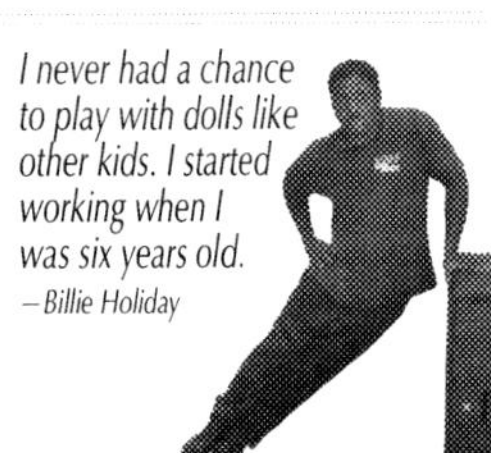

DATE

Steps Walked:
Cardio Workout:
Strength Training:
Calories Consumed:
Calories Burned:
Difference:
Weight / Body fat:

Write it down & get it done.

1
2
3
4
5
6
7
8
9
10

Read it, live it, love the results.

Cast aside all excuses.
Excuses are lies used to cover up the truth so you can avoid facing reality. Each time you make an excuse for not reaching a goal or sticking to a plan, write down the excuse. Then write down three reasons as to why the excuse is a lie—and don't ever use it again.

Life's tough, get over it, she did.

Jazz singer and songwriter, **Billie Holiday's** career stemmed from hard times. After being imprisoned for prostitution, she began singing for tips at night clubs. According to legend, penniless and facing eviction, she sang *"Travelin All Alone"* in a club, reducing the audience to tears. Eventually, she was discovered by talent scout John Hammond. Critic John Bush wrote that she *"changed the art of American pop vocals forever."*

*Creativity is allowing yourself to make mistakes.
Art is knowing which ones to keep.*
– Scott Adams

sitting and twisting knee raise

Sit on the front edge of your chair with feet flat on the floor, back straight, angled back, chest out and abs in, with fingertips resting on your neck, elbows out. Contract your abdominals as you twist your upper body, bringing your right elbow to meet your left knee. Hold 2-3 counts, then return to the starting position, keeping the left leg slightly suspended above the floor. Complete 10-15 repetitions on each side.

Steps Walked:
Cardio Workout:
Resistance Workout:
Calories Consumed:
Calories Burned:
Difference:
Weight / Body fat:

DATE

Eating healthy tastes great!

Awesome Chicken Strips
4 chicken breasts, cut into strips
1 onion, sliced thin
$^1/_4$ cup mushrooms, sliced
1 green pepper, sliced thin
1 red pepper, sliced thin
3 tbs olive oil
1 $^1/_4$ tsp paprika
black pepper to taste
Sauté chicken strips and onions in olive oil. When done, add remaining ingredients and simmer 10-15 minutes. Serve hot.

Read it, live it, love the results.

You have everything you need to be healthy and fit.

*"The best six doctors anywhere
And no one can deny it
Are sunshine, water, rest, and air
Exercise and diet.
These six will gladly you attend
If only you are willing
Your mind they'll ease
Your will they'll mend
And charge you not a shilling."*

–Nursery rhyme quoted by Wayne Fields, What the River Knows, 1990

Write it down & get it done.

1
2
3
4
5
6
7
8
9
10

office chair twist

Sit on the front edge of a chair with feet flat on the floor. Lean back as far as possible without touching the back of the chair. With the palms of your hands together and arms straight point fingers toward the ceiling. Keeping your hips and arms stationary, rotate your body to the right, hold for 2-3 counts, return to middle and repeat. Complete 10-15 repetitions on each side.

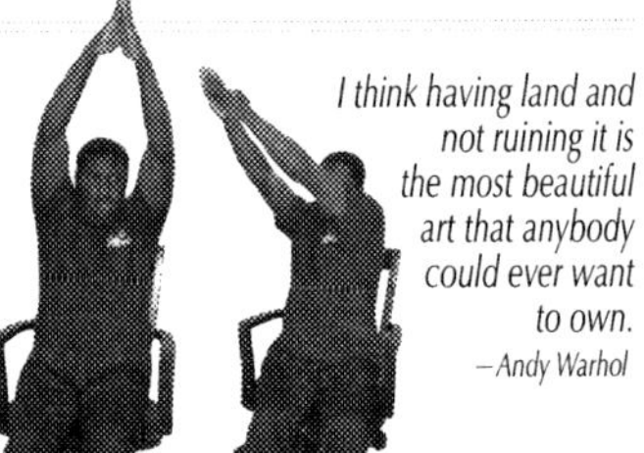

I think having land and not ruining it is the most beautiful art that anybody could ever want to own.
– Andy Warhol

DATE

Steps Walked:
Cardio Workout:
Strength Training:
Calories Consumed:
Calories Burned:
Difference:
Weight / Body fat:

Write it down & get it done.

1
2
3
4
5
6
7
8
9
10

Read it, live it, love the results.

Be where you want to be.
Whether you want to admit it or not, you are self-made. You are exactly where you want to be. You make the decisions which affect and direct your life. If healthy and happy is where you want to be, you must take the steps necessary to get you there. No one can do it for you. If the decisions you make today don't take you towards your goal they are taking you from it, you determine the direction.

Life's tough, get over it, he did!

When in the third grade, artist **Andy Warhol**, suffered from a disease to his nervous system, which rendered him bed-ridden much of his childhood. Here he drew, listened to the radio and collected pictures of movie stars around his bed. Warhol later described this period as very important in the development of his personality, skill-set and preferences. Warhol became famous worldwide for his work.

chair crunch

Sit on the front edge of your chair with feet flat on the floor and legs opened slightly wider than shoulder-width. Lean back as far as possible without touching the back of the chair. With hands folded across your chest, contract your abdominals and bring your knees up to your elbows. Hold for 2-3 counts, then return to the starting position without allowing your feet to touch the floor, or back to touch the chair. Repeat 10-15 times.

Change before you have to. –Jack Welch

DATE

Steps Walked:

Cardio Workout:

Strength Training:

Calories Consumed:

Calories Burned:

Difference:

Weight / Body fat:

Eating healthy tastes great!

Healthy Onion Rings

2 onions, sliced • olive oil
3/4 cup wheat flour • 1 tbs Old Bay®
2 tsp baking powder • 3 eggs/ beaten
1 1/2 cups wheat breadcrumbs

Preheat oven to 450 F. Place onion rings in cold water. Prepare three seperate bowls; (1) flour and baking powder (2) eggs (3) breadcrumbs and seasoning. Coat onion rings with flour, then egg, then breadcrumbs. Bake on greased pan 10 minutes, turn and bake 8 to 10 minutes more until brown.

Read it, live it, love the results.

He who takes medicine and neglects to diet wastes the skill of his doctors. –Chinese Proverb

Don't expect doctors and modern medicine to take care of you. You must take care of yourself. When you give this responsibility to others you lose your independence. You have this one body to care for, make it your top priority. If you're not responsible enough to make it your top priority, do you really think others will?

Write it down & get it done.

1
2
3
4
5
6
7
8
9
10

tricep press

Sit on the front edge of a chair with legs together extended straight out and feet flat on the floor. Place your hands on the chair near your buttocks. Pressing your heels into the floor lift your your body from the chair.Hold this position for 2-3 counts, lower and repeat 10-15 times.

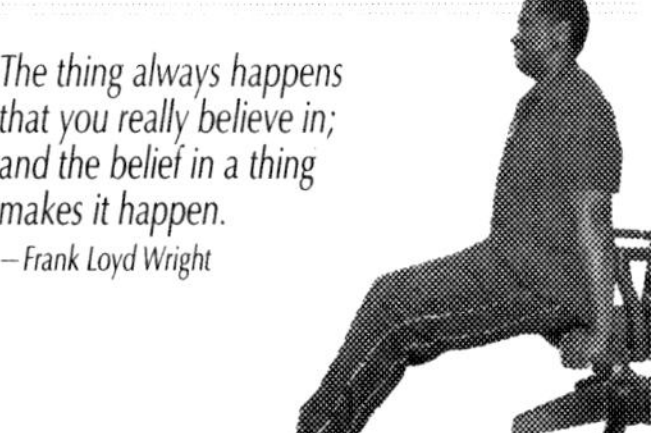

The thing always happens that you really believe in; and the belief in a thing makes it happen.
— Frank Loyd Wright

DATE

Steps Walked:

Cardio Workout:

Strength Training:

Calories Consumed:

Calories Burned:

Difference:

Weight / Body fat:

Write it down & get it done.

1
2
3
4
5
6
7
8
9
10

Read it, live it, love the results.

Help others and you will help yourself.

One of the best ways to improve your life is to help others improve their's. When you support those in need, you are better able to put your own life into perspective. Personal problems shrink and may even disappear completely.

Life's tough, get over it, he did!

Founder of the Marathon of Hope, **Terry Fox**, had been diagnosed with a malignant tumor, which resulted in having his leg amputated several inches above the knee. Three years after losing his leg at age 18, Fox decided to run from coast to coast to raise money for cancer research. He created the Marathon of Hope, and raised over $24 million for cancer research. Sadly, he passed away at age 22, his legacy now lives on to help others who face cancer.

"After after reviewing scores of health books, the most credible share some things in common. 1) They present the real answer: Getting fit and dropping pounds isn't easy; it's work, takes discipline and dedication but doesn't have to be a drudge. 2) They're written in conversational language. 3) They're interactive, presenting programs that are flexible, logical and time-tested. 4) They make the reader accountable to herself, often in writing.
This manual has those elements. It reads like I'm talking to a nutritionist and a personal trainer without paying $50 an hour for each."
– Harry Jackson Jr. • Editor, Health & Fitness St. Louis Post-Dispatch

"This book is a winner. Not just scads of information I didn't know to ask for but the daily journal to keep me in tune with the program."
– Jan Scott Editor, Women's Yellow Pages St. Louis Women On The Move

"With this journal Cindy has made it easy to get fit and stay fit both physically and mentally 365 days a year. This is a book I plan to continue to use year after year."
– Lori A. Johnson, CCP • Chief Human Resources Officer Bryan Cave LLP

"I have reviewed the journal and am extremely impressed with its format and contents. As Director of the Employee Benefits Department of a large company, I would be most interested in incorporating this journal into the Wellness Program we will be launching in the near future."
– Sandy Brown • Director, Employee Benefits Laclede Gas

Wow, the more I read your book, the more I love it. I love the little gems in the success stories. You can exercise and read these little stories just before you go to sleep. Everything is bite-sized in the book so that you can digest it easily. *–Michelle Bryant*

I absolutely LOVE the journal!!!! I just got it Tuesday, and I've already read through it and I write in it every day. Writing my goals and thoughts really helps me as I travel this journey of my lifestyle change. I can't wait to try some of the salad recipes. This book has become my new best friend! *– Ellen DeWitt*

I thank you, Cindy, for taking the time to put your heart and soul into the very book that has changed my heart and mind about exercise, food, and just the overall accountability that it gives me! I wouldn't be able to do it if I had nothing to push me towards my goal...this is just the punch I needed!! Thank you!!
–Meaghan Portell

I used my sick day off yesterday and read your book. I was really impressed with the literacy and the suggestions, pictures (easiest part for me to understand) and everything. You should be proud and now I demand an autograph copy. *–Michael S. G*

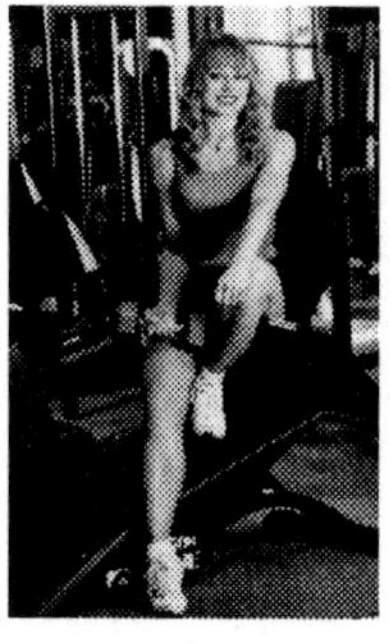

***Cynthia Brenneke** is a fitness club owner, personal trainer and class instructor with a Bachelor of Science in Eduction. She has produced workout videos, has monthly workouts featured on television, gives lectures on health and fitness and was the winner of the 2007 Gateway Naturals Figure Competition. In this book, she as compiled years of research and notes to hep you get into the best shape of your life!*

what others say